Diagnosing Literary Genius

Diagnosing Literary Genius

A Cultural History of Psychiatry in Russia, 1880–1930

IRINA SIROTKINA

The Johns Hopkins University Press

BALTIMORE AND LONDON

© 2002 The Johns Hopkins University Press
All rights reserved. Published 2002
Printed in the United States of America on acid-free paper
2 4 6 8 9 7 5 3 1

The Johns Hopkins University Press
2715 North Charles Street
Baltimore, Maryland 21218-4363
www.press.jhu.edu

Library of Congress Cataloging-in-Publication Data
Sirotkina, Irina.
Diagnosing literary genius : a cultural history of psychiatry in
Russia, 1880–1930 / Irina Sirotkina.
    p.   cm. — (Medicine & culture)
Includes bibliographical references and index.
ISBN 0-8018-6782-7
1. Psychiatry—Russia—History—19th century. 2. Psychiatry—
Russia—History—20th century. 3. Russian literature—19th
century. 4. Russian literature—20th century.
I. Title. II. Series.
RC450.R8 S57 2002
616.89′00947—dc21   2001000581

A catalog record for this book is available from the
British Library.

CONTENTS

This is an untraditional history of psychiatry: besides describing the key period in the formation of the new specialty in Russia, it focuses on psychiatric discussions of writers and of literature. The reason for this approach is the central role of literature in Russian culture, for doctors as well as for many other people. Literature created the image of Russia both inside and outside the country; it dramatically shaped expression of fears and aspirations. Foreigners came to see the Russia of Tolstoy and Dostoevsky, and Russian men and women modeled themselves on literary characters, from the romantic Tatiana Larina to the laid-back Oblomov.

The institutionalization of psychiatry in Russia coincided with one of the most eventful periods of the country's history, marked as it was by rapid economic, scientific, and cultural changes as well as by wars and revolutionary upheavals. The second half of the nineteenth century is known as the golden age of Russian literature, when writers and literary critics exercised a powerful influence over people's minds. By writing about literature, psychiatrists wanted to contribute to cultural and political life as well as use the universal love for literature to spread support for their medical activities.

Psychiatrists in many countries willingly claimed that they provided insights into human nature similar to those rendered by writers. In Russia, given literature's exceptionally high standing, such self-presentation was extremely flattering. By comparing their work with the portrayal of human moral failings and pathologies by such famous writers as Gogol and Dostoevsky, psychiatrists embellished their professional image. They went further in using literature to enhance the authority of their views, however, when they attributed the peculiarities of Gogol's and Dostoevsky's characters and writings to mental illness. Russian psychiatrists eagerly adopted the genre of pathography—medical biography of famous people, which mixed clinical case study with moral fable and art criticism.

The psychiatrists' encounter with literature was not merely an attempt to "label" famous people. In the Russian case, at least, the relationship between psychiatrists, writers, and the general public was much more subtle and interesting. The genre of pathography met with an ambivalent response from the Russian public. Indeed, when they discussed the supposed mental illnesses of famous writers, some psychiatrists altered their diagnoses in order not to offend the feelings of lovers of literature. And it is noteworthy that the genre of "psychiatric criticism" of literature flourished shortly before and after the 1917 Revolution; further into the Soviet era, pathographies, in their own turn, became a target of criticism.

I begin, in the Introduction, by describing the background to Russian psychiatry and the nature of the enterprise of pathography. The first three chapters deal with psychiatric "diagnoses" of Gogol, Dostoevsky, and Tolstoy; one key consequence of these discussions was the eager acceptance of different forms of psychotherapy. The fourth chapter describes the treatment that psychiatrists gave to so-called decadent literature in the context of a developing interest in mental hygiene. In the last chapter, I trace the story of pathography into the early Soviet decades, when there was a strange but significant interest in genius. Taken together, this is the first book-length narrative in English of the history of Russian psychiatry over a half-century decisive for medicine and society alike. My hope is that, by developing the theme of the links between psychiatry and literature, the book will attract historians of Russia and cultural historians as well as those with a more specialized interest in medical history.

While working on this book I had the generous support of several institutions and received help and encouragement from many colleagues. I wish to acknowledge the support of the Wellcome Trust, which awarded me a research fellowship and enabled me to spend a year at what was then the Wellcome Institute for the History of Medicine in London. The Science, Technology, and Society Program at the Massachusetts Institute of Technology hosted me for an academic year, and Loren Graham offered his friendly support over a much longer period. The Maison des Sciences de l'Homme in Paris generously awarded me a fellowship and provided a setting in which Serge Netchine and Gabrielle Netchine-Grynberg introduced me to the French language, culture, and scholarship. Thanks to the support of Régine Plas and the Université Paris V (René Descartes), I was able to return to Parisian libraries and archives at the concluding stage of work on the manuscript. I also had a period of support from the University of Manchester, where I benefited from contacts with Peter McMylor, Wes Sharrock, and other colleagues in the Department of Sociology. In Russia, the late Dr. S. D. Dusheiko, director of the Public Museum of the Preobrazhenskii Hospital, kindly made available to me the materials from the museum. My warm thanks go to Roger Smith, who helped me throughout the project, from the initial stage to commenting on the entire manuscript and working on my English. An earlier version of Chapter 2 appeared as "The Notion of Illness in the Works of N. N. Bazhenov" in *History of Psychiatry* 9 (1998): 135–49; an editor of the journal, Roy Porter, encouraged me to pursue my work.

In transliterating Russian titles, quotations, and names, I have used the Library of Congress system—except in the case of well-known persons (such as Dostoevsky) whose names are familiar in other spellings.

Diagnosing Literary Genius

Introduction

The philosophy of the history of the Russian intelligentsia is also in part a philosophy of Russian literature
. . . The conditions of life of the Russian intelligentsia
turned out to be such that the fire, which had been
forcibly extinguished elsewhere in a soggy and sordid
public life, burnt only in literature . . . Love and hatred,
political struggles, deep ethical demands—all shone
brightly in literature . . . Russian literature is the Testament of the Russian intelligentsia.
—R.V. Ivanov-Razumnik

To remove the veil of mystery from a great man, to solve
the puzzle of his soul, to uncover the greatness of his
deeds, to penetrate into the secret conceptions of his
artistic thought . . . should become an object of urgent
search and a duty for the contemporary generation!
—I. A. Sikorskii

"Without a medical evaluation you cannot understand anybody. It is intolerable to see men and their actions judged by linguists and other armchair
pundits. They have no inkling that more is needed than moralizing and the
average knowledge of people."[1] The German neurologist and psychiatrist
Paul Julius Möbius, who was interested in the diseases of famous figures,
addressed these words to lay biographers and critics. Möbius himself also
wrote medical biographies of the great, and he coined the term *pathography*
to describe the genre.[2] By writing pathographies, he intended to achieve a
better understanding of great men than did lay biographers who lacked med-

ical knowledge and based their interpretations on common sense and moral evaluation.

A twentieth-century historian might interpret Möbius's statements as a physician's claim for the superiority of medical expertise over lay judgment. Indeed, some historians have argued that nineteenth-century medicine attempted to explain literature by reducing it to medical terms; when physicians and in particular psychiatrists dwelt upon writers' ailments, they produced an image of creative writing as pathology. The most cited example is the Italian psychiatrist and criminal anthropologist Cesare Lombroso (1835–1909), who suggested that genius is connected with, if not caused by, epilepsy and is therefore a sign of degeneration. Moreover, his heirs still attempt to locate artistic and scientific talent in nervous structures and correlate it with psychological traits.[3] As a result of these activities, it appears, literature was turned into a product of disease, "an epiphenomenon, something that could be understood by scientific medicine."[4]

In the 1960s and 1970s, attempts to diagnose writers' disorders and to explain literature as a product of pathology were reinterpreted in terms of deviance theory and theories of social control. According to these theories, powerful professions attempted to control groups or individuals by "labeling" and "stigmatizing" them as deviant or abnormal. Thus deviants were redescribed as the "victims" of a process of stigmatization.[5] Deviance theorists identified experts in general and the medical profession in particular as powerful instruments of social control.[6] Within this framework, pathographies can be interpreted as instruments of stigmatization, as was done, for instance, by George Becker in his book *The Mad Genius Controversy: A Study in the Sociology of Deviance*.[7] He argued that, at the beginning of the nineteenth century, the notion of genius was transformed as a result of medical stigmatization. He recounted the story that the ancients attributed the source of poetic inspiration to "genius," which they imagined as a spirit or a "demon" in selected people. Then, in 1836, a French physician, Louis-François Lélut, interpreted Socrates' "demon"—his "inner voice," an alleged source of his wisdom—as literally a hallucination. Lélut's *Démon de Socrates,* according to Becker, was the first pathography. Ten years later, Lélut pronounced a similar judgment on Blaise Pascal.[8] Thereafter, the controversial genre of pathography flourished in France, supplying medical lives of the Marquis de Sade, Lord Byron, Edgar Allan Poe, Gustave Flaubert, and others.[9]

Interpretation of a supposed confrontation between Romantic and Victorian notions of the artistic genius provided another example of stigmatization. According to this view, the Romantics used the ancient notion of "divine illness," Plato's *enthusiasmos,* to emphasize the spontaneity, emotionality, irrationality, and intuition of the artistic genius. By contrast, the Victorians, who endorsed the values of morality, reason, and self-discipline, perceived these traits as infantile and irresponsible and pronounced "irrational" artists to be in need of control. In this account, artists themselves appeared to be responsible for creating the image of the artistic genius that later was turned into a social stigma. The redescription of the artistic genius therefore could not be explained as a simple process of stigmatization. In response, historians and sociologists suggested a refinement of deviance theory and stated that, by consciously choosing a "deviant" identity, the "victims" could initiate a labeling process.[10] Becker remarked that "what is significant about the genius-madness controversy . . . is . . . that the genius was clearly not the helpless 'victim' of philistine labelers—he not only contributed heavily to his 'victimization,' he even, to a degree, instigated it." In these terms, the declaration by the Romantics that "divine illness" was a source of artistic genius seems a risky statement. As Roy Porter ironically comments, when the Romantics announced themselves "mad," they did not think about the consequences. These consequences were that nineteenth-century physicians were able to transform both "divine illness" and artistic genius into medical categories.[11]

Becker admitted that physicians did not initiate labeling, but to the question "who were the people to promote the image of mad genius?" he unambiguously responded that most of them were members of the medical profession. Later, however, both sociologists and historians emphasized that deviance is constructed by the efforts of more than one group and that social control usually has multiple sources. Pursuing this point, one can claim that the medical profession did not, any more than any other single group of experts, either initiate or lead the process of labeling. Recent historical writing shows the limitations of the concept of medical stigmatization.[12] Though this concept has its time and place, from the perspective of historical research it must be treated as one dimension of a wider picture. The present study shows that the notion of stigmatization hardly does justice to the rich cultural history of pathographies.

In contrast to the proponents of sociological theories that describe the activity of professional groups in terms of their claims to social power, historians may wish to address the culture of a particular professional occupation. They may seek to clarify the kinds of projects in which the profession was involved, which social attitudes and values it adopted, and which it rejected. For the history of pathography, it is important to know who the authors were, the extent to which they formed a particular occupation, their professional and personal goals, and how the project of pathography was integrated with other activity. To write cultural history is to engage with the contextual meaning of psychiatrists' claims, and this meaning is not encompassed by theories of social control. Thus the Möbius statement that begins this Introduction was in fact directed to nonmedical biographers and literary critics who, in his view, exaggerated the mental problems of their subjects.

As the historian Francis Schiller comments, Möbius began to write pathography partly out of a desire to correct unjustified statements about famous people's illnesses. By producing what he hoped would be exemplary studies of Jean Jacques Rousseau, Arthur Schopenhauer, and Johann Wolfgang Goethe, Möbius wanted to counteract the influence of profane biographies. In his pathographies, he "did not degrade his subjects," and his attitudes towards the artists were "sympathetic rather than debunking." Möbius at the same time admitted the existence of a "desire common to psychiatrists (and am I not a bit of one?) to consider everybody insane, particularly so as to tarnish shining lights with medical comments." But he did not wish his readers to find in his own endeavor "a further example" of this desire. Möbius's ambition in psychiatry was to diminish the distance between the normal and the pathological and to show that in most cases "insanity" does not separate people from the rest of humanity and, conversely, that many more people have minor mental disturbances than is usually believed. He intended to demonstrate this in his pathographies. He wrote further that "we have to abandon the prevalent old division into healthy and sick minds . . . Everybody is pathological to a certain degree . . . The more so the more elevated his standing . . . Only myth and cliché have it that a person must be either sane or crazy."[13]

In this book I argue that pathographies provided a stage for physicians who wanted to express a world-view, make moral as well as professional claims, and thereby integrate their special interests with a wider culture. Like the genre of nineteenth-century biography, which aimed to describe good and dignified lives, the genre of pathography had a moral standpoint. Victorian psychiatrists believed in progress, reason, and civilization, and these beliefs equally underlined the ideology of asylum psychiatry, the theory of degeneration, and the writing of pathographies. Moral concern shaped the Victorian psychological physician's identity to the extent that, as Michael Clark points out, "it was his exercise of moral-pastoral functions, rather than any practice of medicine as such, which entitled him to claim professional status and authority." Like their Western counterparts, Russian "Victorians" perceived the genre of pathography as the opportunity to address social issues. As a matter of fact, it was in the early 1890s that a professor of psychiatry in

Khar'kov, P. I. Kovalevskii, wrote the first Russian-language pathographies—of Ivan the Terrible and other crowned autocrats.[14]

Both the incentive to write pathography and the meaning of this genre were culturally and temporally specific. When psychiatrists in England and Russia emphasized their belief that literature was an invaluable resource for their profession, their seemingly identical claims had different purposes. Compare, for instance, two similar statements, one by the British psychiatrist Henry Maudsley in the late 1860s, the other by the Russian psychiatrist M. O. Shaikevich almost four decades later. In his *Physiology and Pathology of the Mind* (1867), Maudsley wrote, "An artist like Shakespeare, penetrating with subtle insight the character of the individual, and the relations between him and his circumstances, discerning the order which there is amidst so much apparent disorder, and revealing the necessary mode of the evolution of the events of life, furnishes, in the work of his creative art, more valuable information than can be obtained from the vague and general statements with which science, in its present defective state, is constrained to content itself." The Russian psychiatrist made an apparently similar statement: "However valuable what has been acquired by scientific methods and however wonderful the future which the proponents of experimental psychology promise, still, because the activity of mind has an exceptionally subjective character, without intuitive understanding much will remain unclear. That is why literature and art will always supply us psychiatrists with valuable material."[15]

Both the British and the Russian psychiatrist praised literature at the expense of science for strategic reasons. Nonetheless, their purposes differed. For the well-established Victorian and Edwardian physicians, as the historian of medicine Christopher Lawrence suggests, the interest in literature, especially the classics, was a way to confirm their elevated position within the medical profession. It highlighted their gentlemanly status and distinguished them from the newcomers, physicians with rigorous scientific training and technical skills. By emphasizing their own wide education in opposition to the narrow technical education of the newcomers, the elite hospital physicians, it is argued, defended their privileges. The literary scholar Helen Small expands on this interpretation: for psychiatrists, "literary reference was merely decorative . . . a mark of accomplishment, a guarantee of the doctor's credentials as a gentlemanly physician."[16]

By contrast, Shaikevich worked at a time when psychiatry had already established itself and was facing new tasks. He wrote his eulogy of literature in 1904, in the period when psychological laboratories began to emerge in Russian universities and medical schools. At that time, the application of psychological experiment to mental patients was linked with the name of the German psychiatrist Emil Kraepelin, who developed a "formal" approach to diagnosis and a new classification of mental illness. The Kraepelinian approach was taking over in Russia, where French psychiatry had previously enjoyed wide popularity. Shaikevich's reference to literature emphasized his doubts about the relevance of experimental psychology to clinicians as well as his suspicions about the Kraepelinian psychiatry, which fostered the new psychological approach. Underlying his rejection of both experimental psychology and Kraepelinian psychiatry was a dislike of the naturalistic, positivist view of the world. At the turn of the century, positivism, challenged by neo-Kantian philosophy and the idea of the *Geisteswissenschaften,* was no longer at the height of its influence. When they became interested in these approaches, psychiatrists sensed in literature a different "model of reasoning," an alternative to the naturalistic way of thinking.

One could argue more generally that Russian psychiatrists drew on literary resources more intensely and in more diverse ways than did their Western counterparts. That literature had more than "merely decorative" meaning and was used for multiple purposes is understandable given the place of literature in Russian culture. It has become a commonplace of historical writing to observe that in nineteenth-century Russia, with no other outlet for political and public life, literature was the most important cultural resource. In a much quoted passage, a most influential literary critic of the 1860s and 1870s, N. G. Chernyshevsky (1828–89), argued that in Russia literature stood in for philosophy and what now would be called the human sciences and that it was almost the only medium for expressing public opinion:

In countries where intellectual and social life has attained a high level of development, there exists, if one may say so, a division of labor among the various branches of intellectual activity, of which we know only one—literature. For this reason, no matter how we rate our literature compared to foreign literatures, still in our intellectual movement it plays a much greater role than does French, German or English literature in the intellectual movement of their countries, and there rests on it a heavier responsibility than on any of the others . . . That which Dickens says in England, is also said, apart from him and the other novelists, by philosophers, jurists, publicists, economists etc., etc. With us, apart from the novelists, no one talks about subjects which comprise the subject of their stories. For that reason, even if Dickens need not feel it incumbent upon him, as a novelist, to bear direct responsibility for serving as spokesman for the strivings of his age, in so far as these can find expression in fields other than *belles lettres,* in Russia the novelist cannot have recourse to such justification.[17]

Richard Pipes has attributed this view to the so-called utilitarian school of criticism, which was dominant between 1860 and 1890. Indeed, the leaders of this "school," D. I. Pisarev (1840–68) and Chernyshevsky, carried the view that writers should "put their pen at the disposal of the people's social and political aspirations" to an extreme. Yet the discussion about the social mission of art started much earlier in the nineteenth century. As Victor Terras comments, after the poet and revolutionary K. Ryleev remarked "I am not a poet, I am a citizen," the demand that literature should be both a mirror and a builder of society reappeared in public debate and persisted throughout the century.[18] Another literary historian observes that when the literary critic N. A. Dobroliubov (1836–61) wished to make a political point by tracing Russia's social development, he did so in a critical article on the literary heroes of the period; when the literary critic Chernyshevsky wished to propagate his ideal of a rational society, he wrote a novel, *What Is to Be Done?*[19] The Russian intelligentsia perceived literature as the pulse of the nation's inner life. In Alexander Solzhenitsyn's words, literature formed the "second"—alternative—government when it came to working for society by working against the official ideology.[20] In response, the authorities also took literature seriously and established a huge machine for censorship.

At the turn of the century an observer of Russian culture wrote, "Not to know literature, not to be interested in it, and not to love it meant to be an outsider, a useless member of society and nation, a narrow-minded, ignorant, and selfish man."[21] Writers became the central figures in Russian society and history "whom everybody listens to," and psychiatrists were no exception. They argued that the aim of psychiatry was not dissimilar to the literary project of exploring the human soul and reflecting on the psychological ailments of the age. Psychiatrists claimed therefore that some characters in novels could be used directly to illustrate psychiatric literature,[22] and they called belles lettres "a real textbook" for their profession.[23] One observer remarked that long before certain mental diseases acquired a place in psychiatric classifications, they had been portrayed by writers and in particular by native Russian geniuses such as Alexander Pushkin, Lev Tolstoy, and Fyodor Dostoevsky.[24] Another psychiatrist believed that Dostoevsky "made mental illness understandable for the general audience . . . and attracted public attention to it better than any scientific popularization could have done."[25] In his opinion, Dostoevsky's humanistic writings prepared the road for the reform of madhouses and helped mitigate the life of prisoners. To emphasize that psychiatry and literature were involved in the same kind of social and moral project was the best way to gain the sympathy of the general audience. By describing writers as great "psychopathologists" and predecessors, psychiatrists gained powerful allies; and by intervening in discussions about literature, they both strengthened their social standing and felt they were enriching national culture.

Some psychiatrists, however, perceived writers as rivals and attempted to assert the uniqueness of their own expertise. A professor from Dorpat (now Tartu, Estonia) who wrote monographs on Dostoevsky and Ivan Turgenev thought his own authority was needed to confirm the "absolute truthfulness and striking precision of the descriptions of pathological phenomena" in their works.[26] Similarly, some decades earlier, a British alienist wrote about *King Lear*, "At every stage of this wonderful play we find evidence . . . of Shakespeare's great medical knowledge, a knowledge scarcely possessed by any even in our day, except those few who devote themselves to this special department of medical science."[27] One of his Russian colleagues announced that the lay public could not by itself uncover the real meaning of Nikolai Gogol's "mentally ill" literary characters, while another persuaded his readers that "the complete understanding of Dostoevsky's characters can be achieved only with the psychiatrist's help."[28]

One could argue, however, that although psychiatrists declared the superiority of their own expertise over lay judgment, what they in fact wrote about literature strongly correlated with the opinion of literary critics. Thus Russian radical critics, who adopted the doctrine of the social mission of art, castigated late Gogol for "social escapism." To explain why Gogol "betrayed" the democratic ideals of his youth in favor of "reactionary" religious beliefs, the literary critic V. G. Belinsky (1811–48) suggested that Gogol was insane. Subsequently, psychiatrists applied their own expertise to Gogol's case and also diagnosed mental illness. At the beginning of the twentieth century, when the doctrine of the social mission of art began to lose its position in Russian literary criticism, Gogol's diagnosis was reconsidered. "The Gogol case," as I discuss in Chapter 1, demonstrates how closely nineteenth-century psychiatry was tied up with the moral projects of literary critics and Russian society in general. The chapter also examines how both literary critics and psychiatrists altered their views on literature with the coming of the "psychological," as opposed to "moralistic," twentieth century.

In contrast to the view that when psychiatry and literature interact, literature is merely an object of psychiatric studies, some historians have pointed out that psychiatric diagnoses can in fact be modeled after literary characters. Within the body of scholarship on "literature and medicine," there is a growing tendency to study the impact of writers and their literary characters on psychiatry.[29] Several decades ago, Henri Ellenberger could mention only the affinity between psychiatric case histories and contemporary novels, but recently Mark S. Micale devoted an entire monograph to the role of Flaubert's *Madame Bovary* in the origin of the diagnosis of hysteria.[30] Similarly, Dostoevsky's characters, many of whom were given symptoms of "falling sickness" (reportedly Dostoevsky's own disease), provided psychiatrists with material to use in their discussions about the diagnosis of epilepsy.[31] Dostoevsky's contemporaries, however, were reluctant to talk about the writer's own illness, because at that time epilepsy was regarded as a sign of degeneration. Respectful of Dostoevsky's talent, Russian psychiatrists hesitated to label him as mentally ill. One of them, N. N. Bazhenov, wrote apologetically that if he had dared to examine Dostoevsky's illness, he did it "not out of a sort of scientific vandalism, but rather out of deference."[32] Though he characterized decadent writers and poets as degenerate, Bazhenov avoided applying this characterization to the respected writer. In order to come to terms with Dostoevsky's disease, psychiatrists had to reconsider the concept of degeneration, and as a consequence they elaborated the alternative idea of "progeneration." Geniuses of Dostoevsky's standing, even in the opinion of psychiatrists, did not show symptoms of decline but rather signs of the progressive evolution of humanity. In Chapter 2 I describe how the encounter with established writers challenged psychiatric views of degeneration.

As in the case of Gogol, when Russian radicals criticized Tolstoy, psychiatrists again echoed their judgment. The radicals reproached Tolstoy for not going far enough in his opposition to autocracy and for propagating nonviolence and self-improvement instead of revolution. They pronounced Tolstoy a brilliant writer but a bad, prejudiced thinker. This judgment had been repeatedly quoted before it was confirmed by psychiatrists who "diagnosed" Tolstoy's condition as neurosis or even "affective epilepsy." While telling the story of diagnoses of Tolstoy, Chapter 3 also examines how the writer, metaphorically speaking, "fought back," in other words, how his philosophy, literary works, and personality challenged psychiatrists to reconsider their doctrines. It is significant that this happened simultaneously with the introduction of psychotherapy in Russia. Tolstoy's philosophy, when adopted by some physicians, provided a favorable climate for the reception of psychotherapy and psychoanalysis. His concern with "the education of the soul" helped psychiatrists develop their own ideas about psychological cure. Tolstoy's criticism of narrow-minded specialists converted some psychiatrists to a belief in healing by "personal philosophy" rather than by ready-made theories, a view that encouraged them to accommodate a variety of conceptions of psychological cure rather than choose one particular doctrine. It also stimulated the development of small clinics and sanatoria for neurotics as secluded places, like "lay monasteries," where physicians were free to pursue their own versions of psychotherapy. Tolstoy, who strongly disapproved of conventional psychiatry, "sanctioned" nervous sanatoria by taking refuge in one of them.[33]

By writing pathographies and discussing literary characters, psychiatrists shared in the Russian tradition of debating political issues in the form of literary criticism. Like their British and American counterparts, Russian psychiatrists were fascinated by Shakespeare's plays, especially *Hamlet*. Their understanding of Hamlet was, however, structured by a particular context. Projecting their own political concerns, Russian psychiatrists explained Hamlet's indecisiveness and passiveness by his oppressive environment. Whether in Hamlet's or their own times, psychiatrists argued, repression distorted the personality and produced an "incomplete psychological type." They found a Hamlet-like weakness of the will in the oppressed and neurasthenic Russian intelligentsia. When the first Russian revolution in 1905 changed the political landscape, psychiatrists discovered a new type of patient. Unlike the indecisive Hamlet, he was a man of action, a "pathological altruist," modeled after the odd but vigorous main character of Miguel de Cervantes' *Don Quixote*. When psychiatrists conceptualized their patients in terms of literary characters and read out the causes of their diseases from the *Zeitgeist* rather than from their brains, they created a psychiatry with an explicit social meaning, a psychiatry within the *Geisteswissenschaften* based on a value-laden approach to mental disease. This was characteristic of the period of cultural turmoil on the eve of the October Revolution, as I argue in Chapter 4.

The Russian Revolution was followed by an explosion of quasi-utopian projects. Some of them later became real, such as the project of preventive psychiatry, which produced a network of neuropsychiatric dispensaries, basic institutions for mental health care in Soviet and post-Soviet Russia. In contrast, a parallel project for dispensaries for geniuses remained unfulfilled. The author of the latter project, the psychiatrist G. V. Segalin from the Urals, believed that mental illness stimulated talent; he suggested that mental illness should be cultivated and ill geniuses should be protected in state institutions. Underlying both the fulfilled and unfulfilled projects was the tendency to unite public, state, and psychiatric control, concentrating it in institutions of a special kind. In retrospect, one can see in these tendencies some of the institutional foundations for the later use of psychiatry in the persecution of intellectuals.[34] Segalin's project again demonstrates that psychiatric views on literature and writers tended to confirm existing attitudes and to follow established public opinion. Before the Revolution, it was the radical intelligentsia who shaped this opinion. In the Soviet period, the voices of opposition were silenced and public opinion coincided with the establishment. This explains why, during different periods of Russian history, psychiatrists have identified with different social forces. Chapter 5 traces the relationship of psychiatrists to literature into the early Soviet era.

The enormous growth of literature on the history of psychiatry has not yet produced a comprehensive history of psychiatry in Russia. The two major Russian-language contributions in this field provide basic information about the history of psychiatry: D. D. Fedotov's study focuses on the institutionalization of psychiatry before the reforms of the 1860s, and T. I. Iudin's influential history takes the development of psychiatry further, up to the Soviet period.[35] Written in the 1950s, these histories need updating in the light of recent research, developments in medical historiography, and the political changes in Russia.[36] Within the body of English-language scholarship, the works by Julie Vail Brown are the most illuminating. She concentrates on the period from the 1860s to the October Revolution, focusing on the professionalization of psychiatry set against a complicated political background. By contrast, Kenneth Dix has studied the earlier period and described public attitudes towards mental illness in Russia. In his "critical history" of Russian psychology, David Joravsky touches upon some developments in psychiatry from the eighteenth century until the end of Stalin's rule.[37]

Existing historical accounts link the appearance of the first separate institutions for the mentally ill in the reign of Catherine II (1762–96) to her reform of local government. In 1775 she established Departments of Public Welfare in each region and made them responsible for constructing madhouses.[38] By the mid-nineteenth century there were over forty madhouses in Russia, and they were commonly regarded as places of horror to be avoided. During the reign of Nicholas I (1825–55), the government established a committee to reform asylums, but progress was extremely slow. In the course of the great reforms of the 1860s, the responsibility for education and public health was assigned to the local self-governments, *zemstva* (singular, *zemstvo*), created in 1864. In 1875 the government obliged *zemstva* to provide accommodation for all individuals in need of mental care, and it funded the expansion of existing structures and the construction of new facilities.

The reform of medical education, which followed Russia's disastrous experience in the Crimean War (1853–56), also boosted the development of psychiatry. In 1857 the Medical-Surgical Academy in St. Petersburg established the first department (*kafedra*) of psychiatry. I. M. Balinskii (1827–1902), the head of the department, was also a founder of the first professional association of psychiatrists in Russia (1862). The first national congress of psychiatrists convened in 1887, and the Union of Russian Psychiatrists and Neuropathologists was founded in 1911. In 1883 the first psychiatric journals were launched: one by Balinskii's successor at the Medical-Surgical Academy, I. P. Merzheevskii (1838–1908), and the other by P. I. Kovalevskii (1849–1923) in Khar'kov (Ukraine). Khar'kov University was the second to establish a department of psychiatry, under Kovalevskii's directorship. In 1885 Merzheevskii's former student V. M. Bekhterev (1857–1927) was appointed head of a newly established department of psychiatry in Kazan'. In comparison with St. Petersburg, Khar'kov, and Kazan', Moscow was late in establishing a department of psychiatry, which formally separated from the department of neurology only in 1893. But by the last decade of the nineteenth century, most Russian universities had programs in psychiatry.

These innovations created a career structure for the profession. They also stimulated interest in Western models of mental health care, and psychiatrists traveled abroad to examine asylums in Belgium, Great Britain, France, Germany, and Switzerland. Returning to Russia from these "psychiatric excursions"—the title they usually gave to their reports—*zemstvo* physicians (those working in health care for the poor, mainly peasants) pushed local governments (*zemstva*) and the central administration to reform mental health care. They were not satisfied with the results. Though the number of asylums increased severalfold during the final decades of the nineteenth century, the proportion of the population institutionalized was smaller than in many Western countries. Moreover, the position of psychiatrists, sandwiched between the requirements of the state and the needs of the population, contributed to the growth of a professional consciousness in very important and distinctive ways. Russian psychiatrists declared themselves advocates for Russia's insane population, even against state interests. They lobbied to introduce such institutional innovations as countryside colonies and family care for the mentally ill, and they opened private clinics and sanatoria. Negotiating with the government, psychiatrists constituted themselves as both a professional and a political force. Whatever side—radical or conservative—they took, on the eve of the great changes in Russia almost all of them were involved in political, social, and literary debates.

The present study deals with the period from the late 1880s to 1930. This period saw major transformations in psychiatry: the achievement of professional standing, a search for new forms of practice, the introduction of psychotherapy, and the crucial changes that followed the Revolution. The arrival of psychoanalysis in Russia has attracted much attention from historians, and it is important to see that this occurred as part of a larger shift towards psychotherapy in general.[39] In the absence of a comprehensive history of psychiatry in Russia, this book provides insight into what was perhaps the most eventful period for this profession. Viewing this period through the genre of pathography is justified by the centrality of literature in Russian culture. The focus on pathographies and on psychiatry's relationship with literature in general clarifies our understanding of the projects in which psychiatrists were engaged and of their place in society. Sharing the values of the Russian intelligentsia, psychiatrists regarded literature as both an indicator of the nation's mental health and an integral part of its wellbeing. When, for instance, psychiatrists emphasized the significance of literature for educating and civilizing Russian youth, cultivating its feelings, and hardening its will while awakening the nation's dignity, they made writers allies in their own struggle. The history of this vibrant period of Russian psychiatry is crystallized in the discourse about literature.

Gogol, Moralists, and Nineteenth-Century Psychiatry

People are under the misapprehension that the human brain is situated in the head: nothing could be further from the truth. It is carried by the wind from the Caspian Sea.   —N. V. Gogol

Until recently, the psychiatrist thought about mental illness as a phenomenon . . . caused by deep changes in the anatomy of a handicapped brain, and he sought for confirmation of his statements and assumptions there. This search . . . for physical alterations, which cannot yet be found, leads the psychiatrist to a theory of functional, molecular, chemical, and other changes . . . [but it] does not allow the study of the phenomenon from the point of view from which he has the best chance to learn something about it—from the mental or psychological point of view.   —I. D. Ermakov

Nikolai Gogol's contemporaries were puzzled by what they saw as an extraordinary turn in his life when, at the height of his career, admired for his talent as well as for his social criticism, he stopped writing fiction and became exceedingly religious. "The enigma of Gogol" mystified his contemporaries until they explained it by illness, which supposedly transformed a brilliant writer and ardent patriot into a religious maniac.[1] They made the judgment on moral grounds, and it did not require a medical certificate. Following radical literary critics, Gogol's contemporaries believed that a writer, in order to produce good and sound work, should devote himself to a social cause. But psychiatrists, whose voice in society was growing stronger, eventually intervened. Fifty years after Gogol's death the psychiatric profession became involved in an intense discussion of the writer's supposed illness. In 1902 two pathographies, by N. N. Bazhenov and V. F. Chizh, offered authoritative confirmation of the prevalent nineteenth-century opinion that Gogol suffered from a mental disorder. The two psychiatrists used medical resources to endorse the popular opinion that art ought to have a social mission.

Chizh was especially forceful in suggesting a medical underpinning for the moral evaluation of Gogol. In his life project as a moralist, Chizh integrated his writing about Gogol with psychiatry and experimental psychology. With the beginning of the new century, however, literary critics' opinion of Gogol shifted. On the eve of the 1905 revolution against autocracy, they perceived him as a victorious genius, not as someone confused in his purposes and mistaken in his commitments. Subsequently, Chizh's views came under attack from his younger colleagues, who were eager to reconsider the moral project of "the long nineteenth century" and to reassess Gogol's supposed insanity in the light of the new, revolutionary vision. They brought into the discussion of Gogol new conceptual resources—the idea that geniuses were advancing the development of human beings rather than revealing signs of degeneration—and they called for the replacement of the psychiatric labeling of geniuses by studies of their psychology.

Nikolai Vasilievich Gogol

Although there are as many versions of Gogol's life (1809–52) as there are biographers, the most widespread version sharply divides his life into two parts. Gogol's first books gained him wide popularity and his readers' genuine love. Full of light humor, in contrast to the usual Russian seriousness, they described peasant and gentry life in Gogol's native Ukraine. During the first part of his literary career, he also wrote a comedy, *The Inspector General* (1836), in which he aimed to render the official life in Russia contemptible and ludicrous and to portray the corruption universal in the civil service and the alternating arrogance and servility of men in office. This comedy brought him great success with the public and criticism from the authorities; hence the liberal opposition regarded him as a leader. In order to escape from official criticism, Gogol went to Italy. Here he continued to work on *Dead Souls* (1842), his main novel, in which he told the story of an adventurer who travels around Russia making fictitious purchases of "dead souls," that is, of serfs

who have died since the last census, in order to pledge his imaginary property to the government. The novel, seen as a polemic on Russian provincial
life, enhanced Gogol's reputation as a satirist who attacked social problems,
made people laugh at them, and in this way brightened the dark sides of
Russian life.

Gogol lived in Italy throughout the 1840s, returning to Russia only for
short stays. After a long period of silence, he published *Selected Passages from
Correspondence with Friends* (1847), which had an explosive impact on the
Russian audience.[2] Its prophetic tone contrasted with everything he had
published before. Gogol wrote *Selected Passages* for himself, after he became
"grievously ill; death was near," as a preparation for a Christian death, as well
as for his readers, whose "slumbering souls" he hoped to awaken. The book
contained his "Testament" and a collection of letters and essays on religious,
political, and historical questions. Gogol's mainly aristocratic audience was
appalled, however, by the parts of the book in which he instructed a governor how to govern a province, a married couple how to live in marriage,
and a landowner how to run his estate. Gogol had no personal experience in
any of these matters. The comic writer and satirist had turned into a pre-
sumptuous preacher; to make this impression worse, state officials promptly
publicized *Selected Passages* as proof of Gogol's support for the status quo in
Russia.

Many of Gogol's former devoted readers turned away from him, and some
even suspected that he published his book in order to obtain personal benefits
from the tsar. The conservative party of Slavophiles celebrated *Selected Passages* as the only worthy book by Gogol, and they claimed a triumph over
the Westernizers who had ascribed a content of social and political protest
to *The Inspector General* and *Dead Souls.* Both sides, however, were shocked
by what seemed to be Gogol's toadying to the government of Nicholas I. A
review in the *Literary Gazette* (*Literaturnaia gazeta*) proclaimed that Gogol
"died when he published his last work [*Dead Souls*]. His physical death is much
less important."[3]

The discussion around *Selected Passages* reached its apogee in an open letter to Gogol from the literary critic V. G. Belinsky (1847). Belinsky, previously
one of Gogol's principal admirers, had earlier praised the writer as a founder
of a new literary movement, the so-called Natural School, which had succeeded in turning the attention of writers towards everyday reality. In the
1830s and early 1840s, he defended Gogol from those critics who blamed
the writer for choosing inferior topics and using an "ignoble" language; Belinsky's sharp and witty polemic contributed considerably to the writer's im-

mense popularity. "I loved you," he now wrote to Gogol, "with all passion with which a man, bound by ties of blood to his native country, can love its hope, its honour, its glory, one of the great leaders on the path toward consciousness, development and progress. And you had sound reason for losing your equanimity at least momentarily when you forfeited that love." He claimed that Gogol, who now invested all his hopes for the betterment of the Russian people in religion, deeply misunderstood their problems and needs: "you failed to realize that Russia sees her salvation not in mysticism or asceticism or pietism, but in the successes of civilization, enlightenment and humanity."[4]

One of the "letters" in *Selected Passages,* addressed to "the Russian Landowner," especially provoked Belinsky's anger. In this letter Gogol advised the landowner to preach the Gospel to his peasants and, if somebody did not listen, to "give [him] a good scolding in front of everyone; say to him 'You, you unwashed bum! You have always lived in such grime that your eyes no longer see . . . who does not call on reason dies like a dog.'"[5] Belinsky was outraged: he called Gogol a "proponent of the knout, apostle of ignorance, champion of obscurantism and Stygian darkness, panegyrist of Tatar morals." He was the first to suggest publicly that madness could be the only dignified explanation of Gogol's actions: "Either you are ill—and you must hasten to take a cure, or . . . I am afraid to put my thought into words!"[6]

Written in the safe Austrian town of Salzbrunn, out of reach of the Russian police, Belinsky's letter contained, alongside the criticism of Gogol, a spirited attack on the tsarist regime. Publication of the letter was not possible in Russia, and distribution of copies was illegal—it was for the distribution of Belinsky's letter that Dostoevsky received the death sentence (commuted to exile to Siberia). Yet the letter made a deep impact on Russian revolutionary consciousness. Even more noticeable was Belinsky's influence on the perception of art and its place in society. Insisting that literature should have a social role, Belinsky condemned "pure art" on moral grounds.

The long-running conflict between proponents of the social mission of art and those who supported the idea of "art for art's sake" became *the* issue in Russian literature and literary criticism well into the twentieth century.[7] Belinsky made heavy moral demands on writers, requiring continuity and coherence between the writer's life and his literary work. This position became established as a tradition, identified by Isaiah Berlin as particularly Russian, in which the line between life and art is not clearly drawn. In this tradition, the same judgments apply both to art and to the artist's everyday life, so that "praise and blame, love and hatred, admiration and contempt are freely expressed both for artistic forms and for the human characters drawn, both for the personal qualities of authors and for the content of their novels."[8] Gogol became the test case for this tradition, and he was judged again and again by several generations of critics, historians, and readers who shared, in Berlin's words, the "Russian attitude."

Belinsky died of tuberculosis in 1848 and became a hero of Russian liberals and revolutionaries, and his idea of "two Gogols"—one a flaming patriot, the other a traitor to freedom and democracy—was reinforced in the minds of Russians.[9] Gogol himself perceived the polemic around the book as "a slap in the face" and felt as if "the living body of a man still alive was subject to such a terrible anatomy, which could draw cold sweat even from a man with a stronger constitution." In private he attributed his mistakes to "a morbid and constrained state of mind" while he was writing *Selected Passages*, but he never doubted the values embedded in it and refused to believe it could be harmful to the public.[10] He denied that he had undergone a sudden transformation and claimed that *The Inspector General, Dead Souls,* and *Selected Passages* were guided by the same intention: to portray the corruption of souls so that readers would take steps to improve themselves. In 1848 Gogol accomplished his old plan of making a pilgrimage to Jerusalem, and soon thereafter he became a devotee of an Orthodox priest and ascetic, Father Matvei (Matthew). The priest persuaded Gogol that secular art was a sin, and in early 1852 the writer burned the manuscript of the second volume of *Dead Souls*. Father Matvei also encouraged him to fast during Lent, and Gogol, who previously enjoyed food almost to an obsessive degree, ate nothing and knelt before the icons.

Vladimir Nabokov, finding sentimentality distasteful, hesitated to describe the last days of Gogol's life.[11] The doctors summoned to Gogol by his anxious friends could not agree about the diagnosis, and they subjected the physically exhausted Gogol to heroic medicine and hypnosis. One of them later remembered the events:

In the evening Sokologorskii [one of the doctors] came to magnetize [Gogol]. When he put his hand on [Gogol's] head, then under his shoulder, and began to make "passes," N[ikolai] V[asilievich] moved and requested, "leave me."—Later in the evening Klimenkov was called and struck me with the arrogance of his behavior. He began to shout out at [Gogol] as at a deaf and insane person [*bezpamiatnyi*], forcibly held his hand while asking where he felt pain. It was clear that it annoyed the patient and he was losing consciousness. Finally, he begged, "leave me," turned away and hid his hand. Klimenkov advised bleeding him or wrapping him in cold sheets; I suggested waiting till next morning.—Yet, the same evening, they skillfully inserted a soap suppository when the patient was turning over, which caused again cries and screaming.[12]

The next day Gogol was plunged into a warm bath and his head soused with cold water, after which he was put in bed with a half-dozen leeches affixed to his nose. This treatment, together with purgatives and bloodletting, was thought to have accelerated his end.

Medical Accounts of Gogol's Life

Gogol's death provided an opportunity to reinterpret his life. His friend M. P. Pogodin expressed the alternatives in a necrology. He rhetorically asked whether Gogol's destruction of the second part of *Dead Souls* was "the greatest deed of Christian self-sacrifice . . . or . . . a fruit of deeply hidden self-seduction, or whether only a cruel mental illness acted here." The radical critic N. G. Chernyshevsky suggested that before one "definitely decides to blame Gogol . . . for playing a role," there should be further investigation into his life. According to Chernyshevsky's own version, Gogol, an honest and sincere man, at the end of his life acted "against his own will" in a "bizarre delusion." Even sympathetic contemporaries emphasized Gogol's strangeness: "What an intelligent, queer, and sick creature," Ivan Turgenev wanted to exclaim when he saw Gogol not long before his death, and he reported that "all Moscow" shared the opinion that Gogol was "an extraordinary man of genius whose mind had somehow been affected." The first biography of Gogol, by the Ukrainian writer and ethnographer P. A. Kulish, was designed to investigate such painful changes: of the two volumes of this biography, the first dealt with the period before 1842, supposedly the year of the criminal turn, and the second one covered the short later period.[13]

A subsequent biographer, V. I. Shenrok, fully shared the contemporary moral judgment: "If Gogol had had a happy guide and had been able to limit himself to the modest task of revealing social ulcers with satire and not pursuing colossal utopias, the fruits of his literature and life would shine as a bright star for his descendants." Shenrok explored the idea that Gogol was unable to act adequately and suggested that he had exhausted himself working on the first volume of *Dead Souls:* "this . . . led to the illness which brought him ultimately to the mystic path . . . where he must have buried his talent." Occasionally Shenrok called Gogol's illness "madness" and "mental derangement," yet he did not approve of the doctors' final treatment of him, when, unable to enter Gogol's inner world, they "pitilessly poisoned his last hours, which should have been destined for his preparation for the great moment."[14]

One of the first medical versions of Gogol's life came from Italy. In his *Genio e follia* (1863), Cesare Lombroso took Gogol as an example of the connections between genius and illness. For him, all Gogol's habits and illnesses, alongside the writer's talent, were merely stigmata of his degenerate constitution. The writer, according to Lombroso, "after suffering from an unhappy love affair, gave himself up for many years to unrestrained onanism, and became eventually a great novelist." When Gogol reached the summit of his fame,

a new idea began to dominate him; he thought that he painted his country with so much crudity and realism that the picture might incite a revolution . . . He then thought by his writing to combat western liberalism, but the antidote attracted fewer readers than the poison. Then he abandoned work, shut himself up in his house, giving himself up to prayer to the saints and supplicating them to obtain God's pardon for his revolutionary sins. He accomplished a pilgrimage to Jerusalem, from which he returned somewhat consoled, when the revolution of 1848 broke out, and his remorse was again aroused. He was constantly pursued by the visions of the triumph of Nihilism, and in his alarm he called on Holy Russia to overthrow the pagan West . . . In 1852, the great novelist was found dead at Moscow of exhaustion, or rather of *tabes dorsalis,* in front of the shrine before which he was accustomed to lie for days in silent prayer.[15]

The anticlerical Lombroso, like his Russian contemporaries, did not approve of Gogol's mysticism, and he brought a new medical touch to the accepted version of Gogol's life. The Russian doctors also took for granted the critics' version of Gogol's life and, like Belinsky, reproached him for betraying liberal values; like Chernyshevsky and Shenrok, they suggested that Gogol's talent was destroyed by illness.

The first physician to step into the discussion of Gogol's illness was a well-known psychiatrist in Russia, N. N. Bazhenov. In December 1901, on the eve of the fiftieth anniversary of Gogol's death, Bazhenov gave a speech at an annual meeting of the Moscow Society of Psychiatrists and Neuropathologists; an extended version of the talk appeared as a book a year later.[16] Bazhenov believed Gogol was severely ill, but his illness was misdiagnosed and he was given the wrong treatment: "they ought to have done just the opposite of what they in fact did with him—that is, to force-feed him, and, rather than letting blood from him, . . . to have fed him intravenously." But, he claimed, the physicians should be excused because "in medicine, as elsewhere, the path to truth passes through many mistakes."[17] Because medicine had much improved since Gogol's time, Bazhenov intended to give his own diagnosis, based on a thorough study of biographical materials; he obtained some of these materials privately from Shenrok, who was then preparing a major biography of Gogol for publication.

Bazhenov did not accept the conclusion arrived at by one of the main witnesses, Dr. Tarasenkov, who had followed Gogol's illness until the fatal end. Shocked by what he saw at Gogol's deathbed, Tarasenkov later came to believe that the causes of Gogol's sufferings were "spiritual":

Judging the visible symptoms without paying attention to all the details of his life, like his way of thought, his convictions, his aims, all the atmosphere around him, it is, of course, easy to put the problem aside by calling his illness *typhus, gastro-enteritis, mania religiosa,* as has been done; but, it is enough to know only those details that could be observed in his house for it to be difficult to pronounce such a superficial verdict. There was such a variety of conditions here, as if his end were predestined, that the right conclusion can be drawn only from recognizing their combination. A spiritual element was the dominant cause of his illness. A seeker as a writer, he was not satisfied with reproducing Russia's life, but attempted to solve the task of how to influence everybody with his poetic images so that everything would change for the better.—He disliked the existing order; he mourned for it and hoped to guess what a better order, better people, better life would be.[18]

Tarasenkov also reported an episode in Gogol's life when, on a cold and dark February night, the writer took a cab to the other end of town, to the Moscow City Psychiatric Hospital (Preobrazhenskii). He got down from the sleigh and walked back and forth at the gates, but finally drove away. Tarasenkov, like some other friends of Gogol, supposed the writer might have wanted to consult a patient there, Ivan Koreisha, who had a reputation as a soothsayer.

Bazhenov, however, shared neither of the old doctor's speculations. He suggested that the uncompleted visit to the hospital could "be explained easily if one is aware that the Preobrazhenskii at that time, and much later, was the sole public institution in Moscow for the psychically ill. We may assume that Gogol knew this and, typically for those suffering from his illness, when he felt a psychic catastrophe threatening him, rushed for help, but, in an equally typical manner, stopped in indecision before the gates of the hospital." Yet he had to admit that in Gogol's time alienists would not have been able to offer appropriate help and that the very illness from which, as Bazhenov supposed, Gogol suffered—periodical psychosis—was not introduced into psychiatric classification until two years after his death. The physicians at the Preobrazhenskii in particular would have been no good for the ill writer, because, as Bazhenov had a chance to witness himself, even thirty years after Gogol's death it "was no hospital but a home for the demented on the gates of which one could justifiably have written the inscription of Dante's Hell—'abandon hope, all ye who enter here.'"[19]

Since Gogol's time, Bazhenov claimed, psychiatry had progressed and the writer's disorder could now be diagnosed in a scientific way. Although Bazhenov did not doubt that Gogol had a mental disorder, he criticized Shenrok's comment about the writer's "madness," for it implied the existence of such strong symptoms as violent delirium, delusions, and absurd acts, which Gogol did not exhibit. Moreover, Shenrok "was absolutely incompetent to judge either the degree of Gogol's ailment or what is to be called mental derangement in general"; this was the prerogative of a specialist, and a specialist armed with the knowledge of modern psychiatry.[20]

Bazhenov did not take for granted Shenrok's assumption that the writer took a crucial turn in the middle of his life. Instead, he shared the opinion of some of Gogol's friends and critics that Gogol always held the same attitudes, which only became stronger towards the end of his life. The psychiatrist believed that Gogol had always had confused ideas: as a great talent, he wrote progressive works, whereas his everyday attitudes did not go beyond a commonsense conservatism.[21] Bazhenov claimed that even in his promising years, Gogol was already "a neurasthenic with hypochondria"; he suffered from headaches, anxieties, and switches of mood and acted in an odd way. The psychiatrist suggested that the writer inherited, especially from his mother, "unquestionably a woman of psychopathic temperament," a predisposition to mental illness: "In this persistently nervous psychological soil, Gogol's real illness developed . . . During almost the entire second half of his life, Gogol suffered from the form of psychic illness which we in our scientific terminology of today call periodic psychosis—more specifically, periodic melancholy."[22] The bouts of this periodic illness explained the writer's periods of decreasing productivity and increasing religiosity.

Though Bazhenov's essay was well documented and his demonstration that Gogol had a mental illness was persuasive, the conclusion sounded much milder than Lombroso's statement that Gogol was a "degenerate type." Bazhenov believed that neither Gogol nor other geniuses should be regarded as degenerate; he argued instead that they should be classified in the more advanced, "progenerating" part of humanity. Progeneration, a progressive development of the human species, is achieved in geniuses who, though ill, possess qualities that average people do not have. (Bazhenov's idea of "progeneration" is discussed in Chapter 2.) At the time when he published it, Bazhenov's opinion was highly controversial. Its supporters appeared a few years later, when the general climate in politics and literary criticism in Russia had dramatically changed. In 1902, however, there were more opponents than defenders of the view of Gogol as a "progenerating" genius.

A few months after Bazhenov had made his points about Gogol in his talk to the Moscow Society of Psychiatrists and Neuropathologists, his colleague Chizh in Dorpat (now Tartu, Estonia) gave a similar speech at a university meeting (published in 1904). Although the two psychiatrists had different backgrounds (Bazhenov's is described in Chapter 2), they pursued similar didactic purposes, as became clear from Chizh's introduction. Chizh thought it his duty to explain "why our great satirist wrote so little, ended so early his career which was needed by Russia, why he spent his most productive years abroad, why he was not engaged in public activities." He therefore set out to "divide sanity from insanity in the works and acts of the writer who is our national pride" and came to the conclusion that it was Gogol's illness, which he diagnosed as melancholia, that "took him away from Russia."[23] Chizh's pathography of Gogol was closely tied to the moral project of nineteenth-century psychiatry.

Vladimir Fedorovich Chizh

V. F. Chizh (1855–1922) was born into the Ukrainian gentry. His father, a general, owned an estate near Poltava, in a prosperous agricultural region—the same region where Gogol set his first sunny and cheerful work, the *Evenings on a Farm near Dikan'ka* (1831–32). Chizh, however, was not able to absorb much of the region's cheerfulness; he was born when the family lived in the Russian town of Smolensk and was sent to Petersburg to study.[24] After graduating from the prestigious Medical-Surgical Academy in 1878, he became assistant physician at the Navy Hospital in Kronshtadt, an island fortress in the Baltic Sea. In 1881 he moved back to Petersburg, where he was appointed physician at a police institution, the Shelter for Primary Care for the Insane. He also worked as an assistant physician at the Prison Hospital. There he faced more questions than his medical education had prepared him to answer. One of them was a puzzling question about the connection between crime and insanity, a question that Chizh shared with his contemporaries, including a man of similar class background and intellectual occupation, the literary critic and historian D. N. Ovsianiko-Kulikovskii (1853–1920). Ovsianiko-Kulikovskii confessed in his memoirs that from his early years he had an ambivalent interest in the abnormal, an interest combined with repulsion. Ovsianiko-Kulikovskii wrote that by upbringing he "belonged to the category of people for whom there are two great misfortunes—to go mad and to kill, especially the latter. But in my intimate self-feeling they were bound so tightly together that the moral horror of a murder expanded towards madness. And, out of all kinds of madness the most horrible was so-called 'moral insanity' which caused in me an unbearable disgust, intolerable mental sickness."[25]

Criminal anthropology provided the answers to these questions. It sought for organic causes of what Chizh, Ovsianiko-Kulikovskii, and others believed was the willful transgression of God-given innate knowledge of right and wrong. It argued that the cause of crime "is not an 'evil' or 'criminal' will, but the criminal's entire imperfect organization, physical as well as psychic."[26] Ovsianiko-Kulikovskii recalled that when he first read Lombroso, his doctrine "immediately had a tremendous appeal to me—as if I were prepared to accept it . . . The existence of the criminal type (at least a psychic one) which reproduced atavistically the psyche and 'morals' of the primitive man was for me not to be doubted. I imagined this type, together with similar phenomena of mental and moral degeneration and feeblemindedness, as a fatal evil, a grave human illness transmitted from century to century and threatening to distort completely all the best initiatives and achievements of culture."[27] Ovsianiko-Kulikovskii then embarked on an academic career with an emphasis on philosophy, literature, and psychology, whereas Chizh looked for answers to the same questions in psychiatry, criminal anthropology, and experimental psychology.

The majority of Russian psychiatrists and criminal anthropologists supported the social point of view in the public debate about "heredity or milieu." At the 1889 Congress of Criminal Anthropology in Paris, Russian delegates followed with great interest the "duel" between the main speakers in support of each viewpoint, Lombroso and the French alienist Valentin Magnan. Bazhenov, who wanted to explore the issue firsthand, spent hours with Lombroso and the French anthropologist Léonce Manouvrier looking in the Sorbonne's anthropological collection for a particular cranial hollow that, so Lombroso claimed, was typical of the skulls of criminals.[28] With rare exceptions, the Russians joined the French side against Lombroso, who, they finally decided, defended "unhealthy tendencies" and had "extremely unscientific ambitions."[29] V. P. Serbskii (1858–1917), who taught forensic psychiatry at Moscow University, wrote that "society regards as criminals only the most unhappy and inferior people, while 'superior' criminals, not seen in the prisons, are regarded as honest people or even sometimes join society's crème de la crème."[30]

Unlike many of his fellow physicians in Russia, who criticized Lombroso's notion of the criminal type, Chizh compared the Italian psychiatrist with Charles Darwin—Lombroso emphasized that not only is crime hereditary but the "born criminal" is an evolutionary throwback.[31] He called Lombroso "a genius," explaining the contempt in which contemporaries held this "undoubtedly outstanding scientist" as caused by envy.[32] He also read the literature on psychological medicine, especially the works of the Scottish prison doctor James Thomson and the English alienist James Cowles Prichard, whose notion of moral insanity he enthusiastically adopted. In Chizh's view, the notions of moral insanity and inborn criminality coincided; thus he believed a morally insane person would "necessarily commit a crime."[33]

Chizh's conservative morality and equally conservative political views were not accompanied by active religiosity, so criminal anthropology appealed to him because of its scientific approach. In criminal anthropology, which provided an unemotional language for describing potentially traumatic observations, Chizh found a rationalization of the horrors that he observed as a prison physician. He never reported any of these cases, however. On the contrary, he wrote about the almost complete insensitivity of criminals in whom he did not notice "anything resembling repentance, shame, reproaches of conscience." The majority of them "pictured themselves as unfortunate victims of enemies, police agents, court's errors" and appeared thoughtless and indifferent to their sentences and their lives in the future. But the main support for his conclusions Chizh found in literature. He called Dostoevsky a genius who "alone is able to understand [the criminal's] soul."[34] Dostoevsky's fictional criminal characters, although intelligent and clever people, also "demonstrate that their minds are absolutely inefficient and that they are not capable of any serious vocation, any regular activity." Chizh thought Dostoevsky's observations in prison, in his *Memoirs from the House of the Dead* (1860–62), supported the main assumptions of criminal anthropology. Dostoevsky wrote about some of his fellow prisoners: "such a brutal cruelty . . . is undoubtedly not possible [in normal people]. It is a phenomenon and not merely a crime; it must be some constitutional defect, some bodily or moral deformity that science does not yet recognize."[35] Later Dostoevsky's work made the same impression on the British scholar Henry Havelock Ellis, who believed Dostoevsky gave the best literary illustrations of "the moral insensibility of the instinctive and habitual criminal, his lack of forethought, his absence of remorse, his cheerfulness."[36]

When he moved back to Petersburg in 1881, Chizh enrolled as a doctoral student in his alma mater, the Military-Medical Academy (the Medical-Surgical Academy was so renamed in 1881), where he studied with I. P. Merzheevskii. Merzheevskii's clinic was a major center for postgraduate training in psychiatry and neurology, with more than two dozen students preparing their dissertations in a supportive and enthusiastic atmosphere. One of them later recalled, "What a lovely, flourishing time it was for the Petersburg psychiatric clinic! The laboratory was crowded into two rooms next to the professor's study, and it was packed with a lot of students working in there. Solely histological studies prevailed, but . . . very often the cries of animals—victims of experiments—were heard in the back room."[37] For his dissertation, which academic rules required to be completed and defended within two years, Chizh chose a conventional topic, a histological study of alterations in the spinal cord during progressive paralysis. Yet, parallel with his dissertation, he succeeded in addressing the topic that was his main interest—mental deviance—and completed two papers, one on a sexual perversion and the other on the effects of drugs (morphine, atropine, silver nitrate, and potassium bromide) on the nervous system.[38]

As a rule, after receiving a degree, promising Russian students were given stipends for traveling abroad, to complete their education in the laboratories and clinics of eminent European scientists. Chizh, who obtained the funds from the Ministry of the Interior (which supervised prisons and the prison hospital where he had worked), had an additional mission: to study the impact of solitary confinement on health in Western prisons. In the 1880s, when it was debated whether lengthening the period prisoners spent in solitary confinement helped in dealing with crime, psychiatrists were called on to give expert opinions.[39] Some of them, especially those who accepted the traumatic origin of mental illness, supposed that a longer confinement led to so-called prison psychoses. Those who believed in inner organic causes of mental illness denied that prison psychoses were a separate category.[40] Chizh was expected to weigh the evidence in support of each point of view and give a clear answer to the authorities. Before his trip he assumed that solitary confinement was harmful and, following Merzheevskii, believed that the Slavs were even less fit to tolerate it than other peoples.[41] What he saw abroad between April 1884 and October 1885, however, made him reconsider his belief and confirmed what he knew from books about the "moral insensibility" of criminals: "I have inspected prisons with solitary confinement in Belgium, Germany, and France, and have worked for three years in Petersburg prisons, but have not found sufficient evidence in support of some observers' statements about the harm of solitary confinement. One can only be surprised how easily the convicts endure physical and moral suffering caused by imprisonment, fear of punishment, and awareness of a ruined life. Observations of such persons convince me that the impact of morality on mental health is insignificant."[42]

Though he visited Belgian, French, and German prisons, the longest stops he made during his almost two-year trip were in Paris, where he attended Jean-Martin Charcot's lectures at the Salpêtrière, and in Leipzig, where he worked with the psychologist Wilhelm Wundt and the neurologist Paul Flechsig. Along the way, Chizh attended the hypnotic ssessions of Hippolyte Bernheim in Nancy and Joseph Delboeuf in Brussels and visited Richard von Krafft-Ebing in Vienna. He was eager to learn more about scientific studies of pathology, including moral pathology. French experiments with induced pathology interested him no less than Flechsig's histological methods and Wundt's psychological experiments. Before going on this scientific tour, Chizh had experimented with drugs, using himself as the subject, and found that the destructive impact of drugs on mental functions started with "moral feelings": even when intellect, memory, and perception remain normal, he noted, a drugged subject becomes "morally insane."[43] It is therefore not surprising that the names of Jacques-Joseph Moreau and Charcot attracted him to Paris. Moreau, after accompanying a rich patient to Palestine and Syria, started propagating the use of hashish in the treatment of mental diseases and as a means of psychological investigation. Charcot, while a young intern at the Salpêtrière under Moreau, agreed to subject himself to experiments with hashish.[44]

Chizh was not the first Russian to travel to France in pursuit of knowledge about the physiological effects of drugs. His fellow student from Merzheevskii's clinic, S. P. Danillo (1848–97), was already in Paris assisting Charles Richet in experiments with hashish and coca.[45] Sigmund Freud, who was also interested in the physiological effect of coca, arrived in Paris to study with Charcot in October 1885, a month before Chizh returned to Russia. Danillo observed in his self-experiments with hashish that a sudden thought that somebody might attack him on the streets when he went home late at night caused an uncontrolled movement to check the gun in his pocket. His interpretation was that hashish produced "a state of automatism in which the poisoned person is not able to inhibit and regulate his voluntary impulses, so that every thought immediately expresses itself in a corresponding action." Danillo and Richet reported that the drugged animal, "lacking the power of inhibition, . . . becomes wild."[46]

The medical history of drugs illustrates many of the interconnections between medical and moral judgment.[47] In the nineteenth century, drug addiction had the double meaning of "a disease *and* a vice," and "addicts" became stigmatized by law and public attitudes.[48] Aware of this, scientists who used drugs as a research method, a kind of "mental microscope," drew a line between their studies and the everyday attitude towards drug addicts. In their research, they avoided "treading upon the ground . . . of morality."[49] Yet, in spite of their efforts, evaluations were embedded in the interpretation of experimental results. Physicians and physiologists used language that was already value-laden, as the historian Roger Smith demonstrates for the concepts of inhibition and hierarchy in nervous functions. When surgeons began to use anesthetics for their patients, they noticed that the loss of mental activity started with the powers of will, attention, and reason, progressing to the point where only organic functions remained.[50] The British neurologist John Hughlings Jackson suggested that the earlier the function appeared in evolution the more stable it was, whereas relatively recent functions were more vulnerable. Bringing these ideas into a system, the French psychologist Théodule Ribot formulated a "law of evolution of mental functions," which seemed to be applicable in the cases of drugged animals and people. Thus, when Chizh claimed that moral sense, as the latest achievement of civilization, was the first to be affected in drug experiments, his conclusion was in the mainstream of contemporary science.[51]

Chizh was one of the first Russians to study and work with Wilhelm Wundt.[52] Wundt's approach was quite different from the long-standing French pathological tradition, which considered illness, natural or induced by hypnosis or drugs, the best psychological experiment.[53] In Russia, where French influence was significant, Wundt's views appeared "essentially different from the accepted ones," because he rejected "hypnotic experiments" on the ground that the hypnotic state excluded controlled introspection.[54] Wundt's refusal to call hypnotic experiments psychological in the proper sense seemed strange to those who thought only "experiments on animals and hypnotized subjects" were "truly objective."[55] Wundt indeed equipped his laboratory in order to study the structure of normal consciousness and discover laws of psychological causality parallel to laws of physical causality. As Kurt Danziger has demonstrated, he distinguished between actual introspection, or self-observation (*Selbstbeobachtung*), and "internal perception" (*innere Wahrnehmung,* i.e., simple judgments about stimuli). Wundt criticized introspectionists who tried to develop broad, systematic methods of self-reporting; in his institute, he attempted to limit introspection to simple reports of *innere Wahrnehmung*.

The data records collected in Wundt's institute consisted mostly of measurements made with kymographs or chronoscopes, not of verbal introspective reports. Introspection became the ultimate method of psychological study later—for example, with E. B. Titchener, who developed his own research program.[56]

Wundt's students and successors, liberally interpreting the framework established by their teacher, used laboratories to pursue their own purposes. Although Wundt had excluded higher psychological processes from experimental investigation, others developed his techniques to study memory, aesthetic judgment, and thought.[57] James McKeen Cattell and Emil Kraepelin (1856–1926) separately began to use reaction-time experiments to gather information about differences in individuals rather than studying the general structure of mind. Cattell, at the time when Chizh was experimenting with drugs in Petersburg, tried all kinds of stimulants—from hashish to chocolate—on the other side of the Atlantic.[58] Kraepelin, a young enthusiast of psychological experiment, for a short time in 1882 was an assistant to Paul Flechsig in the psychiatric clinic of Leipzig University, where he set up a psychological laboratory and conducted experiments with drugs. Then he occasionally worked in Wundt's laboratory. Wundt generally set certain restrictions on the kinds of psychological experiments in his institute, but he did not object to Kraepelin's plan "to expand [his] tests with drugs, coffee and tea and to measure the mental reactions of psychiatric patients to get a better idea of the mental changes." As Kraepelin wrote in his memoirs, Wundt let him proceed with his plans and even supplied him with materials to construct his own apparatus when he left Leipzig.[59]

Although some historians have argued that the history of psychological experimentation on the mentally ill was the result of sheer coincidence—that is, Kraepelin, a Wundtian, also happened to be a psychiatrist[60]—there was more to it than being simply an outgrowth of Kraepelin's personal history. Like Kraepelin, Chizh became enthusiastic about the project of reforming psychiatry with the help of experimental psychology. In Wundt's laboratory in Leipzig, Chizh conducted orthodox experiments on the time of simple and complex reactions,[61] but he also carried out reaction-time experiments on mental patients, with the aim of finding psychological differences between them and normal subjects.[62] Any suspicion that Wundtian experiment was less objective than "pathological" experiment disappeared and was replaced by the hope that, if the insane were to become subjects of Wundtian experiments, as previously they had been subjects of hypnotic investigations, psychiatry would start a new page.[63] At a meeting of the Moscow Psychological

Society in 1887, the psychiatrists G. I. Rossolimo (1860–1928) and A. A. To-karskii (1859–1901) held the attention of the audience by demonstrating both Wundt's experiments and a hypnotic session.[64] In 1895, the same year in which British psychologist and anthropologist W. H. R. Rivers showed reaction-time experiments to his fellow psychiatrists in England and argued that the method could be expanded to study children and the insane, Tokarskii set up a psychological laboratory in the psychiatric clinic of Moscow University in order to teach future psychiatrists about what he thought had become a nec-essary instrument in their work.[65]

Experimental psychology had a prestigious scientific image for many psy-chiatrists, and it satisfied their desire to escape from hospital routine. But by arming psychiatry with sophisticated measuring devices, as Mitchell G. Ash has argued, they acquired more than just scientific respectability. Together with those psychologists who operated outside hospital walls, psychiatrists participated in reshaping what they studied. Mental and moral capacities were transformed into psychical functions that acted or failed to act in a measur-able way.[66] It was the possibility of studying moral feelings scientifically that attracted Chizh and, probably, Kraepelin to Wundt's laboratory. While work-ing hard in Wundt's laboratory, Kraepelin "had written a generally compre-hensive essay on the roots of morals."[67] His moral concern dictated his choice of subjects for study—the influence of alcohol, drugs, and fatigue. He in-cluded the normative quality "working capacity" in the list of basic attrib-utes of the personality and regarded his research on this topic as his major achievement in psychological medicine.[68]

Nevertheless, Kraepelin and Chizh ultimately pursued different goals. Krae-pelin's main ambition was to reform psychiatry by replacing the old phe-nomenological classification with a new one based on the etiology of dis-eases. He undertook his psychological research hoping to find the underlying structures of diseases—patterns that would consist of anatomical and psy-chological symptoms tied to one another.[69] Advancing steadily along this path, Kraepelin created his own classification of diseases (nosology), which remains the foundation of modern psychiatric systems, with the famous diag-nostic categories of manic-depressive psychosis and dementia praecox at the center. Though Kraepelin subsequently abandoned psychology and concen-trated on clinical research, his attempt to uncover the correlation of psycho-logical phenomena with diseases became well known, in Russia as elsewhere.

Chizh, who did not share the aim of perfecting psychiatric classification and never accepted the Kraepelinian category of dementia praecox, had dif-ferent hopes for psychology. His ambition was to find, through comparative psychological studies of insane, criminal, and normal people, the foundation of moral feelings. As in his earlier experiments with hypnosis and drugs,[70] he sought in psychological experiments to prove that the mentally ill and criminals had a biologically determined weakness of moral feelings and will. He highly valued the concept of *active apperception*, which Wundt made responsible for attention and will, precisely because Chizh saw in this concept the psychological foundation of morality. He assumed that the mentally ill must have defective attention and will, and he looked for evidence of their weak apperception. With Wundt's and Flechsig's authorization, Chizh conducted his first series of reaction-time experiments on the mentally ill in Flechsig's clinic. He found that the reactions of insane patients were much slower than those of normal subjects. This was undoubtedly caused, he concluded, by weak apperception. When a subject with progressive paralysis had quicker reactions with associations to familiar stimuli, Chizh explained this in the same way, by weakness of apperception: associations not controlled by attention would require less time.[71]

Kraepelin was interested in nuances of psychological processes in different mental illnesses and hoped psychology would help provide, to use modern language, a differential diagnosis. By contrast, because Chizh's interest was in the foundation of morality, he was seeking a "general factor" of insanity rather than differences between mental diseases. He was not interested in varieties but in degrees of insanity, which, in his view, depended on how well active apperception was preserved in a mentally ill person. "Choosing patients for research," he wrote, "I completely ignore the forms of illness; at this stage the mentally ill interest me only as different stages of insanity . . . I study given pathological states, not forms of illness."[72] A self-experiment on assessing the inner sense of time completely persuaded him that will and character were independent of sensorial processes. Every night for a whole year, before going to bed, Chizh gave himself a command to wake up at a particular time. Mostly he succeeded, and he found the results revealing about his character. "To be always earlier, never late" was an individual feature that he preserved even when asleep. His punctuality, self-discipline, and will made him, he wrote, an excellent subject for experiments in Wundt's laboratory.[73]

These qualities apparently helped Chizh with his career, too. On his return to Russia in 1885, he was appointed head psychiatrist in the St. Panteleimon Hospital in Petersburg. There he organized a psychological laboratory equipped with the instruments and apparatus brought from Leipzig, and he proceeded to conduct a series of experiments on the patients.[74] To his opponents who could not comprehend psychometrics, he answered with Plato's words, "everything beautiful is difficult."[75] He followed the development of experimental psychology in the West, periodically reported on it in Russian journals, and edited Russian translations of Theodor Ziehen's *Physiological Psychology* and his own lecture notes from Wundt's course on ethics.[76] He became an authority in the area, and his name (occasionally transliterated as Woldemar von Tchisch) was mentioned by reviewers alongside the names of Wundt, F. C. Donders, and Sigmund Exner.[77] Chizh's career advanced steadily: in 1886, he lectured on nervous and mental diseases at the Military-Medical Academy, and two years later he became *Privatdozent* (a nonsalaried teacher, receiving pay only from students' fees) in forensic psychiatry in the department of law at St. Petersburg University. He suggested the use of psychological experiment in forensic psychiatry as a very sensitive instrument that could detect the first signs of insanity long before they overtly manifested themselves. A delayed reaction time, he believed, was an undeniable sign of a developing insanity. Chizh was also the first in Russia to apply psychological experiment to criminals, and he concluded that their "narrow span of attention," in combination with "an absence of moral education and deteriorated moral feelings," caused their criminal conduct.[78] In 1891 Chizh received the professorship at the University of Dorpat that had been held by Kraepelin since 1886. Their paths crossed for the second time.

Kraepelin would not have chosen Dorpat if he had been offered a professorship in Germany. Though Dorpat (Derpt) was a German-speaking university, it was located within the borders of the Russian Empire and was cut off from the main German academic centers. While teaching there, Kraepelin was burdened by the hospital's financial problems and frustrated by the language barriers with his mainly Estonian- and Russian-speaking patients. Psychological experiments, as he wrote, maintained his academic spirit. He "carried out tests on aphasic and other suitable psychiatric patients and on manic patients" and later set up "a school of psychology in Dorpat," luckily having found "self-sacrificing students prepared to devote many, many months' work solely to their doctorate thesis."[79]

Kraepelin remained in Dorpat until political reaction, which followed the murder of Alexander II in 1881, began to affect the universities. The government set out to limit academic freedoms and increase the powers of its inspectors over student and faculty bodies. The Higher Education Law of 1884 transferred the authority to nominate professors from the universities to the Ministry of Education.[80] Later in the decade Dorpat was given a Russified name, Iur'ev, and the university was renamed the Imperial Iur'ev University. Foreign professors were required to take an oath to the tsar, and those who refused—Kraepelin among them—were fired.[81] His career, however, did not suffer, as he had already been called to a chair in Heidelberg.

In 1891, then, Chizh inherited Kraepelin's laboratory and his students, to whom he started teaching physiological psychology. Soon thereafter he launched a campaign to introduce the course into medical curricula nationwide. It is worth noting that the first Wundt-style laboratories in Russia emerged in psychiatric clinics and the first courses in physiological psychology were introduced in medical departments.[82] Traditional psychologists, who were affiliated with chairs of philosophy within departments of history and philology at Russian universities, were left behind. While they argued that real knowledge of mind could be obtained only through self-observation and that experimental psychology was but an introduction to a true science of mind, their colleagues from medical schools were buying apparatus for measuring reaction times and were practicing hypnotic experiments. When G. I. Chelpanov (1862–1936), a psychologist from Kiev and later the founder of the Moscow Psychological Institute, wrote about a "psychological institute" at Moscow University, organized from private funds on a Western model, he was referring to the laboratory at the university's psychiatric clinic.[83] Only in 1896 was the department of history and philology of Moscow University to introduce experimental psychology into the curriculum.[84]

At that time psychological experiments were still associated with "balances, laboratory glasses, ovens, jars, knives, pitiful victims of vivisection," and a layperson could "ask in confusion whether it is really possible to weigh the soul, to put it in a jar, to heat [it] over a fire, to dissect it."[85] Proud of psychiatrists' reputation as pioneers of laboratory psychology in Russia, Chizh vehemently protested when N. N. Lange (1858–1921), a doctoral candidate in philosophy, in defending his thesis on experimental psychology ignored the work already done by psychiatrists.[86] With time, however, Chizh's experimental zeal weakened, and in 1902 he stopped teaching his course.[87] Fewer and fewer students—who, anyway, were now distracted by events outside the university walls—were at his disposal to conduct time-consuming experiments. The last thesis came from his laboratory in 1904, on the very eve of radical changes in Russian life.

In 1904 Russia entered a war against Japan. The tsarist government thought "a little victorious war" could distract the masses from rebellious intentions, but the hoped-for events did not follow. The war, which saw the Russian fleet destroyed and territory and thousands of lives lost, proved a disaster, and its extreme unpopularity contributed to the rise of revolutionary aspirations. Together with other medical professionals, psychiatrists were heavily involved in the Russo-Japanese war. It was the first occasion on which the Russian army established a special psychiatric service. Chizh apparently lost some of his students to the army.

Chizh now turned away from psychological experiment and towards literature, which alone, he thought, could express the nuances of the psychology of criminals and the mentally ill. An established professor, he no longer needed to secure his reputation as a rigorous scientist; by expressing an interest in literature and art, Chizh could better communicate his superior status as a professor of clinical psychiatry. He now stressed the limitation of the experimental as opposed to the clinical approach, claiming that "efforts to know patients by the same means as we know . . . the objective world, are not sustainable."[88] Clinical psychiatry was both science and art, he argued, and this explained why the best clinicians, such as Russian physicians S. P. Botkin and N. I. Pirogov, were good writers and Charcot was a connoisseur of the arts. References to Henri Bergson's *intuition* and Theodor Lipps's *Einfühlung* (empathy) gradually replaced psychometrics in Chizh's works. He perceived their methods as similar to those employed by a novelist or a portrait painter: in a similar way, a good clinician attempted to go below the surface, deep into the "core of personality."

Chizh had continued his exploration of literature, started in 1885 with his book on Dostoevsky. In 1898 he published a similar study of I. S. Turgenev (1818–83), in whose characters he found excellent illustrations of insanity. But now, even more than in his book on Dostoevsky, Chizh judged literature with the tone of an expert: he believed that his "duty, the duty of a Russian psychiatrist, [was] to acknowledge the absolute correctness of the descriptions of mental pathology in Turgenev's works."[89] He especially valued Turgenev's observation that the mentally ill had strangely shining eyes. Chizh himself was remembered for identifying a "particular symptom of epilepsy," a lead-gray metallic shine in the eyes of the mentally ill.[90]

Chizh next wrote an essay on the poet Alexander Pushkin (1799–1837) for Pushkin's centenary in 1899. Pushkin was favored by many generations of readers, and the leading critic, Belinsky, called him "the sun of Russian poetry." Pushkin's contemporaries, including Tsar Nicholas I, regarded him as one of the brightest men of his time. His joie de vivre attracted the hearts of many friends and women, and his concern for his country made him the archetypal "poet-citizen" in Russian eyes.[91] After the famous speech by Dostoevsky at the unveiling of the monument to Pushkin in Moscow in 1880, the poet had become a figure onto whom anyone who wished to make a political claim projected his attitude. Different groups within the Russian intelligentsia used his emblematic figure in order to articulate their values, the poet acquired a mythical status, and the Pushkin centenary grew into an important social and political occasion. As a result, Pushkin became above criticism, including criticism in the form of psychiatric diagnosis. For the same reason that British Victorians thought it "impossible for the mind to conceive of a mad Shakespeare,"[92] Russian intellectuals could not conceive of a mad Pushkin. Chizh indeed argued that the poet was an embodiment of mental health. Pushkin possessed, together with his poetic genius, a "rich, harmoniously developed nature." His "drive towards truth, goodness, and beauty" strikingly contrasted with "the insane person's inability either to love or understand truth, goodness, or beauty."[93]

To recognize the beauty and greatness of human nature and to be filled with the "good" emotions of admiration, love, and hope was a requirement for the "good" person in the Victorian period.[94] Darwin defended the superiority of love and self-sacrifice for one's fellow-creatures by identifying these virtues with "natural social instincts" that push an animal to act for the good and welfare of the community rather than for its personal happiness.[95] His followers, Chizh included, believed that moral perfection required perfect health: "the higher, the more perfect is psychic organization, the more man is able to love humankind." Though, Chizh argued elsewhere, hysterical patients could feel compassion, they could not distinguish between good and evil, and their love therefore was directed by caprice and whimsy rather than by sublime moral feelings.[96] The mentally ill had irretrievably lost their higher "intellectual feelings"—curiosity, intellectual honesty, and love for truth. Even if some of them, "pretended inventors and reformers," claimed to have a passion for knowledge, they in fact were not striving for truth.[97] Unlike the irreproachable Pushkin, many outstanding figures, lacking the necessary qualities to be essentially sane persons, failed to pass Chizh's test. Gogol was one of these: "Alfred de Musset, Edgar Poe, Baudelaire, Verlaine, Flaubert, Gogol were strikingly indifferent towards public issues . . . Gogol did not like science."[98]

Revolution and Morality

Russia entered the new century pregnant with political conflicts. Every level of society had reasons to oppose the regime: peasants suffered from regular famines, workers from unlimited exploitation, educated classes from political repression, and all Russians from restricted access to power under the absolute monarchy. The opposition movement, led by the professional intelligentsia and the radical part of the gentry, demanded an end to autocracy and establishment of representative government.[99] The last decade of the nineteenth century, with its cholera epidemics, impoverishment of the peasantry, and workers' strikes, provoked a rise in political consciousness. Physicians, many of whom worked for *zemstva* (local governments, the sites of opposition to autocracy) and were exposed to social problems in their everyday work, became deeply involved in the struggles of the day. The majority of Russian physicians carried heavy duties as state employees: they were required by law, without being paid, to witness corporal punishment and capital executions, place their expertise at the service of courts, carry out autopsies, and respond to epidemics. The growing radicalization of the medical profession placed it in the vanguard of the opposition movement.[100]

Psychiatrists were as much involved in politics as was the medical profession in general.[101] Political attitudes and degree of involvement varied widely from individual to individual: while some hid activists, rebellious students, and illegal literature in mental hospitals, others were perceived as proponents of "police" psychiatry.[102] Yet nobody could avoid the issues of the day. Chizh, though known for his loyalty to the regime and his nationalist attitudes, at least once protested publicly when his fellow psychiatrists were removed from their positions for political reasons.[103] His own intention, however, was to stand aside from political battles and to carry out his professional obligations. Nevertheless, even when he discussed only literature, he still felt constantly dragged into political debates.

In 1902, fifty years after his death, Gogol was remembered countrywide. Always ready to say a psychiatric word at a writer's anniversary, Chizh published a small article on one of the characters in Gogol's *Dead Souls*. For Russian readers, this comic character—whose name, Pliushkin (different from Pushkin!), was derived from *pliushka* (a roll)—was a synonym for avarice. Chizh, however, argued that Pliushkin was "not the type of an avaricious man, but rather the type of senile dementia." Pliushkin's apparent greed was not a passion, as he had lost "even the simplest selfish feelings" and retained nothing beyond aimless and meaningless habits, but was a pure pathology. As soon as Chizh's article appeared, his former student Ia. F. Kaplan challenged his opinion. Kaplan argued that Pliushkin, though "petty, miserable, and disgusting," was not a product of illness but the result of normal changes in old age. He proved his point with Gogol's remark about Pliushkin, that old age is "horrifying, oppressive and inhumane." Chizh, who was much older that his critic, argued back that a sane man, even in his old age, would not, like

Pliushkin, have "become so undignified, could not have lived outside of society, could not have loved nothing but wealth."[104]

When other psychiatrists intervened in the discussion, it became clear that something more than a diagnosis was at stake. One of them, Iulii Portugalov, took the role of an arbiter in the Chizh–Kaplan polemics. He thought both psychiatrists were mistaken when they applied their professional expertise to a literary character. He wanted to put what he called the "psychopathological method in literary criticism" under the control of literary critics and sociologists.[105] Almost certainly, Portugalov claimed, psychiatric analysis should not be applied to Gogol, who was distinguished first of all as a social writer. Any psychological or psychiatric interpretation of Gogol's characters that ignored their significance as social types would be irrelevant to the author's plot. Pliushkin, Portugalov thought, symbolized an accumulator of wealth, and he was therefore to be understood as a type of the precapitalist era. He was created as a counterpart to the main character of the novel, Chichikov, in whom Gogol pictured a new type, the capitalist entrepreneur. Analyzing Pliushkin's pathology, both Chizh and Kaplan misunderstood the meaning of the novel, which portrayed the emerging capitalist era. Portugalov's message was that on the eve of momentous social changes, nobody, including psychiatrists, could ignore the social meaning of the novel.

Other psychiatrists agreed that by psychologizing and pathologizing Pliushkin, Chizh and Kaplan succumbed to a "false tendency—to explain social defects and social crime by nervous and mental diseases."[106] Another psychiatrist, accepting that politically neutral psychiatry was not possible, wrote that "psychopathology, both in theory and in the practice of art and life, can only be a subservient instrument, a source of counterevidence in solving religious, moral, and philosophical problems."[107] By insisting that the psychiatric analysis of literature should always be informed by social and literary criticism, psychiatrists signaled their willingness to take part in political struggles. In unprecedented circumstances, psychiatrists, acting against their usual tendency to expand the claims for their expertise, accepted that their competencies were limited. Convinced that control over mental health in a country with an oppressive regime and a starving population was beyond their power, psychiatrists accepted that social problems should be adequately dealt with, whether through reform or revolution. At the meeting of the Pirogov Society (the Society of Russian Physicians in Memory of Pirogov) in 1904 and the Second Congress of Russian Psychiatrists and Neuropathologists in 1905, both groups stated in their resolutions that political reforms were a necessary step to the nation's mental health. The radical majority expressed their disappointment with those psychiatrists who, like Chizh, wanted to be above the battle.

In 1903 Chizh gave a talk on Gogol (published as a newspaper article, a journal article, and a book) in which he discussed the writer's own mental health.[108] Without responding to the criticism of his article on Pliushkin, he produced a variation on Belinsky's theme that it is better on moral grounds to consider Gogol insane rather than a traitor. Having set out in his new essay to describe Gogol's insanity, Chizh decided that the writer suffered from and died of melancholia. For several reasons, the book was badly received. Even Chizh's fellow physicians criticized him for instigating a psychiatric diagnosis of a writer dear to people's hearts. In particular, a Dr. Kachenovskii cared to preserve Gogol's reputation as a sane person and blamed Chizh for "the chaos that he produced in readers' heads, for they will hardly understand that a mentally insane person could create a work of genius . . . and could be a great altruist." From his point of view, Gogol's oddity was entirely within the range of normal conduct and could be explained by a somatic disease. He believed that Gogol, who did not as a child receive proper education, which would have prevented him from indulging in slackness, was not able to repress his bad temper when he suffered physically. While seeking to excuse Gogol's failures by his weak health, Kachenovskii also challenged psychiatrists, who, he thought, gave an exaggerated picture of Gogol's pathology, with the words of Christ: "Why beholdest thou the mote that is in thy brother's eye, but perceivest not the beam that is thine own eye?"[109]

But there was another kind of criticism from Chizh's contemporaries, which showed that the time for accepting Belinsky's judgment of Gogol had passed. As Chizh might have discovered with surprise, the view prevailing throughout the nineteenth century that literature necessarily had a social mission was going out of fashion.

Gogol's Rehabilitation in the Twentieth Century

Critics drew attention to the fact that the principal grounds for the diagnosis of Gogol's insanity had really been moral, not aesthetic.[110] This became a problem for the generation inspired by Friedrich Nietzsche. Critics, philosophers, and artists reported that "morality has ceased to inspire . . . it is perceived as a hindrance to the creative energy of existence," and they debated the creative drive and unconscious roots of art. "If social duty was the highest virtue of an earlier generation," a historian remarked, "now intellectuals strove toward the goals of self-discovery and self-realization."[111] Gogol, whose case was a foundation stone of Belinsky's moral vision of literature, was the first candidate for reassessment in the atmosphere of "transvaluation of values." In what would become a manifesto of the Russian Nietzscheans, the philosopher Lev Shestov demolished the moralistic view that the value ascribed to Gogol's works should be preserved at the expense of his reputation as a person: "When Gogol burned the manuscript of the second volume of *Dead Souls,* he was declared insane—otherwise, it would have been impossible to rescue ideals. But Gogol was more correct when he burned his precious manuscript (which could have provided immortality on earth to a whole score of 'sane' critics) than he was when he wrote it. This is something idealists will never tolerate; they need 'Gogol's works,' but they are unconcerned with Gogol himself, with his 'great misfortune, great ugliness, and great failure.'"[112]

During the late-nineteenth-century religious revival in Russia, Gogol's search attracted sympathetic attention from Lev Tolstoy, Dmitrii Merezhkovskii, and other religious thinkers. They demonstrated the importance of Gogol's Christian beliefs for any meaningful discussion of his works and attempted a reconciliation or a synthesis of Gogol's supposed contradictions, claiming that they were inherent in his nature. Merezhkovskii argued that Gogol's critics failed to understand that in *Selected Passages* Gogol "went along the same path as ever," that he had always been religious and had not experienced any inner turmoil. They reconsidered the belief in his insanity and doubted the criteria of normality and pathology that psychiatrists had earlier applied to him. A young psychiatrist from Petersburg, M. O. Shaikevich, asked rhetorically whether "only sane and sound people are able to love freedom, truth, humanity, to hate injustice, to seek the light, to ease the sufferings of others." He mentioned counterexamples of much loved writers and dignified people who suffered from mental illnesses.[113]

In tune with Shestov, the psychiatrist G. Ia. Troshin (1874–1938) opposed the view that Gogol should be judged by nonliterary people, including psychiatrists: "the personality of the brilliant satirist, taken without his creative consciousness, is an artificial target to which any label can be applied . . . Previously the Slavophiles and Westernizers targeted it, now psychiatrists take over the battlefield. All of them think that 'the best that can be said is to call him insane.'"[114] Troshin was one of a number of physicians who combined genuine commitment to medicine with love of the arts, and he was a musician and wrote poetry. As a young man he had reflected on the psychological effects of music in an essay "Musical Emotions" (1901), and two years before his death he published a book, *On the Influence of Music on Creativity* (1936). In the year when he defended his doctoral thesis with Bekhterev on the reflexes of the brain, he published the book *Literary and Artistic Emotions, Normal and Pathological* (1936).[115]

Troshin agreed that the contradiction between Gogol's beliefs and the character of his work needed an explanation, but he claimed that it was to be found in the "writer's method, in the psychology of laughter, and in the unconscious factor."[116] He suggested replacing the reductionist psychiatric interpretation, which missed out the intimate Gogol, with a psychological interpretation that gave priority to the writer's self-perception and to the unconscious factors of creative processes: "Gogol himself interprets the moments [of his inspiration] as God's deed, while psychiatry replaces God by ideas of grandiosity; psychology of creativity needs neither. It starts from the assumption that intellectual and emotional factors alone are not sufficient for creative processes, and that a third—unconscious—factor is necessary. The work of the last factor is in many senses mysterious to us."[117] Troshin hoped for a "psychology of creative work," more imaginative, less moralistic, and more suitable for literature and writers. It would reject the Lombrosian assumption that genius was a product of disease or an atavism, a sign of degeneration of the human species. The new psychology would start from the assumption that genius was above the rest of humanity. Like Shestov, Troshin believed that Gogol, Dostoevsky, and Nietzsche were prophets of a new humanity.[118]

To fight the belief that Gogol was "degenerate," Troshin used the term *progeneration,* which Bazhenov had coined a few years earlier in speaking about the "supreme sanity" of geniuses. Following Bazhenov, Troshin thought genius represented a forthcoming, "progenerating" human type rather than a declining one. Other psychiatrists also developed similar ideas. A psychiatrist from Kiev, I. A. Sikorskii (1845–1918), found that although artists, writers, poets, and some scholars had a peculiar mental organization that differed from the normal, this difference was not in the direction of decline or degeneration. Quite the opposite: this was "a highly progressive phenomenon caught in the moment when its development has not been completed [and this is] a step towards man's ideal evolution."[119] Sikorskii illustrated his thesis by referring to a recently published novel in which the hero, a young and conscientious physician, exemplified this type; though the character is disharmonious, he is evolving in the right direction.

Other psychiatrists, however, pointed to the discrepancies in Bazhenov's and Troshin's speculations about the superiority of ill geniuses. Bazhenov, in the words of one critic, M O. Shaikevich, had collected abundant material that was more than sufficient to confirm Gogol's mental illness, but he regrettably "had not followed the case till the end" and had muddled the final diagnosis. The very term *progeneration* was extremely confusing. Shaikevich objected, "Let us suppose that a man suffering from either periodic psychosis or epilepsy . . . is endowed with artistic talents . . . If his positive, useful qualities had had more weight, he would be called a progenerate, if negative ones—a degenerate. It is much more convenient in such cases to keep to the old term, the higher degenerate." The same point was made against Troshin, who admitted that Gogol had much stronger reactions to ideas than did normal people, but refused to assess Gogol from the point of view of what is normal, because, as he wrote, "the emotions of great creators differ in scale from ours."[120] Shaikevich doubted that Gogol's disease, which he believed was periodic psychosis, could be considered a simple disharmony or instability determined by the progeneration of a higher psychic type.[121]

At the time this discussion was taking place, it was everybody's impression that Russia stood on the threshold of an unknown future. In 1905 the wave of opposition to autocracy reached its peak. The year began with Bloody Sunday (January 9), when an unarmed procession of workers went to the Winter Palace in Petersburg with a petition to the tsar. They pleaded with their "little father" to abolish punishments for those who suffered for their religious and political convictions, to proclaim civic freedoms, to introduce universal public education and an eight-hour workday, and to change the taxation system in favor of poorer people. To emphasize their peaceful intentions, a number of workers took their families along; the procession was headed by the priest Gapon and carried icons and sang hymns. The crowd was met by gunfire and the day ended in a massacre. Bloody Sunday was followed by an increase of violence and provoked what was later called the first Russian revolution.

During a subsequent uprising, the All-Russian Union of Medical Personnel joined other professional associations in the Union of Unions, a militant force in support of the revolution.[122] Both the meeting of the Pirogov Society in 1904 and the Second Congress of Russian Psychiatrists and Neuropathologists in 1905 included in their final statements a demand for representative government. Left-wing psychiatrists argued that "the policies of the Russian government are a direct cause of the increased number of cases of mental disturbance."[123] Their opposition to the policies of the tsarist government was also implicit, as the historian Julie Vail Brown remarks, in the widespread movement to "democratize" the profession from within and, in particular, to change control of the asylums.[124] The director usually ruled each asylum almost single-handedly, and rank-and-file psychiatrists, not to mention unqualified personnel, had almost no power over the asylum's daily life. The nursing staff was in a particularly bad situation: working in overcrowded asylums, nurses and wardens were underpaid and often did not have accommodation other than in the asylum's wards.[125] Like the Russian Empire itself, the asylum was built on the principle of absolutism, and like the Russian Empire, it was thought to be in need of reform.

The psychiatric department of the St. Nicholas Hospital in Petersburg, where Troshin was assistant physician, was known as one of the poorest, most overcrowded, and most poorly managed public asylums. With the beginning of the revolution, the staff, dissatisfied with the director's dictatorial policy, asked for participation in decisions. The director rejected their suggestion of "collegial administration," and one day the workers, led by junior physicians, broke into his office and carried him from the building in a wheelbarrow. Having removed the hospital's chief officer, they began to release some of the prisoners, including "political" ones, who were incarcerated in the institution. The staff and workers were arrested and taken to court. All were sentenced, including Troshin, their leader, who was imprisoned for sixteen months.[126]

Chizh and Troshin, the proponents of the two different points of view on Gogol, stood now on opposite sides of the barricade. Unlike the majority of psychiatrists, who had liberal or radical attitudes, Chizh always remained loyal to the tsarist regime. Following in the steps of the French historian and philosopher Hippolyte Taine, Chizh treated revolutionaries as "anarchists and political criminals" whose "destructive drive, anxiety, and dissatisfaction . . . depend on their pathological organization."[127] The revolutionary crowd during the events of 1905–7 appeared to him to be full of alcoholics and the insane; the revolutionary leaders, he believed, were degenerates.[128] Both criminal anthropology and experimental psychology, in which he sought at different times for an adequate expression of his views, proved too scholastic for his purposes. In opposition to what he had believed for decades, Chizh now criticized criminal anthropologists who, operating with "scientific" methods, had completely forgotten "the method of individual observation," which writers like Dostoevsky possessed in abundance.[129]

At the beginning of the revolution, psychiatrists published reports on the supposed increase in the incidence of mental disease, which they believed was the result of street violence.[130] Unlike his radical colleagues, who held the government responsible for the increase in violence, Chizh suggested that violence came from both sides. He cited cases in which rebels tortured a policeman and a priest, with traumatic consequences for the victims. When psychiatrists invented a category of "revolutionary psychosis," he rejected it, as earlier he had rejected the categories of "prison psychosis" and, during the war with Japan, "war psychosis."[131]

Chizh believed, first, that insanity was certainly the result of inner organization rather than outside influences and, second, that his fellow psychiatrists shaped their views about the traumatic etiology of mental illness to suit their political sympathies. He reproached his contradictory colleagues when "at the first congress [of psychiatrists in 1887] they admitted that liberation had a bad effect on mental health, and at the second congress [in 1905] they stated that the limitation of freedom had a bad effect on mental health." When, in the aftermath of the revolution, psychiatrists warned about the threat of the repressive atmosphere for mental health, Chizh argued that "respect for the fighters is incompatible with the idea that they could become mentally ill as a result of political failure."[132] Arguing that revolution by itself was neither healthy nor harmful, Chizh called for the separation of psychiatry from the struggles of the day. As in the polemics about Pliushkin, psychiatrists who found it impossible to stay outside the political battle questioned Chizh's neutrality. Psychiatrists also knew that at the time when they were fighting for abolition of the death penalty, Chizh served as an attending physician at the executions of political prisoners. Not surprisingly, his radical colleagues ostracized him as a staunch supporter of the regime.[133]

In 1915 Chizh left Iur'ev to become chief physician of the West Front Division of the Russian Red Cross, based in Kiev. When the Bolshevik Revolution arrived he was still in Kiev, where he died in 1922.

Conclusion: Psychological Man

In 1909 a newly founded almanac, *Landmarks* (*Vekhi*), continued what Shestov and others had started before the 1905 revolution: it became a voice for artistic, private, noncivic concerns. Its editor called for "the theoretical and practical priority of spiritual life over the external forms of society, in the sense that the inner life of the personality is the only creative force in human existence and is . . . the only firm basis for any social reconstruction."[134] In the year when this manifesto appeared, the literary world as well as "all educated Russia" celebrated Gogol's centenary. It was clear that any straightforward medical interpretation of the vicissitudes of Gogol's life and work had become much more difficult.

For a while, neither medical nor nonmedical accounts of Gogol's life and death gained the upper hand; instead, they simply coexisted. On one side, in a jubilee essay on Gogol, the writer V. G. Korolenko praised Bazhenov for his "excellent work" in which he gave Gogol's illness a "scientific diagnosis— depressive neurosis." Korolenko even collected his own evidence that Gogol's supposed inherited vulnerability was not from his mother's side, as Bazhenov guessed, but "was an exact copy of the illness from which his father died."[135] Speculating about its causes, he wrote that "physicians give a physiological explanation to spiritual depression without obvious reason: the blood vessels that feed the brain become narrow so that blood cannot reach the area that is responsible for mood. This is, so to say, a purely mechanical [cause]. Gogol inherited this apparatus already damaged, and as a result he was prone to melancholia, and often depressed and sad." Yet spiritual discourse competed with the medical one in this account: "The writer of genius, descending to the bottom of Russian life and rising to its heights, was painfully seeking a way out for himself that at the same time would be a way out for his unfortunate country. He died in 1852 from a deep and constantly increasing spiritual depression, not from any particular illness . . . he dwindled like a candle, and, finally, extinguished like one, when nothing remained that could maintain his life." Both "the joy of creative work" and "unfavorable organic influences" emerged with equal rights in Korolenko's account, like "two contradictory forces [that] fought in the writer's fragile constitution."[136]

Further into the "psychological century," the accent shifted towards interpretation of Gogol's inner world as a battlefield of contradictory tendencies. A new generation portrayed Gogol as "a genius tormented by the absence of self-confidence and inner stability, who sought to free himself and to feel strong and powerful."[137] Psychoanalysts found confirmation for the idea that inner conflict is resolved through creative work in Gogol's own reflection on his talent and illness.[138] The younger generation of psychiatrists believed that a new psychology would be based on the Nietzschean vision of the Superman, as "opposed to 'modern' man, to 'good' man, to Christians and other nihilists, . . . as an 'ideal' type of a higher kind of man, half 'saint' and half 'genius.'"[139] In contrast to the nineteenth-century moral man, the new one was to be a "private man, who turns away from the arenas of public failure to re-examine himself and his own emotions."[140] The new disciplines, psychology of creative processes and psychotherapy, were created for this new man. Chizh would hardly have been comfortable with these changes. A man of the "long nineteenth century," he perceived Gogol's pathography essentially as a way to express his concern with morality.[141]

Dostoevsky

From Epilepsy to Progeneration

Listen, I don't like *spies* and *psychologists,* at least those
who poke into my soul.   —F. M. Dostoevsky

Dostoevsky . . . is the psychologist of psychologists.
                                    —Stefan Zweig

Dostoevsky made mental illness comprehensible for a
general audience . . . He demonstrated to everybody that
. . . the insane can be found not only among the inmates
of asylums, but that they mix in everyday life together
with sane people.   —V. M. Bekhterev

When he was a young man, Fyodor Mikhailovich Dostoevsky (1821–81) was
an adherent of socialist ideas. After years of suffering and reflection he became more conservative, and his later novels contained bitter and profound
criticism of the extreme policies of the radicals. In return, radical literary critics emphasized the "nervousness" of Dostoevsky's talent, and some of them
even argued that his interest in human suffering came close to being a perverse, sadistic predilection. After Dostoevsky's death, a rumor about his epilepsy was added to such characterizations. Inspired by the writer's masterful
descriptions of psychological dilemmas and mental pathologies, psychiatrists
attributed his special talent to his own experience of illness. The joint efforts
of critics, psychiatrists, and some literary historians gradually transformed
Dostoevsky into, to use Joseph Frank's expression, "a tormented genius exist-

ing on the edge of madness and creating novels of hallucinatory power out of the fantasies of his semidemented psyche."[1]

Around the turn of the century, N. N. Bazhenov, a psychiatrist with a strong interest in literature and the arts, approached Dostoevsky from this point of view, seeking to show how the writer's falling sickness was reflected in his literary works. Nineteenth-century psychiatry took epilepsy to be a sign of degeneration. Bazhenov, however, hesitated to apply so belittling a judgment to a writer whose talent he revered. When he analyzed Dostoevsky and other writers, he altered his psychiatric perspective and introduced a notion of "progeneration," by which he meant a progressive development of humanity, which reaches its final point in artistic genius. Instead of labeling Dostoevsky a "higher degenerate," Bazhenov made him into the prototype of the future perfect human being. Similarly, other turn-of-the-century psychiatrists, inspired by a Nietzschean revival of Romantic values, rejected the postulates of the degeneration theory and reformulated "the suffering" of great artists in terms of creative illness.

"A Cruel Talent": Psychiatrists and Radical Criticism of Dostoevsky

The more V. G. Belinsky, in the 1840s, was disappointed with Gogol's betrayal of the sacred mission of art, the more he praised the young Dostoevsky for his promising first novel, Poor Folk (1846). Belinsky perceived this novel as a long-awaited portrayal of society's ailments and a call for compassion for the poor. He pronounced Poor Folk Russia's first "social novel." But Dostoevsky's subsequent works puzzled the critic. "A strange thing! An incomprehensible thing!" he exclaimed, confused by the Hoffmannesque tale, The Landlady (1847); and he dismissed The Double (1846), a psychological investigation into the problem of split personality, as a portrayal of madness for its own sake.[2] In contrast to Belinsky, the critic Valerian Maikov, another of Dostoevsky's contemporaries, believed the latter story—about Golyadkin and his double—had a universal meaning. Maikov demanded, "Ask yourself: isn't there in you yourself something of Golyadkin, to which no one wants to confess?"[3]

Though both liberal and radical factions drew attention, at a very early stage, to what became notorious as Dostoevsky's "psychological" manner, they attached different meanings to it. While the liberals regarded it as a strength, the radicals considered it a failure. When Maikov compared Dostoevsky's art of penetrating the human soul to "the experience of a man of inquiring mind who has penetrated into the chemical composition of matter,"[4] it was a positive appraisal. By contrast, when Belinsky and his heirs, who demanded that artists should tackle the problems of the day, said that Dostoevsky was only a "psychologist" and that his works were psychological sketches, it was a condemnation. Dostoevsky himself recognized the derogatory meaning of "psychologist," saying in protest that he was a "realist" not a psychologist. Yet the ambivalent label of "psychologist" stuck firmly to him.

The two views of Dostoevsky's *The Double*, represented initially by Belinsky and Maikov, gradually became emblematic of the rejection or acceptance of Dostoevsky's highly polemical work. Those who, like Belinsky, argued against Dostoevsky's point of view tended to find the characters in his novels mad or pathological, thereby dismissing the writer's moral and psychological quest as irrelevant to their own concern with social and political matters. On the opposite side, those who admired and cherished Dostoevsky's work tried not to use the label of "insanity." Either they saw his characters as normal people open to moral temptation and psychological suffering, or they attempted to explain his characters and therefore justify their ailments.

Belinsky, whom Isaiah Berlin held responsible for what he called the "Russian attitude,"[5] cultivated in his readers' minds an expectation that there should be coherence and continuity between a writer's life and work and that the writer's personal traits were largely responsible for the distinctiveness of his literature. When Belinsky wrote about the "nervousness" (*nervichnost'*) of Dostoevsky's talent and called him "a writer of human suffering," he was understood, according to the "Russian attitude," to be referring both to Dostoevsky's style and to the writer as a person. Dostoevsky's life seemed to confirm what Belinsky foretold at the beginning of the writer's career. When he was twenty-seven, Dostoevsky joined a circle of intellectuals, gathered around M. V. Butashevich-Petrashevsky, who discussed Charles Fourier's socialism. Dostoevsky's participation in the reproduction of Belinsky's "Letter to N. V. Gogol" (see Chapter 1) led to his arrest, an accusation of sedition and conspiracy against autocracy, and a sentence of death by firing squad. After the trauma of a mock execution, he spent four years in Siberian labor camps, before being required to serve as a soldier in Kazakhstan. It appears that in Siberia he began to experience falling sickness, possibly after corporal punishment, which added to the burden of life as a prisoner and exile.[6]

The new tsar, Alexander II, who came to the throne in 1855, refused to relieve Dostoevsky's suffering, and his prison term continued for four more years. When he did finally return to European Russia, Dostoevsky published *The Memoirs from the House of the Dead* (1860–62), based on his experience as a prisoner. His subsequent works, *The Insulted and Injured* (1861), *Crime and Punishment* (1866), and *The Idiot* (1868), added to his fame as a humanist and defender of "downtrodden people." In later novels, *The Brothers Karamazov* (1879–80) and *The Devils* (1871–72), he reconsidered his earlier faith in radical socialism. A polemicist par excellence, Dostoevsky quickly became a center of political discussions.[7] His *Diary of a Writer* (1873–81)—which first appeared in installments in a popular periodical—brought him even more fame during his life than did his novels. *The Devils*, which he called a "novel-pamphlet" when he began it, was an especially powerful attack on the extremist policies of Narodniki (the Populists), who developed a Russian version of peasant socialism. On its publication, the radicals immediately accused Dostoevsky of falsifying and distorting the revolutionary movement.[8]

A leading ideologist of the Populists, N. K. Mikhailovsky (1842–1904), responded to *The Devils* in a way that was similar to Belinsky's earlier criticism, castigating Dostoevsky for empty psychologizing. But unlike his predecessor, who criticized Dostoevsky simply for wasting his literary talent instead of writing on significant social topics, Mikhailovsky implied that Dostoevsky's exercises in describing pathology were not so innocent. A portrayal of radical socialists as political adventurers with dubious moral standards and unbalanced minds, he argued, was a deliberate attack on the left. The characters of *The Devils,* Mikhailovsky wrote, are "either people who are in an extremely excited state or monomaniacs who are given a chance to think up and preach exceedingly high-flown theories." He accused the writer of "putting the solution of some moral problem in the mouth of a man who is tormented by mental illness," in other words, of dismissing revolutionaries as madmen and ignoring the "really progressive young people"—the Populists.[9]

Thereafter, the radical camp followed Mikhailovsky's criticism of Dostoevsky.[10] The prince-anarchist P. A. Kropotkin (1842–1921) called Dostoevsky's later novels "unwholesome," with every character "suffering from some psychical disease or from moral perversion."[11] Kropotkin contrasted Dostoevsky's antiheroes with the affirmative characters of Turgenev and the even more affirmative ones of N. G. Chernyshevsky. In the 1860s and 1870s, the popularity of Chernyshevsky's novel *What Is to Be Done?* (1863) outweighed that of the writings of Turgenev, Tolstoy, and Dostoevsky. *What Is to Be Done?* pictured a utopia of a rationally organized and therefore happy society and presented a clear program of action for the radicals, such as Chernyshevsky himself, who wrote the novel in prison. A particularly inspiring image in the novel was Rakhmetov, a revolutionary who renounces his aristocratic origin, wealth, and all earthly pleasures and finally tests his endurance by sleeping on a board studded with nails.[12] He is sturdy, robust, educated mainly in science, critical but positive in his thinking, ready to act, not afraid of violence—in short, an exemplary revolutionary. Dostoevsky's characters, "weak, unstable, governed by caprice, given to irrational acts of rebellion," could not compete with the Rakhmetovs.[13]

When applied to Dostoevsky's characters, Mikhailovsky's arguments seemed to remain within the boundaries of literary criticism, though a political disagreement lay behind them. Immediately after Dostoevsky's death, however, when the influential religious philosopher Vladimir Solov'ev pronounced him a prophet and a spiritual leader of the Russian people, Mikhailovsky redoubled his efforts and attacked Dostoevsky personally. Solov'ev perceived Dostoevsky as a Christ-like figure whose prophetic power came from suffering, and this reputation was soon confirmed internationally by the half-French, half-British diplomat and literary critic Eugène Melchior de Vogüé. In a widely recognized study of Russian literature, which won him a chair in the Académie Française, de Vogüé featured Dostoevsky under the heading "A Religion of Suffering."[14] Mikhailovsky argued in response that Dostoevsky's admired humanism did not have holy sources and that his passion for the "humiliated and insulted" bordered on a delight in human degradation. Dostoevsky's humanism had a reverse side, which Mikhailovsky termed a "cruel talent," a talent guided by the pursuit of the sensual pleasure involved in torture: "no one in Russian literature has analyzed the sensations of a wolf devouring a sheep with such thoroughness, such depth, one might say with such love as Dostoevsky, if it is possible in fact to speak of an attitude of having a loving attitude towards a wolf's feelings. And he was very little preoccupied with the elementary, crude sort of wolf's feelings, simple hunger, for example. No, he goes deep into the very heart of the wolf's soul, seeking there subtle, complex things—not the simple satisfaction of appetite, but precisely the sensuality of spite and cruelty."[15] Mikhailovsky followed the "Russian attitude" and sought to explain what he saw as a peculiarity of Dostoevsky's work by referring to the author's personal traits. When Belinsky wrote about Dostoevsky's "nervous talent," his remark, though apparently within the framework of literary criticism, already contained a hint about Dostoevsky's state of mind. Mikhailovsky restated Belinsky's idea in more definite terms, interpreting the abundance of "pathological characters" in the novels as a reflection of the writer's own exaggerated interest in abnormality, which, he implied, is itself abnormal.

Psychiatrists took up as their own cause the completion of the circle, the establishment of a connection between Dostoevsky's supposed interest in abnormality and his own illness. They joined the discussion about Dostoevsky soon after the writer's death and two years after Mikhailovsky's essay appeared. The first step was V. F. Chizh's book *Dostoevsky as a Psychopathologist* (1885) (see Chapter 1).[16] In the "objective" tone of a scientist, Chizh repeated, whether intentionally or not, what Mikhailovsky had argued: that "Dostoevsky's collected works are an almost complete [textbook on] psychopathology." Chizh, however, emphasized not only the sheer quantity of "descriptions of mental illnesses" in Dostoevsky's work but also their quality, "correctness and precision." His declared aim was not literary criticism but popularization of psychiatry, and he found Dostoevsky's works especially good for "didactic purposes." Chizh deliberately presented the supposed illustrations of pathology, chosen from Dostoevsky's work, as "in a psychiatric textbook: from the elementary to more complex phenomena," starting with the etiology of mental diseases as the writer described it.[17]

Though Chizh was full of praise for Dostoevsky as a psychologist in general, his opinions about particular works varied. He found *The Devils* and *The Idiot* less successful from the psychiatric point of view. Like radical critics, who dismissed *The Devils* as a caricature of the revolutionaries, Chizh found the main characters of the novel "artificial" and their frenzies exaggerated. The radicals regarded as a failure Dostoevsky's attempt to create a "conservative" positive hero, Prince Myshkin in *The Idiot,* in opposition to his "radical" characters. Similarly, Chizh found Prince Myshkin "extremely idealized." Radical critics attacked another of Dostoevsky's affirmative characters, a quiet and reflective believer, Alyosha Karamazov; "the personality of Alyosha . . . is extremely pale, unnatural, undefined, and incomprehensible," wrote one critic, "it is simply an invention of the author, a fantasy."[18] By the same token, Chizh argued that "Dostoevsky tried to make [Alyosha] very attractive, almost a hero. This time, I will allow myself to disagree with the author: Alyosha, as I think, can only provoke empathy like any weak and sickly creature. If he had not yet done anything bad, it is no more than chance; people like him are too soft a wax in the hands of others, their conscious self is very poor and weak. What else indeed can one expect from a man who even at the age of eighteen was absolutely alienated from any conscious strivings for scientific or public activity!"[19] Yet, when comparing it with *The Idiot* and *The Devils,* Chizh was much more content with *The Brothers Karamazov,* a novel in which he found "an epic tableau of a mentally ill family, a family with degenerate traits." Following Chizh's lead, the neurologist V. A. Muratov (1865–1916) analyzed the novel and confirmed that almost every character in it suffered from some kind of pathology and that the whole novel was an inventory of "degenerate types."[20]

Chizh concluded that Dostoevsky revealed an "amazing depth of understanding," describing little-known diseases and even "foreseeing" those that contemporary psychiatry had not yet discovered. He found Dostoevsky's portrayal of abnormalities so sophisticated that "only a very gifted psychiatrist would discover the real and complete meaning of this novel."[21] In the concluding paragraphs of his study, he addressed the question of the possible sources of Dostoevsky's penetrating capacity. Chizh believed Dostoevsky's knowledge had not been acquired from psychiatric books; he mistakenly thought Dostoevsky had not read any.[22] In Chizh's opinion, Dostoevsky could have drawn his knowledge from two sources: his observations in prison, where many inmates were insane, and his own illness. Nevertheless, at the time when Chizh was writing his book, the persistent gossip and speculation about Dostoevsky's epilepsy remained unsupported by any published medical records. Dostoevsky periodically spoke about his falling sickness with his friends, and in his letter to the tsar asking for permission to return from exile, he had mentioned his illness as a reason to move to Petersburg or Moscow, where medical aid was available. And as he later informed the authorities when asking permission to travel outside the country, his trips abroad were motivated by the need to consult European specialists in nervous diseases.

Though Chizh's work appeared before Dostoevsky's physician published the memoirs in which he described Dostoevsky's condition as epilepsy, Chizh pointed to the writer's epilepsy as a well-known fact. Albeit cautiously, he suggested the disease was accompanied by mental disturbances. In Dostoevsky's semi-autobiographical works *The Diary of a Writer* and *The Peasant Marey* (1876), Chizh found evidence that the writer had hallucinated. Yet Chizh limited his speculations about Dostoevsky's illness to one paragraph, referring to the lack of medical evidence. Though he doubted that sufficient medical evidence could be obtained after Dostoevsky's death, he made it clear that if case records were available, the diagnosis would prove to be as he had supposed. He concluded with the ambivalent statement that "a respect for Dostoevsky's personality and his sufferings restrains even a physician from saying much," a hint that in other circumstances more could be revealed about Dostoevsky's illness.[23]

More conservative than liberal in his attitudes, Chizh could hardly share Mikhailovsky's view and did not have any intention of joining the Populists and using Dostoevsky's illness as a political argument against him. In fact,

Chizh was much closer to Dostoevsky's admirers than to his critics. His book indeed received an unfavorable review from one of the latter, supposedly a person from the radical camp, who questioned the correctness of Dostoevsky's "photographs" of psychopathology. This anonymous critic warned against Chizh's blind faith in Dostoevsky's ability to give a valid psychiatric analysis. Apparently following Mikhailovsky's lead, the reviewer explained that Dostoevsky's "striving to write novels about the mad" resulted from his "serious ailment on the border between nervous and psychic illness."[24] In contrast to the crude language of the review, Chizh's book appeared less tendentious. Yet in essence their arguments were not so different: both Chizh and his reviewer made the same link between Dostoevsky's pathological characters and his own illness. Intentionally or not, Chizh's conclusions repeated those drawn by the radicals. With the publication of his book, radical critics obtained unexpected support from a politically conservative psychiatrist in their project of dwelling on Dostoevsky's supposed mental aberration in order to undermine his beliefs.

Though Chizh only hinted at the possibility of writing Dostoevsky's pathography, critics took his words as a promise that such a study would surely be undertaken in the near future. The liberal critic D. N. Ovsianiko-Kulikovskii, who shared the view that Dostoevsky's talent was "cruel," looked forward to the proper "investigation of Dostoevsky's mental imbalance." He quoted Chizh's opinion that Dostoevsky's extraordinary ability to penetrate the human psyche depended on his own pathology. A proper study of the writer's illness, he argued, would reveal "the intimate psychological connection between Dostoevsky's own pathology, the 'cruelty' of his talent, and his religious and moral search." Likewise, Kropotkin found in a work by a medical doctor a proof of his claim that Dostoevsky's literature was overwhelmingly "morbid." Kropotkin dismissed Dostoevsky's novels as "unnatural," "fabricated for the purpose of introducing—here, a bit of morals, there, some abominable character taken from a psycho-pathological hospital." Apparently referring to Chizh, Kropotkin wrote approvingly that "a Russian specialist in brain and nervous diseases has found representatives of all sorts of such diseases in Dostoevsky's novels, and especially in *The Brothers Karamazov*—while being set in a frame which represents the strangest mixture of realism and romanticism run wild."[25]

There is a strong basis for saying that, as in the case of Gogol, in Dostoevsky criticism the works of critics and of psychiatrists influenced each other. Though critics issued their verdict independently of the medical expertise, they certainly looked into psychiatrists' writings, which they often interpreted to suit their own purposes, merely borrowing the authority of the psychiatrists. As a result, "a cruel talent" eventually became a household cliché about Dostoevsky, and psychiatrists accepted it—though not all of them approved of the radicals' attacks on the writer. In the highly politicized situation of late-nineteenth-century Russia, anything said about Dostoevsky immediately acquired political status. Psychiatrists who attempted an examination of Dostoevsky's illness might well have believed they were giving an objective scientific diagnosis, though in fact they became involved in the debates or were used for political ends.

Dostoevsky's contemporaries, including psychiatrists, constantly shaped and reshaped him as either hero or antihero. Constructing these images, they drew upon Dostoevsky's disease, which gradually acquired an inflated meaning. It was made responsible for the writer's prophetic wisdom, and at times almost mystical qualities were attributed to it. Cesare Lombroso found in Dostoevsky a perfect confirming example of the "epileptic genius" in the same way that the Danish critic Georg Brandes detected traces of "clairvoyance and epileptic character" in the writer's works. In his study of Dostoevsky's illness, James L. Rice observes how "Dostoevsky's basic physiological conflict, a struggle against his own morbid physical being, acquired the aura . . . of a spiritual quest or chivalric duel."[26] At other times, the illness was evoked in order to declare Dostoevsky's personal and literary failure and to compromise his views. Even if psychiatrists intended to "demystify" this image and examine Dostoevsky's illness as illness, their writings in fact contributed to the myth.

Transvaluation of Values in Literature and Psychiatry

At the turn of the century the political atmosphere in Russia changed, and this change was accompanied by a shift in Dostoevsky criticism. After the defeat of the Populist political program in the 1880s, Mikhailovsky's long-held authority in the field of literary criticism was also challenged. The new movement, the modernists, or decadents, who later evolved into the symbolists, formed a vanguard in philosophy, literature, and literary criticism. Its leaders, Vladimir Solov'ev, Dmitrii Merezhkovskii, Lev Shestov, and others, wrote extensively about Dostoevsky. The early radical critics interpreted Dostoevsky's love for the "downtrodden people" as a social protest; the Populists, disappointed in their expectations, condemned it as a perversion, a "pathological cruelty." By contrast, the decadents and symbolists viewed it as mainly apolitical though intimately connected with Dostoevsky's (and their own) vision of human nature.

The ideal of human nature that the modernists sought to establish, with the help of Dostoevsky, was profoundly intimate, controversial, and tragic. This ideal was based on the Christian message that suffering and evil were embodied in human life. In contrast to the Populists, whose great ambition was to find a social cure for suffering, the modernists were deeply pessimistic about the value of social activism. Dostoevsky could hardly have been more helpful in their confrontation with positivism and social optimism. He disapprovingly compared socialists with physicians in their belief that the world and human beings could be reformed. Dostoevsky stated his own creed in expressing the meaning he found in Tolstoy's *Anna Karenina*: "It is clear and intelligible to the point of obviousness that evil in mankind is concealed deeper than the physician-socialist supposes; that in no organization of society can evil be eliminated; that the human soul will remain the same; that abnormality and sin emanate from the soul itself, and finally, that the laws of the human spirit are unknown to science, so obscure, so indeterminate and mysterious, that, as yet, there can be neither physicians nor *final* judges, but there is only One, He Who said: '"Vengeance is mine; I will repay," saith the Lord.'"[27]

The radical critics considered Dostoevsky unable to picture a "healthy," rational, and morally unconfused human being. A positive hero, they believed, should be sturdy, upright, strong-willed, and able to sacrifice everything for a rational cause; Dostoevsky's weak characters were unfit for this role. Even when he attempted to describe affirmative characters, such as Prince Myshkin in *The Idiot* and Alyosha in *The Brothers Karamazov,* they could not stand comparison with the robust heroes of the radicals. But, as Rufus W. Mathewson argues, Dostoevsky created his characters in order to challenge the positivist ideal, not to compete with it. Dostoevsky brought out hidden, intimate, irrational dimensions of the human being. Rather than rationality and civic values, his characters defended the values of intimacy and personal freedom.[28]

In his pivotal collection of essays, *On the New Causes of the Decline and the New Trends in Contemporary Russian Literature* (1893), D. S. Merezhkovskii (1865–1941) confronted the radical realist critics in order to win Dostoevsky for his own camp. He claimed that the characterizations the "poor realist critics" applied to Dostoevsky—"a humanitarian preacher," "a cruel talent," or "a literary Torquemada"—demonstrated their inability to understand the writer's complexity and grandeur. Unlike the radicals, who found a source of Dostoevsky's failure in his penchant for pathology, Merezhkovskii praised the quality that enabled the writer to read "the secret thoughts which you would hesitate to voice . . . even to yourself." Like the radical critics, however, Merezhkovskii could not escape the "Russian attitude," which considered literary work a direct continuation of the writer's life, and he argued that Dostoevsky's strength as a writer was rooted in his own suffering. Dostoevsky's "soul is woven of contrasts, of contradictions, of entangled and unresolvable knots," Merezhkovskii wrote, and that gave him an almost mystical knowledge of people's minds, made him a "seer of the soul." "More our own, closer to us" than most contemporary writers, Dostoevsky was a prophet of the new age, which was bound to be, Merezhkovskii believed, the age of spirit.[29]

A decade later, in his path-breaking work *Dostoevsky and Nietzsche: The Philosophy of Tragedy* (1903), Lev Shestov challenged Mikhailovsky's views as outdated. "The critic's judgment . . . is based on the assumption that humanity is unquestionably better and more lofty than cruel," Shestov wrote, and asked, "Unquestionably?"[30] Populist critics wrongly believed that positivist science and the improvement of social conditions would automatically promote humankind to its original "lofty" state. In Shestov's view, they treated suffering as a contingent feature of the human condition, believing overoptimistically that reason and morals would help get rid of it. The radicals constructed a utopian vision of a rationally organized society in which future generations would not know suffering. The consequence was, however, that the present generation would sacrifice itself in battles with the existing regime for the sake of a bright future.

By contrast, Dostoevsky called for human charity in the present and therefore for the acceptance of life whatever it is. As Shestov wrote, Dostoevsky brought from his penal servitude "the 'conviction' that man's task consists, not in . . . dreaming of a future in which no one will offend anyone else, and where everyone will spend his days in peace, joy and pleasure, but in being able to accept reality with all its horrors . . . Penal wisdom caught up with Dostoevsky after many years, when he was living a long way from Siberia— in Petersburg in the midst of positivists—and forced him to acknowledge it, to serve it." Shestov juxtaposed a cheap and deceptive social optimism with a true, tragic attitude to life. Referring to Nietzsche's *The Birth of Tragedy,* he contrasted the positivists, radicals, and realists—these "little people" or "people of commonplaceness"—with "people of tragedy." The "little people" would never be able to understand the tragedy of human existence: "*they have no respect* for great misfortune, great ugliness, for great failure!" They would never be able to understand a Dostoevsky or a Nietzsche because "Dostoevsky's novel and Nietzsche's books speak only of the 'ugliest' people and their problems."[31]

Turn-of-the-century psychiatrists were not immune to the modernist vision of the human being, and they joined the ongoing rehabilitation of Dostoevsky. The reassessment was accompanied by major conceptual changes in psychiatry, which involved rethinking notions of the normal and abnormal, the connection between genius and degeneration, and the idea of the destructiveness of illness. All the main assumptions that the medical profession shared with the positivists—the sharp boundary between the normal and abnormal, a definition of the normal through reason and morality, and the association of progress with normality and decline with abnormality—were questioned during the discussion of Dostoevsky.

Psychiatrists of the older generation were not comfortable with these changes. Though Chizh was far from engaging himself in Populism, he shared its positivist outlook and therefore agreed with Mikhailovsky's evaluation of Dostoevsky's heroes. In fact, it is possible to imagine both Chizh and Mikhailovsky as incarnations of the "socialist-physician," the figure Tolstoy and Dostoevsky created as a personification of positivist beliefs. The difference between the critic and the psychiatrist was that Mikhailovsky invited social changes on a large scale, whereas Chizh's idea of social reform was limited to asylums. Chizh viewed psychiatry primarily as the instrument for disciplining and correcting deviant behavior; he even once suggested that Dostoevsky's character Dmitrii Karamazov should be subjected to social engineering: "the only possible way to make a tolerable member of society out of Dmitrii is to treat or, to say more correctly, to reeducate him in a hospital."[32]

Some psychiatrists, by contrast, were willing to make the leap and accept a new vision of human nature. Bazhenov was the most important. Like Chizh, he belonged to the generation of founders of Russian psychiatry, but in his views he was closer to the younger generation. He mediated between the older generation, whose main preoccupation was asylum construction, and the turn-of-the-century psychiatrists, who gave up the faith in custodial treatment and invested their hopes in active methods of mental cure. Bazhenov reassessed the outdated postulates of degeneration theory, and he patronized the pioneers of psychotherapy in Russia even though he did not always share their views. Broad-minded, artistic, and open to new ideas, he addressed the question of Dostoevsky's illness and articulated the new understanding of it. Previously Dostoevsky had been made to conform to the pattern of epileptic genius, but now the ideas of the day—neurosis, creative illness, "progeneration"—were applied to both the writer and his heroes.

Nikolai Nikolaevich Bazhenov

N. N. Bazhenov's (1856–1923) sensibility to art was not rooted in his family background—at least, not on his father's side (his mother died when he was nine years of age). Bazhenov senior was a gendarme officer who advanced to the rank of major general. Rejecting the family tradition of military service, the younger Bazhenov entered Moscow University intending to become a physician. The students of his year, as he reported, were the first to attend a separate course on psychiatry, previously taught as a part of other courses. While still at the university Bazhenov chose psychiatry as his métier, partly under the influence of his teacher and friend S. S. Korsakov (1854–1900), partly because psychiatry most satisfied his interest in social and psychological matters. He read widely on these topics, and even as a student he began a correspondence with Gabriel Tarde, who was then exploring the phenomenon of social imitation and whom Bazhenov later described as "the most original and brilliant modern sociologist."[33] In 1881 Bazhenov informed Tarde about an episode that the latter could use as an illustration of social imitation. During a performance of *La dame aux camélias* in Moscow, starring the famous French actress Sarah Bernhardt, there was a moment when a special exchange occurred between the actress and her audience: "In the fifth act, at the most dramatic moment, when the entire audience was so silent that you could have heard a pin drop, Marguerite Gautier, dying of consumption, coughed. Immediately an epidemic of coughing filled the auditorium, and for several minutes, no one was able to hear the words of the great actress."[34]

Bazhenov first met Tarde at the Congress on Criminal Anthropology in 1889 and was invited to Tarde's family house in the Périgord. He later recalled with awe the visit to the house on the rock, a *demeure* [dwelling] *de troglodyte,* where the grand maître was discovering the laws of social life in silence and solitude. In the Périgord Tarde completed a sketch of a utopian society governed by the creative minority.[35] In this society, where individual inner perfection was the highest value, the more advanced individuals were admired and not envied. Tarde's "geniocracy" may have inspired Bazhenov's vision of progenerating humanity. According to this "aristocrat of spirit," as Bazhenov called Tarde, a few creative individuals lead society, while the great majority spends its life in a state close to hypnotic imitation. By the time, as a student, he wrote his first letter to Tarde, Bazhenov had already formed a clear idea of the part of humanity to which he was going to belong.

Eighteen eighty-one, the year in which Bazhenov had his first brush with

the police and graduated from the university, was also the year of Dostoevsky's death and of the assassination of the tsar. Bazhenov came to the attention of the police after he was involved in student unrest, in a way that paralleled the beginning of Dostoevsky's adult life. After graduation Bazhenov
went abroad, perhaps with the double purpose of completing his education
and avoiding the eyes of the police. During his first visit to Paris, Bazhenov
met his compatriot Peter Lavrov, a convinced socialist and an ideologist of
the Populist movement in Russia. Lavrov was closely connected with The
People's Will, the political party responsible for the regicide of 1881. He and
other Populists called on the intelligentsia to get to know the lower classes,
mainly peasants, with a twofold aim—to help them and to learn from them.
Bazhenov responded to the Populist slogan to be "closer to the people," and
on his return to Russia in the summer of 1885 he became a psychiatrist in a
provincial *zemstvo* hospital in the town of Riazan', two hundred miles south
of Moscow.[36] During a brief stay in Moscow he headed a group of The People's Will, one of sixteen in Moscow, and was in correspondence with the
émigré leaders—an activity that he continued in Riazan'. In 1886, having
found his address in the apartment of a member of The People's Will, the
police arrested Bazhenov.[37] Fortunately, his brief imprisonment did not have
the disastrous consequences that followed Dostoevsky's arrest, perhaps owing
to his father's intervention. Having spent three weeks in prison, Bazhenov
was freed under secret surveillance and was forbidden to live in Moscow and
Petersburg for three years. Instead, he invested all his energy in the Riazan'
asylum.

Before the asylum could be transformed from a custodial to a therapeutic institution, the numbers of chronically ill inmates had to be reduced. In
1885 the hospital board began the construction of a countryside colony to
receive these patients. Bazhenov supervised the colony and, in addition,
planned to start foster care for the chronically ill in peasant families. In 1886
he organized the first Russian *patronage familial* (based on a Belgian model)
in a village nearby, but it lasted only two years. With the introduction of foster care, the poorer inhabitants of the village obtained an independent income
from the hospital. The wealthier peasants protested, because, according to the
account given by a Soviet historian, they lost cheap labor. The peasants themselves argued that their protest was due to arson supposedly carried out by
the patients. The local *zemstvo* authorities, fearing the government would interfere, provisionally ended its patronage of the project.[38] Bazhenov made
several attempts to renew it, despite the opposition of the *zemstvo* and some
of his colleagues, who found the idea unrealistic and did not believe this kind

of organization was possible outside Gheel, the Belgian village where it originated. Yet he remained convinced that *patronage familial* had a future, and he
drew support from the Scottish doctors he had encountered earlier on a visit
to an asylum in Scotland (see below), who confided to Bazhenov that, in a
similar kind of project, they struggled with similar skepticism.[39]

Nonrestraint was another bold innovation made by Bazhenov in Riazan',
which went as far as unlocking doors in a hospital building where a hundred
patients were accommodated. At the very beginning of his career, Bazhenov
had traveled in Europe with the aim of seeing mental institutions in different countries. These "psychiatric excursions" were common among Russian
medical graduates, who after obtaining their doctoral degree were often sent
abroad to continue their education. Bazhenov later reported that "perhaps,
the strongest impression that I had in my medical activity" resulted from his
visit to a Scottish asylum near Glasgow, which had no separate wards for violent and noisy patients.[40] He set out to introduce the nonrestraint system in
Russian asylums, but this was not easy.

When Bazhenov was absent from the countryside colony in 1889 (attending the psychiatric congress at the International Exhibition in Paris), a patient
drowned in a river. Bazhenov had to respond to the authorities' allegations
of irresponsibility, but he stood firmly for nonrestraint, opposing those who
thought unlocked doors in the asylum were an impermissible luxury. He
wrote to his assistant physician in Riazan', "Either you open the doors with
a risk of an accident or you lock them, put fences everywhere and let the
patients out for a walk only with the watchers. I prefer the former, and I was
already bearing in mind both the idea of the 'open doors' and the risk involved
in it at the period when the hospital was constructed and organized." For the
sake of the idea, he was determined not to generalize from this accident or
from that involving another patient's death in the same year: "I do not doubt
that both misfortunes of this year will evoke certain worries in the Riazan'
public as well as talks at the *zemstvo* meetings, but what can one do? We have
to educate public opinion and to be pioneers. The accident with Silichev [the
drowned patient] belongs to that kind which, in my mind, is as impossible to
predict as it is impossible to predict an accident with any sane person who
went off swimming and has drowned."[41] Bazhenov noted that "for five years
in the hospital with 500 to 600 patients there has been one suicide and four
accidents which ended with the patients' deaths, one accident a year," which
in his estimation was a good result.[42]

During his time at the Riazan' asylum, Bazhenov was under constant surveillance by the police. The documents in his dossier at the Ministry of the

Interior state that Bazhenov rented his flat to riotous students; that he gave a speech moderately critical of the regime at a celebration at Moscow University; that he collected money for the Saltykov-Shchedrin Literary Fund for Young Writers in Need; and that he was forbidden to travel abroad. After defending his doctoral dissertation in 1893 he was formally eligible for a university position.[43] Yet his application to Moscow University was declined three times because he still was deemed "politically unreliable," though by that time the restrictions placed on his living in Moscow or Petersburg had been removed. Between 1898 and 1901 Bazhenov headed a psychiatric division of the hospital in the provincial town of Voronezh. Only in 1902 was the Ministry of the Interior to confirm his appointment as a *Privatdozent* for the chair of the "history and encyclopedia of medicine" at Moscow University, where he was to teach a course on "psychic epidemics," the subject that had fascinated him since the acclaimed performance of *La dame aux camélias* in Moscow.[44]

Later in life, as man of society, Bazhenov discovered a great deal more illustrations of Tarde's epigram, "la société, c'est l'imitation." An ebullient character, Bazhenov was a revolutionary, professor, founder of a Masonic lodge, and famous figure in literary and artistic milieu. Early in the new century he was seen to sit at a table with Tolstoy's sons in the Literary-Artistic Circle attended by the artistic vanguard, as well as "all Moscow." Established by famous writers and poets, the circle also attracted a wealthy bourgeois public to its gatherings with a casino, and the profits from the night gambling provided the circle with a substantial income.[45] For several years Bazhenov chaired the circle's gatherings, though he was not on the best terms with the symbolists who frequented the place. The poet-symbolist Andrei Bely described Bazhenov in his memoirs as a "*savant-chantant,* amateur of can-can and pretty women" and "Epicurean and cynic to the marrow of his bones." Bely disliked Bazhenov's "psychiatric style" and believed the psychiatrist "considered us [members of the circle] his patients . . . thinking that he, a Mason, and man of science is allowed to can-can over his patients' beliefs."[46]

Bely's animosity was a response to Bazhenov's criticism of the vanguard movement. In his essay "Symbolists and Decadents: A Psychiatric Study" (1899), Bazhenov, like many critics of decadence, accused the current trends in literature of impotency and imitation of the French poets Charles Baudelaire, Gérard de Nerval, and Paul Verlaine. He believed that the founders of symbolism succeeded in drawing from insanity extraordinary sensual experiences beneficial for their art,[47] but that their numerous followers and imitators manifested "the scarcity of imagination and thought, superficiality, bizarre and capricious moods, perversion of psychological reactions, moral insanity, pathological associations, and lack of logical thinking similar to what one can observe in heavy and incurable forms of psychoses; and all that is accompanied by unjustified overestimation of their own personality."[48] Bazhenov's essay on the symbolists was included in the collection *Psychiatric Conversations on Literary and Public Questions* (1903), which was awarded a prestigious Pushkin Prize for achievement in literature by the Russian Academy of Fine Arts. For this collection, Bazhenov was mentioned as an author in the turn-of-the-century edition of *Preparatory Sources for the Dictionary of Russian Writers.*[49] He became renowned as a "Moscow attraction." He did not miss any premier, and "artistic Moscow" repaid his visits, gathering at improvised costume balls held in Bazhenov's small townhouse.[50] He wrote for a general audience and gave public lectures and speeches at different occasions, beginning with the Gogol anniversary in 1902 and concluding with Chekhov's funeral in 1904. As one of his colleagues remarked, he felt best when he was wielding the chairman's gavel and when he was on stage.[51] When invited to lecture on the "psychology of theater" to the actors of the acclaimed Moscow Arts Theater, he apparently drew on his own rich experience.[52]

In Moscow his social talents flourished. He ran a private clinic, the oldest in the city, and was appointed medical director of the Moscow City Psychiatric Hospital (Preobrazhenskii), in 1904. A proponent of medical education for women, Bazhenov taught psychiatry at the Higher Women's Courses, and he recruited a number of the graduates as nurses and physicians at the Preobrazhenskii. Usually he spent the daylight hours in the hospital and at the Higher Women's Courses and evenings in his private clinic in the same area of Moscow. His psychiatric views were typical of nineteenth-century alienism, with its custodial care and moral treatment. Besides hydrotherapy, the use of medications at the Preobrazhenskii was limited to bromide and injections of scopolamine. A colleague reported that Bazhenov used to "joke that he did not know how to write out any other prescription but bromide [and] he also used to say that 'in our hospital the walls cure.'"[53] Yet he had to work hard on improving the hospital before it could achieve cures. During his directorship at the Preobrazhenskii, he replaced window grills in the wards for violent patients with strong glass of the type used on ships; though the isolation wards remained, their doors did not have locks.[54] Bazhenov also replaced the junior staff—wardens and female servants—who did not have medical training with interns and students from the Higher Women's Courses. He persuaded two merchants to fund the construction of new facilities, promising to give their names to the building, and four new sections of the hospital were opened in 1910. In 1912 he instituted the construction of three more buildings, work that was interrupted by the First World War.

Bazhenov remained involved in political activity throughout his career. When the liberal Constitutional Democratic (Kadet) Party was established in October 1905, he joined it. The Kadets were a party of intellectuals, mostly from the liberal professions and academia, who thought they represented not the interests of a class or a group but the ideal of political freedom and social justice in its pure and abstract form. "The trouble was," as a historian remarks, "that the pure ideal of political liberty and individual freedom" could not do much "in a situation in which government, people, and privileged classes each regarded violence as a sole arbiter in political matters."[55] Both before and at the beginning of the 1905 revolution, the Kadets grouped with more radical parties on the left, including the Bolsheviks. Bazhenov sheltered and offered a job in his private clinic to a physician-Bolshevik, S. I. Mitskevich (1869–1944), who had recently returned from Siberian exile. At the beginning of the 1905 uprising, his clinic hosted the Bolsheviks' meetings, one of them attended by V. I. Lenin.[56]

As the revolution progressed, and the reliance on violence by both revolutionaries and supporters of autocracy grew, the Kadets abandoned their policy of "no enemies on the left" and began to organize a party that could work with "non-violent means, i.e. by participation in the elections to the proposed consultative *Duma*."[57] As one of the main spokesmen for the Kadets, Bazhenov, in his pamphlet *Psychology and Politics* (1906), warned against the Bolsheviks' call for unlimited mass unrest.[58] Nevertheless, he remained a convinced opponent of the tsarist regime and, in newspaper articles, protested against the police searches for rebels in psychiatric hospitals and the prosecution of physicians who gave medical assistance to the rebels injured during the street fighting. In his contribution to the collection of essays protesting against the death penalty, published by the Petersburg Union of Medical Personnel, Bazhenov argued that awaiting execution is a psychological torture, perhaps the most cruel of all, surpassing the crime itself.[59] Bazhenov's article echoed Dostoevsky's tragic experience as well as the story by Victor Hugo, *Le dernier jour d'un condemné*. Hugo's imaginary diary of a condemned criminal, a most "poignant attack . . . on the horror of capital punishment," had also fascinated Dostoevsky sometime before his own mock execution.[60]

Bazhenov's political activism provoked the anxiety of the Moscow medical authorities, which raised the possibility of dismissal from his position at the Preobrazhenskii. They reproached him for neglecting his duties in the hospital and required him to live in the hospital's grounds. Yet Bazhenov successfully defended himself.[61] In spite of his conflicts with the authorities, his expertise was appreciated to the extent that he was appointed to a government committee for revising the law concerning the mentally disabled. In 1911 he presented the final report on the project for discussion at the First Congress of the (newly founded) Russian Union of Psychiatrists and Neuropathologists, of which he became president in the same year.[62]

Freemasonry was another area of Bazhenov's activity. Popular in Russia at the turn of the eighteenth and nineteenth centuries, Masonry was forbidden by Nicholas I after a large group of nobility, almost all of whom were Freemasons, attempted a coup d'état in December 1825. Bazhenov was ordained in a French lodge, Les amis réunis, while he was in Paris in 1884. At that time there were only a few Russian members of any French lodge, and Bazhenov acted to expand the lodge's influence.[63] Much of his professional and social activity was determined by his contacts with French and Russian Masons, as their number grew. When M. M. Kovalevskii (1857–1916), an academician, Mason, and subsequently an activist of the Constitutional Democratic Party, decided to open the Higher Russian School of Social Sciences in Paris, he invited Bazhenov to be the coorganizer.[64] It is also possible that Bazhenov's liaisons with French psychiatrists were reinforced through Masonry. For a long period, however, he remained one of the few Masons in Moscow, until he founded a daughter lodge of the French Loge du Grand Orient in 1908. The Moscow lodge, named Vozrozhdenie (Renaissance, or Regeneration), was a sign of the revival of Masonry in Russia.[65]

The Masonic concept of a new, regenerating humanity contrasted with the apocalyptic vision of decline or, in a psychiatric version, degeneration of the human species. Both the theory of degeneration and the practice of alienism, in which this theory had its roots, became devalued in the eyes of early-twentieth-century practitioners. There was a decline of belief in custodial care and a parallel rise in interest in other methods—hypnosis, therapy by suggestion, the psychological analysis developed by Pierre Janet, and the psychoanalytic methods of Sigmund Freud—that claimed to cure previously incurable diseases. More and more physicians who chose "nervous disorders" as their specialty worked in private clinics and sanatoria. For them, small private facilities had a number of advantages over the huge mental hospitals: besides attracting wealthy clients, they allowed intellectually exciting experiments with various methods of physiotherapy and psychotherapy.[66] The "old guard" of alienists and proponents of the degeneration theory, tempted by the first successes of psychotherapy, began to reconsider its belief in the incurability of hereditary diseases. Even the neurologist Jean-Martin Charcot reportedly sent some of his patients on the pilgrimage to Lourdes, and his late article "La foi qui guérit" (1892) stressed the role of mental factors in the cure of organic disorders.[67]

Bazhenov was also interested in psychic cures. He went to Lourdes and also to Sicily, where he observed the psychological consequences of the eruption of Mount Etna. After his trip to Lourdes, he gave an enthusiastic talk at a meeting of Moscow psychiatrists on the advantages of emotional therapy.[68] The meeting was one of the regular gatherings of a psychiatric society called Little Fridays, organized by physicians eager to discuss recent developments in psychological treatment, including Paul-Charles Dubois's rational therapy and psychoanalysis. Bazhenov was at the head of these discussions. Though he shared with his contemporaries a reserved attitude towards psychoanalysis, for "one cannot look at the entire universe from a single angle," he did not avoid the hot topic. Together with a younger colleague, the émigré psychiatrist N. E. Osipov, he wrote one of the first monographic surveys of the area, *La suggestion et ses limites* (1911), which was published in the popular series edited by the Parisian doctor Paul-Gaston Meunier.[69] At Bazhenov's lectures at the Higher Women's Courses, "a famous miraculous calculator, . . . a telepathist, and a shaman-sorcerer appeared in turn."[70] Bazhenov's inclination towards psychotherapy resulted in his opening, together with his friend Auguste Marie, a sanatorium for "psychasthenics, neurasthenics, hysterics, drug-dependent and overworked patients" in Choisy-le-Roi, near Paris.[71] However, the First World War and Bazhenov's growing illness (he suffered from a heart disease) restricted this activity.

With the beginning of the war, the Russian Red Cross appointed Bazhenov to organize a psychiatric service in the Caucasus and, later, a similar service for the Russian Expeditionary Corps, France-Thessaloniki. With the help of Marie, he organized psychiatric facilities for Russian soldiers in the location of the Villejuif Hospital in Paris.[72] Bazhenov left Russia in late 1916. As a Kadet, he sincerely welcomed the revolution of February 1917 that terminated the reign of what he called the "degenerate" dynasty and cleared the way for the introduction of constitutional government. The Bolshevik Revolution that followed in October 1917, however, was harder to accept. Bazhenov believed that, though the Bolsheviks claimed to bring to power the poorest classes under the slogan of the "dictatorship of the proletariat," in fact, by playing skillfully on mass psychology, they gained unlimited power for themselves. He thought the Bolshevik regime, far from instituting an ideal of meritocracy (perhaps Bazhenov would have preferred to speak of "geniocracy"), was destroying culture and replacing it with a kind of religious movement. Bazhenov warned that "the Bolshevik folly" was spreading all over the world like Spanish influenza, cutting off the path to the progeneration of humanity.[73]

Bazhenov lived in France and Belgium until 1923, when he unexpectedly made the decision to return to Russia, either to die—he was seriously ill and had already had a stroke—or perhaps with the hope of seeing his country revive and regenerate. His old contacts with physician-Bolsheviks made his return possible; some of his former students accompanied the ill professor on the journey and others met him at the Moscow railway station on a spring day. But several days later he died following a second stroke—in his Masonic language, he "went to sleep at the Eternal Orient."

Rediagnosing Dostoevsky: From Epilepsy to Creative Illness

Bazhenov, who divided his time between Russia and Western Europe during these most agitated decades, was in an excellent position to respond to new trends in both psychiatry and literary criticism. This response involved a substantial reassessment of Dostoevsky. In the background lay Bazhenov's formative years as a psychiatrist in France between 1883 and 1885. He studied with Charcot at the Salpêtrière, worked with Valentin Magnan at the Ste-Anne Asylum, and conducted anthropometric research on sculptured busts of famous criminals and outstanding men in Léonce Manouvrier's laboratory of anthropology at the Sorbonne. His prolonged contacts with Magnan had the consequence that the Moscow Society of Psychiatrists and Neuropathologists, whose president Bazhenov became in the first decade of the new century, was regarded as "Magnanian." The French alienist was himself the only foreign honorary member of the society.[74]

Bazhenov was especially close to Auguste Marie, six years his junior, who was married to a Russian woman. They shared much in common both professionally and personally: like his Russian friend, Marie founded a residential colony for the chronically insane in the countryside, in Dun-sur-Auron in 1892. Both men of culture—Bazhenov wrote poetry and translated French poets into Russian, Marie painted—they shared a deep interest in the art of the insane. Marie, like Lombroso in Turin and the psychiatrists of Bethlem Hospital in London, collected samples of his patients' art, and in 1905 he opened a "mad museum" at the Villejuif Hospital. Both Bazhenov and Marie became involved with a group of scholars who seriously studied the art of the insane. The group included J. Rogues de Fursac, Jean Vinchon, Paul-Gaston Meunier, and Paul Sérieux, and, as the historian of psychiatry J. M. Mac-

Gregor has demonstrated, they were united by a particular approach to the art of the insane.[75] These scholars did not dismiss it as "diseased art," but instead they saw in it a specific language, a representation of another reality, or an artistic expression of the experience of insanity, whatever its aesthetic value. They believed the art of the insane and the art of normal individuals were not separated by an unbridgeable gap and hoped that work by the mentally ill could reveal something about creative processes in general.

The main spokesman for these views was an art critic who wrote under the name of Marcel Réja. According to MacGregor, Réja was the pen name of Paul-Gaston Meunier (1873–1957), a physician with an interest in the psychology of dreams and art. In his *L'Art chez les fous* (1907), Réja/Meunier analyzed patterns in the art of the insane, concluding that "a certain number of stereotyped formulas [are] to be observed in their work, which serve as nuclei for their various digressions."[76] Like Lombroso, he believed the art of the insane represented a less complex, inferior form of artistic expression and therefore reflected earlier phases of the history of art. Lombroso, however, saw it as an entirely negative characteristic, an "atavism" or sign of degeneration. By contrast, Réja, who had a taste for primitive art, discussed the work of the insane in connection with the drawings and sculptures of the prehistoric and Afro-Asiatic peoples as pieces of genuine art. MacGregor argues that the driving force behind Réja's reassessment of the art of the insane was a recognition of its aesthetic qualities, a belief that the energy of creative expression is stronger than illness and that the mentally ill can overcome insanity in their creative work. Though he was aware that mental illness could destroy artistic abilities, Réja was particularly interested in cases in which insanity unleashed creative processes and "the terrible aggravation of suffering . . . [broke] asunder the human faculties, drawing forth tormented sobbing and unexpected flashes of lighting." He concluded that "it is the defects in the spirit of the author which themselves permit him to rise to this intensity of expression."[77] Réja/Meunier formulated his creed that in art the mentally ill person triumphed over his or her illness in relation to the visual arts; Bazhenov articulated the same idea in relation to literature.[78]

As mentioned earlier, Bazhenov's first essay on the topic of art and insanity, "The Symbolists and Decadents," treated the decadent movement as impotent and unoriginal. By contrast, the second essay, "Ill Writers and Pathological Literature" (1903), dealt with the established geniuses—Dostoevsky and Maupassant—whose writing Bazhenov genuinely admired.[79] He valued not only their stature as writers but also their qualities as "psychologists," and he approached them more cautiously and with greater respect than did the decadents. In the French version of his essay (1904) he even apologized for treating the writers as mentally ill: "If I have just applied our means of clinical investigation to literary treasures, such as works by Maupassant and Dostoevsky, I did it not out of a kind of scientific vandalism, but rather out of deference and feelings close to a cult. We have approached them with respect and stopped in front of these superior and still unknown intellectual processes that are grouped under the name of *poetic inspiration*."[80] Bazhenov started his essay with what had already become a commonplace about Dostoevsky, his ability to "penetrate deeply into the inmost recesses of people's hearts and understand clearly extreme and terrifying mental anomalies." The psychiatrist wrote that, as a man of science, he almost envied Dostoevsky's talent to achieve "the understanding that science can reach only through painstaking accumulation of facts, detailed analysis, and step-by-step ascent from delusion to truth."[81] Dostoevsky's psychological gift amounted to an almost mystical power to unveil illnesses that were unknown to psychiatry or had only recently been made objects of science.[82]

Assuming Dostoevsky's insights were rooted in the writer's subjective experience of illness, Bazhenov contrasted Dostoevsky with Emile Zola: he thought the Russian writer was "natural" and intuitive about psychology, whereas the Frenchman simply transferred medical cases from psychiatric literature to his fiction. Bazhenov evoked Belinsky's characterization of Dostoevsky as a "nervous talent." He then set about the task of finding "in Dostoevsky's works, besides the types and forms of insanity pictured by him, those very features that were determined by his infirmity." He intended to do the same for Maupassant, but he did not go far with his controversial analysis. "Everybody knows," Bazhenov started, "that [Dostoevsky] suffered from epilepsy . . . which involves more or less important and profound changes of personality." Maupassant, in his turn, was a hypochondriac and drug addict, who ended his days with progressive paralysis of the insane.[83] Despite the energetic beginning, the results of this search were meager. All that Bazhenov could say about Maupassant was that the writer, though still young and healthy and already famous and rich, felt desperate and deeply disgusted by the dullness of life.

When Bazhenov wrote his essay, he was himself still young and healthy and full of hopes for a better future for Russia and his compatriots. Later, disillusioned by the Bolshevik Revolution, he no longer regarded Maupassant's boredom as pathological. He now quoted with sympathy the same passage from Maupassant that he had once used to illustrate the writer's supposed pathology. Like Maupassant, Bazhenov now believed that revolutions cannot change the face of earth, because "the man is the same, his beliefs, his sensations are the same, he has gone neither forward nor backward a point, nor has he been moved [by anything]. Once having reached his limits, they remain firm, close, unchangeable, he goes round like a circus horse, like a fly in a sealed bottle who flies up to the cork and always hurts itself." This resembled Dostoevsky's verdict that "in no organization of society can evil be eliminated; that the human soul will remain the same; that abnormality and sin emanate from the soul itself."[84]

Though Bazhenov carried out a psychiatric diagnosis of Maupassant, his opinion was much milder than, for instance, that of Max Nordau (1849–1923), who concluded that Maupassant was a "pathological erotomaniac whose brain reflects everything in a wrong light."[85] Moreover, Bazhenov criticized Nordau for his extreme and superficial judgments and demanded a much finer analysis. Similarly, when Bazhenov looked for reflections of Dostoevsky's illness in his novels, he did it in a much more modest way than had those who emphasized the writer's epilepsy. Though he quoted Mikhailovsky's characterization of Dostoevsky as a "cruel talent," Bazhenov did not perceive this distinctive trait to be pathological. Instead, he argued that cruelty was intrinsically attractive to many people, a human characteristic mentioned as early as the fourth-century Indian epics. Dostoevsky, Bazhenov implied, was neither unique in describing ambivalent feelings caused by cruelty nor morbid or monstrous if he had such feelings himself.

To describe ambivalent feelings did not mean that, as one scholar expressed it, one "could no longer distinguish between good and evil, pleasure and pain."[86] In the biographer Joseph Frank's words, Dostoevsky was "in no danger of mistaking one for the other."[87] But a seemingly impossible mixture of good and evil in his characters puzzled his contemporaries. In *Crime and Punishment,* for instance, the writer made the prostitute Sonia, a woman who sacrificed her body, the spokesperson for his own morality. The shocked editors of the literary journal in which the novel first appeared ordered Dostoevsky to rewrite the chapter about Sonia in such a way that "the evil and the good are sharply separated, and it will be impossible to confuse and misinterpret them."[88] But unlike Dostoevsky's contemporaries, the following generation was especially sensitive to "the mysterious, fateful mixture of good and evil in life."[89] Dostoevsky, who better than anyone before him showed that "in a pure soul . . . and in a great self-sacrifice . . . there is a germ of criminality," became their hero.[90] Fin de siècle scholars cast Dostoevsky into a figure that "weakened the line separating virtue from vice" and created an atmosphere in which "the exotic blends of character—the honest liar, the lascivious ascetic, the tender murderer, the pious iconoclast—were no longer irreconcilable contradictions."[91]

The turn-of-the-century audience, including psychiatrists, became fascinated by the art with which Dostoevsky discovered "psychopathologies of everyday life," as the German psychiatrist P. J. Möbius termed it. A few years after Bazhenov published his essay on Dostoevsky and Maupassant, his German colleague claimed that "everybody is pathological to a certain degree." Möbius called on psychiatrists "to abandon the prevalent old division into healthy and sick minds."[92] Like Bazhenov and Möbius, many physicians believed the "psychiatry of everyday life" should be added to asylum psychiatry.[93] Freud opposed the sharp boundaries that conventional psychiatry constructed between illness and health and criticized the fatal diagnosis of degeneration. He mocked conventional psychiatry that could "only say with a shrug: 'Degeneracy, hereditary disposition, constitutional inferiority!'" An admirer of Dostoevsky, Freud decided that Dostoevsky could not have had an organic disease of the brain, because the quality of his work did not decline through his life. "Epilepsy is an organic brain disease independent of the psychic constitution," he wrote to Stefan Zweig apropos Dostoevsky's illness, "and as a rule [is] associated with the deterioration and retrogression of the mental performance." Freud had therefore changed the diagnosis: it was hysteria, not an organic disease.[94]

Just as the diagnosis of Dostoevsky's illness was moderated, so was judgment about the diseases of his characters. In the 1880s Chizh rejected as improbable the ending of *Crime and Punishment,* in which the murderer Raskol'nikov experiences the beginning of self-renewal. According to Chizh's own diagnosis, Raskol'nikov inherited a predisposition to a mental disease that would have made his recovery impossible. Forty years later, a young psychiatrist, D. A. Amenitskii, altered the diagnosis of Raskol'nikov's disorder from inherited disease to a more tractable one, psychasthenia. Amenitskii believed that though obsessed by an idea, Raskol'nikov was curable, and he found the end of the novel plausible. In the same way, Osipov reconsidered the renowned abnormality of Dostoevsky's heroes, arguing that in most cases they could be considered neurotic rather than mentally ill. Moreover, he thought many of their neuroses were in an embryonic stage, having emerged as a result of spiritual struggles and conflicts and not yet fully developed.[95]

As earlier, the discussion of Dostoevsky by psychiatrists echoed the critics' opinions. With the beginning of the twentieth century, the critics became more accepting of Dostoevsky, and this encouraged a psychiatric reassessment. Once again, psychiatrists and critics, quoting each other, formed an alliance. When the idealist philosopher N. O. Lossky rejected the view that "Dostoevsky's work is sickly," he referred to the expertise of his friend, the psychiatrist Osipov. Lossky believed Osipov had persuasively demonstrated that "there are many sane as well as 'positively beautiful' characters in Dostoevsky's work." Osipov's view, that the "madness" of Dostoevsky's characters was caused by the battle of good and evil in the human heart, convinced Lossky that Dostoevsky's "preaching of suffering" served the moral purpose of "purification of the soul."[96]

Thus, despite his intention to examine the influence of Dostoevsky's and Maupassant's illnesses on their literature, Bazhenov's fascination with their art outweighed his opinion as a psychiatrist. In the process of his analysis, Bazhenov ceased to speak in terms of illnesses and used the phrase "great suffering" instead, fully conscious of its ambivalent—spiritual as well as medical—meaning. Bazhenov almost certainly knew about de Vogüé's essay on Dostoevsky, *La religion de la souffrance,* as he was in Paris when it was first published. To consider Dostoevsky's physical and moral suffering as a characteristic feature of his literature and a creative source became common among late-nineteenth-century critics. In Bazhenov's account, both epilepsy and "religion of suffering" worked together to produce Dostoevsky's achievement. It was a "combination of great talent with great suffering of the soul" that made Dostoevsky both an outstanding writer and a psychologist.[97]

Dostoevsky proved to be a perfect touchstone for conventional psychiatric criteria; Bazhenov's analysis led him to the conclusion that the effect of illness depended on the scale of the person. As Thomas Mann summarized it a few decades later, such geniuses as Dostoevsky were the best refutation of an old doctrine that "there is nothing but ill from illness." "Above all things," Mann wrote, "it is important *who* is ill, *who* is mad, who is epileptic or paralyzed—an average fool, in whom the illness diminishes the spiritual and cultural aspects, or a Nietzsche or a Dostoevsky."[98] The view that geniuses are marked by an ability to sublimate "great suffering" and transform it into strength was soon to be developed by psychoanalysis, and it slowly penetrated traditional psychiatry.[99] A psychiatrist of the 1920s expressed the belief that the writer's "illness or pathological tension does not matter, even if the result is only a minute of sensation . . . which is harmonious and beautiful, if it gives a feeling unknown before of wholeness, balance, reconciliation, union with the supreme synthesis of life."[100]

The historian Henri Ellenberger traced the origins of the notion of "creative illness" back to the Romantics. He quoted the poet and philosopher Friedrich von Hardenberg (Novalis) who wrote, "Illnesses are certainly an important matter for humanity, since they are so numerous and because everyone has to struggle against them. But we know only very imperfectly the art of putting them to good use. These are probably the most important materials and stimulants for our thinking and activity." With nineteenth-century positivism, as Ellenberger commented, "the utilitarian, materialist notion of illness as simply and exclusively a disorder of physical origin" to be cured by means of scientific medicine became dominant.[101] The theory of degeneration shared this view of illness as an absolute evil, which destroys the most valuable abilities and weakens humanity's potential for creativity and development. Ellenberger believed that the concept of creative illness was revived only in the mid-twentieth century—in particular, in the work of the German physician and philosopher Viktor von Weizsäker. Weizsäker coined the term *logophania* for the phenomenon in which the disappearance of a physical symptom of illness is followed by the appearance of an idea or philosophical notion. Yet what we know about Bazhenov suggests that psychiatrists and psychotherapists had started the rehabilitation of the idea of "creative illness" fifty years before Weizsäker's work.[102]

A Stradivarius Violin: Genius as Progeneration

The altered notion of illness was not the only result of Bazhenov's study of art in general and of Dostoevsky in particular. Another important innovation was the vision of artistic genius as the highest achievement and final point of humanity's development. The idea itself was not new. In the late eighteenth century, the genius, and in particular the artistic genius, came to be thought of as the highest human type, replacing such earlier ideal types as the hero, the saint, the *uomo universale*.[103] At the beginning of the nineteenth century, however, the Romantics, by emphasizing irrationality, spontaneity, and intuition, "compromised" the artistic genius in the eyes of the sober Victorians. In contrast to the emotional Romantic genius, the perfect genius of the positivist age was an infallible rational thinker with a strong will and good sense of morality. Max Nordau, whom George Mosse describes as a "typical liberal of his age," believed the final point of human development is the genius, but the genius of "judgment and will alone."[104] Nordau found very few real geniuses, and these only among the dead; by contrast, he considered all contemporary writers, painters, and artists to be degenerates.[105]

If the number of "real men of genius" was negligible, genius became an unattainable ideal, merely a regulating idea. Lombroso, who in many ways was Nordau's teacher, contrasted individual real geniuses with the mass of

mattoides—the "semi-insane," occupying the area between "madmen of genius, the sane, and the insane properly called"—to whom a "disease gives all
semblance of genius, without its substance."[106] Compared with rational genius, artistic genius appeared a distortion, a throwback in evolutionary development, an "atavistic retrogression." It was located somewhere in between
the rational genius, the highest development, and degenerating types. Magnan coined the term, *dégénérés supérieurs*, "higher degenerates," for these borderline types, inhabitants of the *pays-frontière*. Henry Havelock Ellis placed
the one-sided genius, whose "intellectual originality is strictly confined to
one field," with the "idiots savants, the wonderful calculators, the mattoides
and 'the men of one idea,'" hoping in this way to "bridge the gulf that divided
idiocy from genius."[107]

The psychiatrists who made these distinctions expected that superior and
inferior human types would be different biologically. Nordau supposed that
geniuses differed from the rest of humanity through possession of special
kinds of "brain tissue" and organs, new or altered, destined later to become
typical of the whole of humankind. He believed that biologically superior
geniuses were related to the average human type in the same way that the
professional piano performance was related to the music from an automaton:
"In the average masses the brain centers are like the mechanical music box;
they play no pieces except those for which they were constructed . . . In the
exceptional man, on the contrary, the brain centers are like virtuosos. They
can play pieces that no one ever heard before." In comparison with the "real"
rational genius, artistic or emotional geniuses are inferior mentally and physiologically, "distinguished from average humanity by the greater force of the
automatic action of their centers, but not by any special original development."[108]

Though Nordau's work was abundantly translated and widely but often
critically read in Russia, his book containing the hypothesis that genius is a
site of progressive biological changes was not published in Russia until 1908.[109]
Yet the idea was in the air: in the nineteenth century everyone knew "what
sort of man he wants evolution to produce."[110] Interestingly, Dostoevsky also
mentioned the idea that the new man would be not only more powerful
mentally but also different physically from the contemporary man. But for
Dostoevsky this was a positivist heresy, which he put in the mouth of Kirillov in *The Devils*. Joseph Frank has drawn attention to Kirillov's most curi-
ous dialogue with the narrator: "Kirillov remarks that history will be divided
into two parts, 'from the gorilla to the annihilation of God, and from the
annihilation of God ["To the gorilla?" ironically interjects the narrator—J. F.]

. . . to the transformation of the earth and man physically. Man will be God and be transformed physically.'"[111]

Bazhenov formulated the same idea—that genius is a prototype of the future perfect man—in 1899. In contrast to Nordau's genius, a model of rationality and will, Bazhenov returned to the artistic genius. His image of genius permitted imperfection—"fallibility, error, and failure"—just like Dostoevsky's characters. Although, he argued, some artists are not "harmonious" and may appear as a chaotic heap of ruins, they are in fact "the material collected by a great architect for the construction of a grand building that has not been built yet."[112] Nordau compared his idea of rational genius to a "precision instrument"; Bazhenov used an artistic metaphor: beautiful, difficult to make and easy to destroy, artistic geniuses resembled a Stradivarius violin. A violin by Stradivarius, though fragile, is perfect; similarly, the fragility of artistic geniuses and their vulnerability to nervous disorders could not be regarded as degeneration. Bazhenov therefore found Magnan's term *higher degenerates* a contradiction in terms: those who were "higher" simply could not be placed in a subordinate position. Instead, he thought one could speak of their "incomplete progeneration" on the way to a future perfect type. He wrote in relation to Dostoevsky and Maupassant, "When we use psychiatric terminology in studying the psychomechanics of geniuses, we commit a logical error of *petitio principii;* as a result, the ideas of illness, ancestral reversion, degeneration immediately follow . . . If we accept, for human psychology, as well as for any category of biological facts, the superiority of the law of progressive evolution, why should we not speak of 'progeneration' rather than 'degeneration' and of 'aposteriorism' rather than atavism?"[113]

On the one hand, Dostoevsky's and Maupassant's illnesses were recognized facts; on the other hand, these writers were established geniuses. The quality of their work was so obvious, both in terms of its direct aesthetic impact and because of common opinion, that psychiatrists could not treat them as degenerates, as would have been done if these men were simply among the mentally ill. Even the milder term *higher degenerates* gradually faded out of fashion. Operating by aesthetic and not only psychiatric criteria, psychiatrists wrote an epitaph to the theory of degeneration, which was already dying at the close of the nineteenth century. They opened a road to new conceptions and practices, more suited to the new turn-of-the-century sensibilities.

THREE

Tolstoy and the Beginning of Psychotherapy in Russia

A patient of sanguine temperament, from a quiet ward. The patient is obsessed by mania that German psychiatrists term *Weltverbesserungswahn*. His madness consists of believing that it is possible to change the life of others by a word. General symptoms: dissatisfaction with the existing order, accusation of everybody but himself, and an irritating talkativeness without paying attention to his listeners. Frequent transitions from anger and irritation to unnatural weepy sensitivity. Specific symptoms: doing unnecessary and inappropriate jobs: cleaning and cobbling shoes, mowing hay, and the like. Treatment: complete indifference of others to what he says; occupations that would absorb the patient's spare energy.

—Case Records of the Inhabitants of Yasnaya Polyana,
Case record no. 1 (Lev Nikolaevich)

In biographies and memoirs, Lev Nikolaevich Tolstoy's (1828–1910) sound mind and robust health became almost emblematic. D. S. Merezhkovskii, in his influential essay *L. Tolstoy and Dostoevsky* (1902–3), juxtaposed Tolstoy's "soundness" and Dostoevsky's "sickness" as two spiritual poles; Stefan Zweig perceived Tolstoy as an embodiment of physical and spiritual strength.[1] Nonetheless, because of his untamed nature, Tolstoy's sanity was questioned. His literature, philosophy, and everyday life went beyond any ordinarily conceivable standard and did not fit ready-made classifications. The issue became prominent especially when in the late 1870s Tolstoy, as his contemporaries perceived it, suddenly stopped writing belles lettres and began to philoso-phize. He provoked the anger of many opponents: the government held him to be a revolutionary; the Church excommunicated him for preaching his own version of Christianity; the radicals criticized him for not going far enough in opposing the regime; and literary circles reproached him for aban-doning literature in favor of moralizing. As with Nikolai Gogol, psychiatrists followed the lead taken by critics and provided a medical diagnosis for Tol-stoy's "disorder." Yet, again as with Gogol, their views differed. Some per-ceived Tolstoy as neurotic, others argued that he possessed the supreme san-ity of a genius.

Tolstoy, in both word and deed, "fought back." When his critics pro-nounced him insane, he pronounced the whole world "mad." For many of his contemporaries, his criticisms of existing society and his positive teach-ings were more powerful than those of his opponents. Physicians, including psychiatrists, were not spared from feeling the effects of Tolstoy's philosophy, literature, and reformed way of life. Some of them even used Tolstoy's life philosophy in their own struggles with therapeutic nihilism and custodial psychiatry and in support of the introduction of psychotherapy and psycho-analysis. The social space in which psychotherapy developed, in Russia as elsewhere, was provided by private "nervous clinics" and "nervous sanato-ria," which proliferated at the turn of the century. Though many of these institutions had a commercial purpose, some physicians saw nervous clinics and sanatoria as the places in which to practice a simple, industrious, and spir-itual communal life in accordance with Tolstoy's late ideals. Together with numerous followers of Tolstoy, psychiatrists penned tributes to the writer, praising him as "a great psychologist," a master in the portrayal of psycho-logical conflicts and their cure. "The purification of the soul," which Tolstoy preached in his literary and philosophical work, became the creed of a new generation of psychotherapists. Through the career of Nikolai Osipov, a pio-neer of psychotherapy and psychoanalysis in Russia, we can trace Tolstoy's influence well into the 1930s, by which time many of that generation of psy-chiatrists had left the country and, like Osipov, lived and worked in exile.

Tolstoy's Neurosis

When, in 1897, Cesare Lombroso arrived in Moscow for the Congress of Physicians, he asked Tolstoy's permission to see him in Yasnaya Polyana. The Moscow authorities, however, made it clear that the government would not be pleased with a visit to the disfavored writer, so Lombroso had a conversation with the general charged to persuade him not to go. When Lombroso rejected all the arguments, the general made one last attempt, asking, "Don't you know that Tolstoy's head is not all right?" But Lombroso, as he reported, immediately turned the situation to his own benefit: "That is why I want to see him: I am a psychiatrist," he said, to the general's delight.[2]

The official attitude towards Tolstoy worsened when the writer stopped limiting himself to fiction and began to write philosophical and political pamphlets. Many of his later works were censored and publication was forbidden. In 1891, publication of *The Kreutzer Sonata,* which was due to appear in the thirteenth volume of Tolstoy's *Collected Works,* was stopped by the Church censor. The Ober-Procurator of the Holy Sinod wrote in a letter to the tsar:

Tolstoy is a fanatic with his own mad views, and, unfortunately, he seduces and leads into madness thousands of naïve people . . . Mad people who believe in Tolstoy are obsessed, just like himself, by the spirit of untamed propaganda, and they want to transform his teaching into action and inspire the peasants . . . The most striking example is Prince Khilkov, an officer of the guard, who settled in Khar'kov district, distributed all his lands to the peasants and, living on a farm, is preaching Tolstoy's *Testament* which is based on socialism and denies the Church and marriage. One cannot hide the fact that in recent years mental unrest has increased drastically, and it threatens to disseminate bizarre, perverse ideas on faith, Church, government, and society. This negative direction of thoughts is alien not only to the Church, but also to the nation. It is as if an epidemic of madness was gripping people's minds.[3]

It was not just the authorities who occasionally used the language of "madness" when speaking of Tolstoy's political views. "God knows what is in his head," remarked the liberal N. A. Nekrasov, poet and editor of *The Contemporary,* the literary journal in which Tolstoy's first novel was published. N. G. Chernyshevsky agreed with Nekrasov that Tolstoy should free himself from his "mental rubbish," and Ivan Turgenev found Tolstoy's tendency to philosophize "unfortunate."[4] Tolstoy's contemporaries reacted with suspicion when, approaching his fifties, this wealthy aristocrat, world-famous writer, and happy father of a big family felt that his life had lost its meaning and was tempted to kill himself, and finally found an answer in religion. Many former admirers of Tolstoy the writer protested against his moral program, which, remote from the political fights of the day, resembled the Catechism: "do not lie to yourself, do not fear the truth, do not think that you are right or special, admit your guilt in front of other people, carry on the eternal human duty—work together to maintain your own and other people's lives."[5]

His changed way of life, which included plowing peasants' fields and cobbling shoes, seemed odd even to those closest to him. His wife wrote in a letter to her sister, "Lyovochka works all the time, but, alas, he is writing some religious reflections, reads and thinks till he gets headaches, and all this in order to demonstrate that the Church dissents from the teaching of the Testament. There will be hardly a dozen people in Russia who are interested in it. But, there is nothing to be done: I wish only that it would soon end, like an illness." His son later remembered that, at this time, gossip was spreading around the central town of their province, Tula, that Tolstoy had gone mad.[6] In 1890, a South Russian newspaper published an article titled "Psychopathological Symptoms of Count Lev Tolstoy's New Faith."[7]

The tsarist regime regarded Tolstoy as an opponent, and the radicals welcomed him to their camp. After he had made his philosophy of nonresistance public, however, radicals found it more difficult to call Tolstoy an ally since he opposed the longed-for revolution. They therefore fervently attacked Tolstoy for his "social indifference" and, using Isaiah Berlin's precise phrasing, for his "'aristocratic' cynicism about life as a marsh which cannot be reclaimed." The Populist leader N. K. Mikhailovsky issued a powerful criticism of Tolstoy. Though the Populists shared Tolstoy's belief in a peasant utopia and anarchistic Christianity (Mikhailovsky sympathetically quoted from Tolstoy: "there is more strength, more awareness of beauty and good in the generations of workers than in the generations of barons, bankers, professors, and lords"), they damned his idea of nonresistance. Mikhailovsky once asked Tolstoy whether it was acceptable to stop aggression by force—for instance, to hit a man who was beating a child on the street—but the writer's views remained unshakable. Mikhailovsky believed opposition to the regime was incompatible with the idea of nonresistance, and he decided that what he thought to be a contradiction was also contradictory for Tolstoy. He claimed therefore that Tolstoy must be deeply divided—his "right hand is not aware of what his left hand is doing." At times active and rational, he argued, Tolstoy was at other times passive and fatalistic. Mikhailovsky speculated that this supposed inner contradiction was responsible for Tolstoy's psychological conflict. He concluded that "Tolstoy must have experienced a terrible drama [which is probably responsible for] that gloomy mood that went as far as the thought of suicide."[8]

In the eyes of the Russian intelligentsia, to be divided, not to be able to integrate the personal world and the social mission, was a serious failure. Isaiah Berlin traced this belief back to the 1830s, when the intelligentsia emerged as "a small group of *littérateurs,* both professional and amateur, conscious of being alone in a bleak world, with a hostile and arbitrary government on the one hand, and a completely uncomprehending mass of oppressed and inarticulate peasants on the other, conceiving of themselves as a kind of self-conscious army, carrying a banner for all to see—of reason and science, of liberty, of a better life."[9] This small group of educated Russians had a strong sense of mission and thought of themselves as both citizens and writers. Tolstoy, too, struggled to uphold the ideal that man is one and cannot be divided. When, in the late 1870s, he came to the conclusion that literature was of no use to the working people, he stopped writing fiction and condemned "art for art's sake."

Though Tolstoy, as Berlin remarked, went farther than any great writer in sacrificing his literary talent to his moral creed, he was criticized for not going far enough. Those who criticized Tolstoy for not being persistent in following his mission did not, however, agree about what his true mission was. The liberal and "aesthetic" Turgenev saw this mission in literature; he publicly regretted that Tolstoy stopped writing fiction and called Tolstoy's philosophy of love "hysterical." The radicals, by contrast, believed that his mission was to expose the ills of the existing regime; they therefore reproached Tolstoy for his "passiveness" or his "obscurantism." Yet they shared one point in common with Turgenev: they found Tolstoy's new creed, "Christianity without Christ," bizarre and unrealistic, and they interpreted Tolstoy's views as an escape from the political fight to the world of fantasy. For them, as for Turgenev, Tolstoy was "hysterical." Apparently borrowing the Populist idea that Tolstoy was "divided," V. I. Lenin wrote in 1908 that "the contradictions in Tolstoy's works, views, theories, in his school—indeed cry out . . . On the one hand, [he expresses] a remarkably powerful, direct, and sincere protest against social lies and false beliefs—on the other hand, [he is] 'tolstovets,' a worn out hysterical wimp [khliupik] who is called 'Russian intelligent' and who is saying, beating himself publicly on his breast: 'I am awful, I am disgusting, but I try to improve myself morally, I do not eat meat, I eat rice cutlets only.'"[10] The word hysterical pointed to an interpretive context about which Lombroso and other psychiatrists thought they had something special to contribute.

Before his visit to Yasnaya Polyana in 1897, Lombroso had formed certain expectations: "having for many years studied the pathological basis of genius," he wrote, "I found in Tolstoy's writings so many points relevant to my theory (for instance, inherited disease, caprices and eccentricities in youth, epileptic fits with hallucinations, mental irritation), that I could hope to find evidence of it in the famous artist's life." What he saw in Tolstoy's house, however, disabused him: the sixty-nine-year-old writer invited his Italian visitor to swim and was apparently pleased when the latter, after fifteen minutes in the water, could not keep up with him. Moreover, in response to Lombroso's surprise at his fitness, Tolstoy "stretched his arm and lifted [Lombroso] high off the ground, like a puppy."[11] Their conversation did not go well. Lombroso was upset by the stubbornness with which Tolstoy rejected his own as well as any other theories of criminality on the ground that any punishment is a crime. In response, Tolstoy found his Italian visitor narrow-minded and his theories of little interest. Besides, he had already formed a firm view on inborn criminality, and he later observed in a conversation with a doctor that Lombroso's "point of view . . . failed completely, when serious critics dealt with it."[12] Indeed, a character in Tolstoy's novel *Resurrection* (1899) considers Lombroso's theory out of touch with reality.[13]

Unlike Lombroso, who finally admitted that his expectations about Tolstoy's supposed disease turned out to be wrong, Lombroso's German disciple Max Nordau considered Tolstoy irrecoverably ill. In his famous *Degeneration* (*Entartung*; 1892), Nordau placed Tolstoy, with his "confused ideas about reality," among the degenerates.[14] He argued that when Tolstoy denied progress and called for moral and religious values, he was locked in wishful thinking and out of touch with reality. Nordau called "daydreamers" like Tolstoy "egomaniacs" or "egotists," and he coined the term *tolstoism* for the whole "phenomenon" of escaping from harsh reality into wishful thinking. However scandalous, Nordau's attempt to treat literature and art from the medical point of view had been common in French and German psychiatry since the mid-nineteenth century. Nordau shared with many nineteenth-century liberals a positivist belief in nonteleological thinking. From this point of view, Tolstoy's faith in love was "nonrealistic, uncanny," and his question "wherefore am I alive?" was senseless. Not by chance, Nordau quoted Turgenev's characterization of Tolstoy's "fervent love for the oppressed people" as "hysterical."[15]

This discussion probably motivated a thirty-six-year-old psychiatrist, Nikolai Evgrafovich Osipov (1877–1934), to analyze Tolstoy's psychological problems. In his paper "Tolstoy and Psychotherapy," written several years after the writer's death in 1910, Osipov agreed with the common view that Tolstoy was "divided": "a brilliant writer and psychologist," he was a "genius of destruction." Unlike Lombroso, who had a chance to verify his expectations when he met Tolstoy, Osipov had to confine his observations to Tolstoy's writings. He based his analysis on Tolstoy's autobiographical *My Confession* (1884; written in 1882) and an unfinished novel, *The Memoirs of a Madman,* the main character of which, Osipov believed, was Tolstoy's self-portrait.

Osipov based his analysis on the narrator's story, framing this narrative with comments, so that two voices—the writer's and the psychiatrist's—formed a dialogue. In *The Memoirs of a Madman*, the main character describes being taken to the Provincial Government Board to be certified as insane: "I did my utmost to restrain myself . . . I did not speak out because I am afraid of the madhouse, where they would prevent me from doing my mad work."[16] Osipov commented that this expressed "an obsession with full awareness": though the hero "knew" he was mad, he nevertheless continued his "mad business."[17] "Seeking enjoyments and finding them," the hero continues, "I lived till the age of thirty-five. I was perfectly well and there were no signs of my madness." Then he went to buy an estate in a distant province:

I fell asleep, but suddenly awoke feeling that there was something terrifying. As often happens, I woke up thoroughly alert and feeling as if sleep had gone forever. "Why am I going? Where am I going to?" I suddenly asked myself. It was not that I did not like the idea of buying the estate cheaply, but it suddenly occurred to me that there was no need for me to travel all that distance, that I should die here in this strange place, and I was filled with dread . . .

"But what folly this is!" I said to myself. "Why am I depressed? What am I afraid of?"

"Me!" answered the voice of Death, inaudibly. "I am here!"

A cold shudder ran down my back. Yes! Death! It will come—here it is—and it ought not to be. Had I been actually facing the death I could not have suffered as much as I did then.

"This is typical for obsessive fears," commented Osipov, "which occur from an idea of the object, not from the object itself."

The hero then recounts how he began to read the scriptures and attend services. The next "attack" happened to him when he once again was going to buy an estate:

I got home, and when telling my wife of the advantages that estate offered, I suddenly felt ashamed and disgusted. I told her I could not buy it because the advantages we should get would be based on the peasants' destitution and sorrow. As I said this I suddenly realized the truth of what I was saying—the chief truth, that the peasants, like ourselves, want to live, that they are human beings, our brothers, and sons of the Father as the gospels say. Suddenly something that had long troubled me seemed to have broken away, as though it had come to birth. My wife was vexed and scolded me, but I felt glad. That was the beginning of my madness. But my utter madness began after—about a month after that.

Indeed, Osipov remarked, there was nothing psychotic here yet. In the psychiatrist's judgment, the "obsessive idea" occurred when the narrator attended church: "Then at the exit there were beggars," the hero recounts. "And it suddenly became clear to me that this ought not to be, and not only ought not to be, but in reality was not. And if this was not, then neither was there either death or fear, and there was no longer the former tearing asunder within me and I no longer feared anything." Osipov therefore diagnosed a "typical hysterical delirium" or *Wunschdelirium,* a condition in which the insane person sees not what is there but what he wants to see. He opposed the suggestion made by a literary critic that *The Memoirs of a Madman* was in fact "the memoirs of a seeker": as Osipov argued, there must be something wrong with a seeker who ignores beggars—that is, reality.

In his paper, Osipov, a follower of Freud, brought together the psychoanalytic and the political diagnosis that Tolstoy was in conflict with himself. Whereas Nordau perceived Tolstoy's "confused ideas about reality" as a sign of degeneration, Osipov saw in them neurosis. And, less assertive than Nordau about the application of psychiatric terminology, Osipov feared that his attempt to transform the writer from a prophet to a clinical subject might be vulnerable to criticism. In order to justify his psychiatric analysis, Osipov therefore argued that he was "more experienced than Tolstoy" in several respects: first, he knew about all of Tolstoy's life; second, younger than Tolstoy, he outlived him and saw more; and finally, he was a psychiatrist and was familiar with psychoanalysis.[18]

Osipov's diagnosis, although similar to Nordau's judgment of "egotism," was more informed by contemporary theories. Influenced by psychoanalysis, Osipov related Tolstoy's "destructive power" to the writer's early experience. He referred to an autobiographical episode described in Tolstoy's *Childhood* (1856), when the narrator, as a little boy, led by a strange desire, upended the table on which his brother had placed his collection of rarities. Osipov discovered in Tolstoy a constellation of neurotic symptoms centered around "ambivalent narcissism": Tolstoy "at times loves himself, at times hates himself," is obsessed by his own unattractiveness, is "pathologically shy" and "sexually repressed" ("Tolstoy was longing to love people and was never able to do that"), and exhibits "auto-sadistic acts" (his suicidal thoughts). In addition, Osipov suggested that Tolstoy had an obsessive fear of death.[19] He concluded by describing "Tolstoy's syndrome": a "melancholic state with self-accusatory and self-destructive intentions on the basis of obsessive ideas of his own unattractiveness and fear of death." Osipov mentioned that he had come across "at least two other cases of Tolstoy's syndrome" in his practice.[20]

The psychiatrist's message was similar to the critic's: much earlier, Mikhailovsky had claimed that Tolstoy had an inner conflict as a result of which he nearly killed himself. But, spelled out in a psychiatric language, the message became problematic even for those who shared Mikhailovsky's opinion. Readers of Osipov, and especially of Nordau, thought a psychiatric diagnosis denigrated the writer's honest though confused search for truth.[21] Though a specialist journal published Osipov's article on Tolstoy's neurosis, the editor of a popular magazine did not accept his analysis of I. A. Goncharov's novel *Oblomov*, explaining that "attempts to analyze works of fiction rarely, only in exceptional cases, interest readers without special education." Even Osipov's close colleague, the psychoanalyst M. O. Wulff (1878–1971), reacted cautiously to his examination of Tolstoy; as he wrote to Osipov, "there is no mark of real illness, of neurosis, in Tolstoy as we understand it regarding our patients . . . Geniuses must be measured separately . . . I do believe that their conflicts are not of the same range, and they do not lie on the same plane; instead of resulting from failed adjustment to reality, they result from the impossibility of accepting and reconciling the personality with this reality."[22]

An Ideal Physician

In *War and Peace* (1865–69) Tolstoy ridiculed the doctors' treatment of the young heroine Natasha Rostova, who fell ill after her engagement was broken:

Doctors came to see her, both singly and in consultation, talked endlessly in French, German and Latin, criticized one another and prescribed every sort of remedy to cure every complaint they had ever heard of. But it never occurred to one of them to make the simple reflection that the disease Natasha was suffering from could not be known to them, just as no complaint afflicting a living being can ever be entirely familiar, for each living being has its own individual peculiarities and whatever his disease it must necessarily be peculiar to himself, a new and complex malady unknown to medicine—not a disease of the lungs, liver, skin, heart, nerves and so on, as described in medical books, but a disease consisting of one out of the innumerable combinations of the ailments of those organs. This simple reflection could not occur to the doctors (any more than it could occur to a sorcerer that he is unable to produce magic) because medicine was their life-work, because it was for that that they were paid and on that that they had expended the best years of their lives.[23]

Tolstoy's distrust of specialists, including doctors, was more than just an aristocratic contempt for paid labor. He was brought up on the eighteenth-century philosophes and, like Rousseau, believed that man was born innocent and had been ruined by bad education.[24] "One-sidedness is the main cause of man's unhappiness," wrote the eighteen-year-old Tolstoy in his diary.

Although he observed in himself a nascent "passion for science," he swore, "I shall never surrender myself to it in a one-sided manner, i.e. completely destroy feeling, not concern myself with application, and only endeavor to educate my mind and fill my memory with facts." He had a definite image of what a gentleman of noble origin like himself should know, and he planned to "attain a degree of perfection" in a number of subjects, including practical and some theoretical medicine, agriculture, and some natural science, but only to the extent necessary to be a good governor of his estate.[25] As a wealthy noble, he did not think about an academic career, and he left the university after his second year, partly because he could not allow examiners to tame his young aristocratic honor, partly because he had learned very early that cardinal questions of principle—such as why am I living, what purpose has my existence, how must I live?—required firsthand answers.

Tolstoy's self-education, carried out at home, prevented him from absorbing the current belief in scientific progress, and his literary talent gave him other means to express what he was longing for.[26] This made him very different from most liberals of the 1860s, who were intensely involved in a search for "the intellectual liberation of the individual," a phrase uttered by Mikhail Bakunin, a founding father of anarchism. Bakunin and his followers invested their hopes for the betterment of humanity in materialism and atheism, which they called on to sweep prejudice from their contemporaries' minds. The "nihilists," as Turgenev termed them, propagated natural science as a model for critical and rational thinking and made Herbert Spencer, Auguste Comte, and Charles Darwin the prophets of future society. The nihilists' views, expressed with the boldness of young temperaments, resonated in progressive parts of Russian society and encouraged many young people to choose scientific careers. Nihilism, as the historian Alexander Vucinich has commented, became a fateful phenomenon in Russia, because it combined two tendencies dominant in the 1860s: commitment to destroying the tsarist regime and commitment to the growth of science. Vucinich quotes the historian and literary scholar D. N. Ovsianiko-Kulikovskii: the "progressive" young men of the 1850s and 1860s

strove to enroll in physico-mathematical and medical faculties. Chemistry and physiology were particularly valued . . . The widespread attack on authorities of all kinds did not interfere with the general respect for the scientific contributions of such scholars as Liebig, von Baer and Darwin. At times, these names and the scientific ideas associated with them preoccupied the minds of young men no less, if not more, than such intoxicating words as "people," "freedom," "society," "brotherhood," and "justice" . . . Study of the sciences and the diffusion of materialistic philosophy were considered the most important, if not the only, path to useful work and to a constructive role in the progressive and libertarian movement.[27]

The nihilists laid down a line between "critically thinking" scientists and the rest of the Russian intelligentsia, whom they thought of as unworthy men of letters cherishing romantic illusions. The radical thinkers accused Tolstoy of obscurantism and claimed that his criticism of science played into the hands of reactionaries who wanted to preserve the political regime and Russia's backwardness. Chernyshevsky tried to persuade Tolstoy to write diatribes against the regime, and freshly baked graduates in the sciences wanted to give Tolstoy a dressing down for his denial of science.[28] The description of Tolstoy as a brilliant writer but a bad thinker became a cliché among Tolstoy's numerous critics.[29]

The response from writers was equally powerful. "Cursed Bernards" was the name given by one of Dostoevsky's characters to those blinded by the belief in scientific progress.[30] Tolstoy found the belief in "scientific, evolutionary fatalism . . . even worse than religious fatalism."[31] From his deathbed he warned his children that "the views you have acquired about Darwinism, evolution, and the struggle for existence will not explain to you the meaning of your life nor will they provide guidance in your action."[32] He also asserted in his diaries that the sciences would not increase the goodness of people: it "is just as impossible as making a stretch of water higher in one place than in others." The only answer to questions of human existence came "from increasing love, which by its nature makes all people equal," and from moral self-improvement: "Saint-Simon says: 'What if the 3,000 best scholars were destroyed?' He thinks that everything would then perish. I don't think so. More serious is the destruction or elimination of the best people morally."[33]

Tolstoy was, however, more thoughtful about the issue than his opponents wanted to admit. He thought about science as a social thinker, and in a book-length presentation of his creed, "What Then Must We Do?" (1885), he argued that science could only adapt to the given social conditions, not change them. In an immoral society neither science nor medicine could be moral. He argued that even institutions built with the best intentions, such as *zemstvo* medicine (the system of health care for the poor, mainly the peasants), did not serve their purposes, because they were underfinanced. Thus "science had adapted itself entirely to the wealthy classes and accordingly has set itself to heal those who can afford everything."[34] In an immoral society, science was on the side of power and was used to justify the status quo. When Tolstoy read an article in which the author, a professor of hygiene, argued that alcohol and tobacco, besides other flavoring substances, were necessary for the organism, he burst out in anger: "This stupid, naive article . . . showed me clearly what the hypocrites of science suppose the business of science to be. Not what it ought to be—a definition of what should be—but a description of what is . . . People drink wine and smoke tobacco, and science sets itself the task of justifying the use of wine and tobacco physiologically . . . People believe in nonsense, and teleological science justifies it."[35]

Medicine came under particular attack by Tolstoy because of his own experience. Although a man with a very strong constitution (he was stronger physically than many of his contemporaries), Tolstoy had numerous contacts with physicians. When he was eighteen, he spent a few weeks in the clinic of Kazan' University (where he started writing his diaries, an activity he continued for the rest of his life).[36] He went to a spa in the Northern Caucasus, and he was operated on under chloroform while in the army during the Crimean War. All the same, the more he became preoccupied with a spiritual search, the more critical his remarks on medicine became. In 1876, when the physicians could not help his sick wife, he wrote in a letter, "I do not believe in either doctors or in medicine or in the fact that remedies made by people could in the slightest way alter the state of health, i.e., man's life."[37] Later in his life, however, he often called in the doctors; at sixty-five he wrote in his diary, "I'm afraid I'm beginning to get preoccupied with my medical condition and with treating myself and observing myself, the very thing I condemned so much in [his son] Lyova."[38] He was seriously ill in 1901, and in early 1902 he complained in a letter to his daughter about "stupid philosophizing and manipulations to which the doctors are subjecting me. Owing to my weakness and a desire not to aggravate those surrounding me, I must submit to them."[39] In a similar vein, in *The Death of Ivan Ilych* (1886), the doctors lie to Ivan Ilych, who is dying of cancer. They "put on just the same air toward him as he himself put on toward the accused person" when he was a lawyer in court.[40]

At about this same time (1902), Tolstoy wrote in his diary:

Everything about [medicine] is immoral. Immoral is the fear of illness and death induced by medical aid, immoral is the use of the exclusive aid of doctors, available only to the rich. It is immoral to enjoy exclusive comfort and pleasures, but to enjoy the exclusive possibility of preserving life is the height of immorality. Immoral is the requirement of medicine to conceal from a patient the danger of his situation and the nearness of death. Immoral is the advice and requirements of doctors that a patient should look after himself—his bodily function—and in general should live as little as possible spiritually, but only materially: should not think, should not excite himself, should not work.[41]

Yet, after recovering from this illness, he thought it essential to have a physician attached permanently to the household. Several doctors tried to fill this position, which also involved running a dispensary for the village on Tolstoy's estate, but soon left. Then, in 1904, a Slovak, Dr. Dushan Makovitskii (1866–1921), was employed and became irreplaceable, perhaps not as a physician but as a kind of secretary and literary assistant. A gentle and shy person, he could not stand any discord or argument in the household. When he took a month's leave, Tolstoy complained to a friend, "I tell you frankly, I don't need his medicine, but when I do not see his hat there for a day or two, I somehow or other feel lost. Holy Dushan!"[42] Makovitskii gained the master's unlimited trust and accompanied his patron in his final flight from Yasnaya Polyana.[43]

Tolstoy definitely preferred a humble and "holy" doctor to ambitious specialists with scientific training. Ovsianiko-Kulikovskii drew an analogy between a humble doctor and Tolstoy's ideal of a political leader. In *War and Peace* Tolstoy contrasted M. I. Kutuzov, the Russian general who gained his fame in the war against Napoleon in 1812, an archetype of a man of "natural wit and wisdom," to a narrow-minded specialist who cannot see clearly because of his theories. Tolstoy attributed Kutuzov's success in the war to his "simple, Russian, untutored instinct," owing to which he despised or ignored the German, French and Italian experts."[44] Kutuzov acted according to the everyday wisdom that "an apple should not be plucked while it is green. It will fall of itself when ripe." Tolstoy preferred Kutuzov's strategy of "contemplating the progress of events" to Napoleon's interventionist strategy. The former, in the words of the fictional Prince Andrei, "will not introduce anything of his own. He will not scheme or start anything, . . . but he will listen, bear in mind all that he hears, put everything in its rightful place. He will not stand in the way of anything expedient or permit what might be injurious. He knows that there is something stronger and more important than his own will—the inevitable march of events, and he has the brains to see them and grasp their significance, and seeing that significance can abstain from meddling, from following his personal desires and aiming at something else."[45]

In 1911 Osipov attempted to defend psychiatry as well as scientific medicine in general against Tolstoy's lavish criticism. He began by repeating the cliché that Tolstoy was a brilliant writer but a bad thinker, by describing him as a genius, but a "genius of destruction": "Tolstoy destroys everything that is dear to people—the treasures of life, art, science, or philosophy—through his pitiless analysis, similar to the way little Lyova [Tolstoy as a small boy] turned over the table with his brother's collection of rarities. Tolstoy possesses a genius of destruction, of anarchy . . . It has a wonderful power . . . But after this destruction it is necessary to create something new on the old ruins. Tolstoy begins, but then genius deserts him." Tolstoy, Osipov argued, demanded of medicine impossible results and, when he failed to obtain these results, completely rejected it. Tolstoy did not realize that the physician must compromise and take from science what he needs, choosing the lesser of two evils—the disease or its treatment. At the same time, Osipov approved of Tolstoy's attacks on materialism, which Osipov also believed to be too narrow a world-view for a good physician: "Tolstoy is right when he warns about the danger of one-sided beliefs in general and materialism as the belief in the power of medicines in particular: science allows materialism as a method, whereas materialism in philosophy cannot resist criticism, and Tolstoy is absolutely right to fight. The danger of materialism lies in its extreme narrowness and fanaticism."[46]

Osipov shared with Tolstoy a fear of one-sided beliefs and narrow-mindedness following specialized education, and he was happy to find in Tolstoy's writings what for him became a portrait of an ideal physician. Like General Kutuzov, a man of "natural wit and wisdom," an ideal physician relies more on his own intuition and life philosophy than on any ready-made theory. Osipov saw an ideal physician as a healer rather than a scientist or investigator. An ideal physician has eclectic views because he has to respond to all the needs of his patients, and he should restrain himself from one-sided indulgences in order not to do any harm to the ill person. Tolstoy thought such a physician an unattainable ideal, but Osipov claimed that such a physician already existed and that Tolstoy simply missed him. This ideal was the *zemstvo* doctor.

Osipov knew *zemstvo* doctors very well because his father, Dr. Evgraf Alekseevich Osipov (1841–1904), was one. When he chose medicine as his career, Nikolai Osipov followed his father's example. The father was sufficiently renowned among Russian physicians that his son occasionally "lived on his capital": when Nikolai took his exams at Moscow University (which he had to do because his certificate from a foreign university had to be approved under Russian law), the examiners, after learning he was the son of Evgraf Osipov, did not ask him any questions.[47] Evgraf Osipov worked for the Moscow Region *zemstvo* and was widely known as a founder of community medicine in Russia and as one of the organizers of the Pirogov Society (founded in 1883). The *zemstvo* physicians of the 1870s and 1880s shaped the dominant ethos of the profession, and they were glorified a quarter of a century later.[48] As an author of medical memoirs wrote in retrospect, "if we look at the results of *zemstvo* medicine and at what it has given to simple people, we will remember first of all the glorious figure of the *zemstvo* physician, that physician who in the 1860s and 1870s went to the country to serve the Russian peasants."[49] *Zemstva*—democratic local governments—were responsible for the welfare of the majority of the Russian rural population and the organization of the health care system. Physicians hired by *zemstva* worked on the establishment of new hospitals or on the expansion of existing facilities, and, as village (*uchastkovyi*) doctors, they looked after a vast number of patients. They often had to confront local authorities in their struggle for funds, and they were regarded as the most socially engaged members of the medical profession in late-nineteenth-century Russia.[50]

As Nancy M. Frieden, a historian of Russian medicine, argues, although the *zemstvo* physicians adopted the ideology of servants of the people, they should not be confused with the idealistic medical students who, responding to the Populists' calls, "went to the people" to learn rather than to teach. The majority of *zemstvo* physicians saw themselves as experts, members of a technical elite with highly specialized knowledge, and they "marshaled scientific arguments for their practical goals, trying to apply the latest sanitary and preventive techniques to Russian needs."[51] But in the heated political atmosphere of late-nineteenth-century Russia, it was difficult to stand outside politics. Even a book with the modest title *Medical Assistance to the Peasants* suggested that capitalism in the future should be replaced with a "sanitary type of society" in which "all conditions responsible for suffering and illness would be eliminated."[52] Evgraf Osipov, at least in his younger years, had contacts with revolutionaries and even offered accommodation in his house to Sofia Perovskaia, later one of the organizers of the Populist party The People's Will, which was responsible for the regicide of 1881. Osipov's house in the South Russian town of Stavropol' must have seen heated discussions in which Perovskaia ardently criticized "small deed" liberalism and Osipov's intention "to limit his activity only to the *zemstvo*."[53]

This activity, however, had political impact. Together with three or four other physicians and a few technical workers, Evgraf Osipov inspected thousands of factories in the Moscow Region, where he found appalling hygienic conditions. In the existing political and social circumstances little could be done; the *zemstvo* physicians were trapped and had to admit that the only way out, if their work was not to be senseless and fruitless, was to fight for the removal of the unhygienic conditions.[54] In the years of the 1905 revolution

(1905–7), medical associations issued resolutions in which they demanded the government's resignation as the primary condition for efficient public medicine. We can only guess how Evgraf Osipov would have behaved in these circumstances, as he died in 1904.

In the minds of the younger generation, the image of the *zemstvo* physician showed more similarities to the ideal of a committed intellectual serving the people than to the portrait of a narrow-minded specialist drawn by Tolstoy. By the turn of the century, *zemstvo* physicians had come to almost the same conclusion as did Tolstoy twenty years earlier: science and medicine could do nothing in unfavorable social conditions. The legendary figure of a *zemstvo* physician, as it appeared to Nikolai Osipov and his contemporaries, combined the best features of a professional expert with moral qualities and independent thinking. It was only one step from this image to Tolstoy's ideal of a wise physician who is not dominated by a blind belief in scientific methods or by anybody else's doctrine, but relies on his own intuition and "life philosophy." This image inspired the younger Osipov's generation, even when the political and professional situation changed and the *zemstva* went into decline.

Unlike his father, Nikolai Osipov was never involved in *zemstvo* medicine, and he built his career as an academic and private practitioner. In his student years, he distanced himself from politics and, as he confessed later, "danced a lot and worked a little." Like other students from wealthy and noble families, he wore a luxurious student uniform with a fur collar and white silk lining. Later, his political sympathies did not go further to the left than support for the Oktiabrists, a party of wealthy landlords and bourgeoisie. In February 1899, a student strike began at St. Petersburg University and was joined by several other universities, including Moscow University. Although Osipov was loyal to the authorities, his fellow students elected him to the strike's Executive Committee.[55] He missed the meeting and was not aware of the elections until the following day; nevertheless, he was arrested and spent a few days in prison before being liberated. As a result, he was forbidden to study at Russian universities; in the political jargon of the time, he received a "wolf ticket." He continued his education in Germany and Switzerland, at the universities of Bonn, Berlin, Bern, Zurich, and Basel. In Zurich he renewed his friendship with his father's friend and former colleague in the Moscow Sanitary Bureau, Professor Friedrich (Fedor Fedorovich, as he was called in Russia) Erisman.[56]

Having received his degree from the University of Basel in 1903, Osipov returned to Russia and obtained a position as a demonstrator (*prozektor*) in histology at Moscow University. The professor of histology, V. P. Karpov, was a naturalist-philosopher, a proponent of a romantic view of nature as a whole, which he eventually developed in his book *Main Features of the Organic Under-standing of Nature* (1913).[57] He became one of Osipov's "teacher-friends," and his world-view influenced the young physician, already prone to philosoph-ical reflection, and encouraged him to contemplate an organic as opposed to a mechanistic understanding of nature. Osipov even began to write the man-uscript "Organic Natural Philosophy in Contemporary Russian Science," which he worked on until the end of his life but did not complete.[58] Although he started on academic work, he looked forward to medical practice, partly because it would secure his living. According to Russian law, however, grad-uates from foreign universities had to obtain special permission from the Medical Department before they could be employed in state service. An ex-ception was made to this rule during the war with Japan (1904–5), and med-ical students without the certificate were allowed to replace physicians who had left their clinics and hospitals for the army. In 1904, Evgraf Osipov's friend, the psychiatrist N. N. Bazhenov, became the director of the Moscow City Psychiatric Hospital (Preobrazhenskii), and he invited the younger Osipov to take a temporary position. Here Nikolai Osipov acquired his first expe-rience in psychiatry and began to think of becoming a full-time physician. His choice of psychiatry was also influenced by his mother's illness. She suf-fered, so the family believed, from "hystero-hypochondria," and she was treated, without stable results, by leading psychiatrists in Paris, Berlin, Peters-burg, and Moscow.[59]

After the war the Medical Department certificate was again required for a position in a state hospital, and Osipov had to leave the Preobrazhenskii. Bazhenov invited him to his private clinic, and he was also recommended to V. P. Serbskii, director of the renowned Moscow University Psychiatric Clinic (University Clinic).

Serbskii, who worked as a *zemstvo* psychiatrist at the beginning of his career and organized a *zemstvo* psychiatric hospital in Tambov province, later taught at Moscow University, and in 1901 he succeeded S. S. Korsakov as professor of psychiatry and head of the University Clinic. Like many *zemstvo* physi-cians, he had to struggle to fulfill his professional values. During the events of 1905, he did not stand aside from the political fight. When the police looked for rebels hiding in hospitals, he did not allow them to enter the clinic, and when a mentally ill revolutionary killed himself in prison, Serbskii published an article criticizing the authorities.[60] He was more conservative in questions of clinic management. When, following the common movement for the "democratization" of asylums, the staff of the University Clinic wanted to introduce "collegial management" and bring the junior physicians and workers into running the clinic and taking decisions, Serbskii actively opposed them. He feared that incompetent management would ruin the clinic. The physicians who demanded "democratization" were forced to resign.[61]

The conflict also had a theoretical dimension. The young physicians A. N. Bernstein (1870–1922), S. A. Sukhanov (1867–1916), and P. B. Gannushkin (1875–1933) were followers of Emil Kraepelin, whereas Serbskii was an adept of traditional symptomatological psychiatry and, in particular, argued against Kraepelin's conception of dementia praecox. This conflict fostered a separation between the German-oriented Kraepelinians, who founded their own journal, *Contemporary Psychiatry* (*Sovremennaia psikhiatriia*), and the followers of French psychiatry, who were grouped around the Moscow University Clinic. Serbskii hired new staff, and the anti-Kraepelinian Osipov easily obtained a position as director's assistant in the now emptied clinic.[62] Despite his negative views on Kraepelin, Serbskii was sympathetic towards psychotherapy, the topic that gradually moved to the center of Osipov's interests. He supported Osipov in opening the first outpatient service for neurotics in Moscow at the University Clinic; between 1906 and 1911 Osipov saw hundreds of neurotic patients there.

Osipov's entry into the psychiatric community was complicated by his involvement on Serbskii's side in the conflict, as well as by his reputation as a conservative. Psychiatrists were known as one of the most radical groups in the medical profession, and this reputation was confirmed during the first Russian revolution. At the 1905 meeting of the Pirogov Society, which coincided with the revolutionary events, Osipov was worried that his radically oriented colleagues would jeer his talk. Later, however, Serbskii and his staff proved equally opposed to government policies. In 1911, Minister of Education L. A. Kasso, in response to a student strike, ordered the expulsion of several hundred students from Moscow University. Many professors, Serbskii among them, resigned in support of the students. One day Serbskii met Osipov in the corridor and said, "Well, I pass the clinic over to you. I shall not come back again." But this did not happen: all the clinic's physicians, including Osipov, left together with Serbskii.[63] Professional interests were sacrificed for the sake of political and humane values: the ideal of "noble hearts" still had an influence on young physicians.

The more remote the phenomenon of *zemstvo* medicine, the more it was valued; there was an aura around the names of physicians who had worked for the *zemstva* and organized mental health care in the provinces. Korsakov, the leader of Moscow psychiatrists in the last two decades of the nineteenth century, until his early death in 1900, was especially praised.[64] Osipov, a member of the memorial committee for Korsakov, contributed to the overall admiration with an article written for the jubilee of Moscow University. He called the period of institutionalization a "heroic period in the history of Russian psychiatry" and praised Korsakov and his closest colleagues, Bazhenov and Serbskii, who laid the foundations of mental health care in the country's "deaf corners": "Brilliantly educated and an exceptionally witty man of society, [Bazhenov], nevertheless, went to the provinces and became one of the psychiatrist-fathers, psychiatrist-heroes. When Bazhenov had left to study abroad, Serbskii took his place in the clinic. After a year of work under Korsakov's supervision, Serbskii went abroad, and then became the director of the Tambov *zemstvo* asylum, and also a psychiatrist-father, a psychiatrist-hero."[65] Though Osipov's sympathies were with the generation of the founding fathers, he inherited their ethics rather than their scientism. As he wrote in his memoirs, it was the philosophical rather than the medical side of psychiatry that attracted him. His interest in psychological problems of personality, which began with a biological approach, developed through anatomy, physiology, and pathology to psychiatry, studies of neuroses, psychology, and criminology. As a young man, Osipov expected to find in psychiatry an answer to the "puzzling problem of the soul and the problem of man in general."[66] His fellow psychiatrists also regarded Osipov as one of the most philosophically oriented physicians, someone interested in the epistemology and methodology of psychiatry.

The neo-Kantian philosophers Wilhelm Dilthey, Wilhelm Windelband, and Heinrich Rickert had influenced these interests. In 1894, when Wilhelm Wundt's psychology laboratory in Leipzig attracted dozens of students and visitors from all over the world, Dilthey gave one of his most famous talks in Berlin. In this talk, "The Idea of Descriptive and Analytic Psychology," he criticized experimental psychologists for imitating the natural sciences and explaining mind by physiological processes. His criticism rested on a fundamental distinction between the sciences of nature, *Naturwissenschaften,* and the sciences of human spirit, *Geisteswissenschaften.* The latter, he claimed, have as their subject something essentially different from natural objects—values, sentiments, and systems of meaning—and hence require a different method. In Rickert's words, "reality becomes nature if we consider it in regard to what is general; it becomes history if we consider it in regard to the particular or individual."[67] History and other individualizing—idiographic—disciplines bring the case in question into relationship with values and identify what is most significant for an individual.

Around the turn of the century, the popularity of neo-Kantian philosophy among young and idealistic Russian people, many of whom studied in German universities, was comparable only with the popularity of Marxism. Specialists in different disciplines, including psychology and psychiatry, took the ideas of the *Geisteswissenschaften* as a program for action. Osipov spent a year in Berlin, where Dilthey was a professor, and was deeply impressed by his philosophy of life, especially the thesis that human beings have a special tendency to achieve a comprehensive interpretation, a *Weltanschauung,* or philosophy that combines a picture of reality with a sense of its meaning and value to create a principle of action. Osipov also reflected on the epistemological status of medicine using Windelband's distinction between the nomothetic and idiographic sciences and Rickert's notions of generalization and individualization.[68] In 1911 Osipov opened the meetings of the Moscow Psychiatric Circle, Little Fridays, with a talk titled "On the Logic and Methodology of Psychiatry." The talk, in his own words, was a "paraphrase of Rickert's doctrine." Osipov claimed that psychiatry, though based on the natural sciences, is a clinical discipline that studies the patient as an individual. The psychiatrist should seek "the core value that determines the actual state of the patient."[69]

Rickert had argued that the final result in the idiographic sciences is a concept of the "historical individual." Following Rickert, Osipov claimed in his talk that the result in psychiatry would be a concept of the "psychiatric individual," which the psychiatrist constructs out of clinical observations and knowledge of the patient's past, by writing his case record, his *history*.[70] Emphasizing the unique nature of a "psychiatric individual," psychiatrists bore in mind that they dealt with a variety of illnesses and, so, with a number of "individuals." Osipov argued that medicine takes a middle position between the natural (nomothetic) and the human (idiographic) sciences: on the one hand, medicine is based on systematic investigation in anatomy, physiology, histology, and the other natural sciences, and includes generalizations; on the other hand, practical medicine involves individual cases. In a paper published some years later, Osipov wrote about medicine's "double face," one turned towards science, the other towards the individual patient. He concluded that medicine is more an art than a science and requires the physician to have special abilities. Besides the ability to generalize from different cases, to acquire scientific knowledge, or to do research, the physician should be able to apply his knowledge to each individual case. The physician should have a "double personality," should be both a scientist and a healer.[71]

Osipov discovered a representation of his ideal in Tolstoy's writings. The physician ought to see clearly "the inevitable march of events" and to submit himself to it; like a wise politician, the physician intervenes in the natural course of events only occasionally, in carefully chosen cases. The best he can do is to be aware of the limits of modern science and medicine and to rely on "the simplest direct work of life," trying to develop it in a positive direction. Osipov compared the physician to a slave in an oriental parable who makes a lamp although he does not possess a theoretical knowledge of light. Similarly, the physician does not have a complete knowledge of the organism but, nevertheless, is able to help the ill.[72] Facing the lack of scientific knowledge, the physician relies on his experience and his broad outlook more than on scientific training. "It is not medicine, it is the physician who cures," and he does it by his correct views on human psychology and the nature of illness and, finally, by his personality.[73] Towards the end of his life, in a lecture on neurasthenia—the subject in which he specialized—Osipov remarked with the humbleness of Tolstoy's "holy doctor," "How many neurasthenics have I managed to cure? I will answer: no one. *Medicus curat, natura sanat* [physician treats, nature cures]. Moreover: destiny contributes to the recovery of the nervously ill more than the physician does."[74]

Nervous Clinics and Sanatoria: The Emergence of Psychotherapy in Russia

Tolstoy was vividly interested in mental illness. His children later recalled his invented stories about different kinds of madness, for instance, a tale about a man who imagines he is made of glass. Yasnaya Polyana sheltered, as Tolstoy's daughter remembered, various "strange people"—a dwarf, a former monk who became an alcoholic, a female beggar who wore men's clothes and believed she had a birch tree growing inside her.[75] Partly because he wanted information about his wife's supposed nervous disorder, Tolstoy read widely in modern psychiatry.[76] Yet he believed madness was quite different from how it was described in psychiatric textbooks—it was egoism taken to its final point. He had numerous occasions to observe mentally ill patients. Tolstoy's Moscow estate had a common fence with the garden of the Moscow University Psychiatric Clinic. He liked to converse with the clinic's director, Moscow's first professor of psychiatry, Korsakov. Once, when the Tolstoys were attending theatricals performed by the patients of the clinic, one of them recognized Tolstoy. "Ah, Lev Nikolaevich," he exclaimed, "I am delighted that you are with us!" He thought Tolstoy was a patient, not a visitor.[77]

In spite of his close contact with psychiatry, Tolstoy's remarks about it were as damning as those about medicine in general. Once he intervened in support of an anonymous article describing a case of psychiatric abuse; he found the abuse so horrible and undeniable that he demanded that society and the government prevent it in the future. It was found afterwards that the author of the article was unsuccessfully treated for paranoia in a provincial mental hospital. An insulted psychiatrist wrote in response to Tolstoy's comments, "It is obvious that someone can be a genius of a writer and yet understand nothing about psychiatry."[78] Even after this incident Tolstoy's view of psychiatry remained unfavorable. A few months before his death, he began an essay, "On Madness," and for this purpose visited several asylums near Moscow. As he wrote in the essay, what he saw on his trip were "establishments that people suffering from one common general form of madness organized for people suffering from various forms, the forms not conforming with the general form." He called psychiatry a "comic," "imagined science" and, comparing different classifications of mental diseases, wrote that they agreed only on one clear and comprehensible division: "1. Violent patients . . . 2. Semi-violent. 3. Quiet, and 4. Patients on trial."[79] Supposedly under the influence of Tolstoy's teaching, a Moscow psychiatrist closed down his clinic and left for his family estate in the country, where he then farmed, kept bees, and worked with wood.[80] In contrast to his attack on hospital psychiatry, Tolstoy sanctioned a new development in turn-of-the-century psychiatry—nervous sanatoria—by taking refuge in one of them in 1888.[81]

In the 1880s psychiatry in Russia was already a well-established discipline. Medical students at Moscow University in the 1870s did not have courses in psychiatry and graduated without seeing a single mental patient, but Nikolai Osipov's generation had an opportunity to undergo intensive theoretical training in relatively well-equipped university clinics and small private asylums. Whereas the founding fathers had many administrative obligations and had to negotiate constantly with the authorities, the younger psychiatrists devoted more time to clinical research and private practice.[82] Even in the provinces, this next generation of psychiatrists managed to conduct research and to write reports for psychiatric journals, a number of which were launched at the turn of the century. Political reaction, which began with the demise of the first Russian revolution in 1907, indirectly contributed to a shift toward career-oriented and professional activities, in some contrast to the Populist values of the previous generation. Community medicine went through a crisis during which the *zemstva,* especially those in the most distance provinces, found it very difficult to attract and retain physicians. A contemporary reported that "among *zemstvo* physicians there is . . . suppressed dissatisfaction with their status, the failure of their work, a diminishing of past excitement and a loss of faith in the broad public significance of their work."[83]

Psychiatrists in the 1910s became disappointed with community medicine, partly because of numerous conflicts with local *zemstvo* administrations. One psychiatrist, in a letter to the editor of a Russian psychiatric journal, mentioned six colleagues who "were all forced by some sad turn of events to cut short their useful activities."[84] In 1907 the director of the Voronezh Psychiatric Hospital, N. A. Vyrubov (1869–1918), was fired and exiled from the province, and Bazhenov had similar problems with the Riazan' *zemstvo* administration and had to resign. It is therefore not surprising that in this period many younger psychiatrists sought to secure their income through private practice, which gave older psychiatrists the chance to complain: "Nowadays physicians would rather seek a job in the underequipped laboratories of mental hospitals than carry out their responsibilities in public health care."[85] Former propagandists of community medicine feared that Russian community medicine would become a commercial enterprise, as it was thought to be in European and Anglo-American practice. In 1911, indeed, one-third of Russian psychiatrists (eighty-one of 266) worked in private clinics or made their living from their private clientele; most of these (sixty-one) were in Moscow.[86]

Private institutions for "nervous" patients played an important social role at the time when the new generation of practitioners came onto the stage. A clinic or a sanatorium for those with nervous illness was very different from an institution for the mentally ill—a madhouse or private hospital—as it existed, for instance, in Britain in the first seventy years of the nineteenth century. Despite the techniques of "moral treatment" adopted in Britain, the madhouses were places of forced confinement, where families locked up patients. This "trade in lunacy," as W. H. Parry-Jones has shown, led to a growing disparagement of private madhouses, and their number drastically decreased at the turn of the century.[87] By contrast, the institutions for the nervously ill were modeled on private clinics for internal diseases and were intended for voluntary patients. Established by psychiatrists, who did not have the secure salary of a university teacher or a physician in a mental hospital, these nervous clinics often pursued commercial aims. Yet, unlike private madhouses, institutions for the nervously ill often appeared to sell a medical service to the patients themselves, not to their families. This shifted attention secured a better reputation for nervous clinics and sanatoria.

The prototype of an institution for the nervously ill in Russia was founded in Moscow in 1828, when a physician from the Baltic city of Riga, Hans Johann Loder, opened an "establishment for artificial mineral waters," where patients were treated not only with water but with promenades, music, reading, and conversation. By the end of the nineteenth century Moscow had more than forty private psychiatric clinics and sanatoria. The model for these clinics came mainly from German-speaking Europe, where private clinics for *Nerven- und Gemütskranke* (nervous and psychiatric patients) flourished in the second half of the nineteenth century.[88] The first sanatoria for the nervously ill were opened in the southern provinces of Russia, at the seaside, in the 1880s.[89] By the turn of the century Russia had a number of clinics, sanatoria, and outpatient services for nervous, "overworked," and alcoholic patients. Several nervous sanatoria (Vsekhsviatskii, Podsolnechnyi, Nadezhdino, Kriukovo) were founded between 1908 and 1914; the First World War and the 1917 Revolution, with its restrictions on the private sector, stopped this rapid development.

"Nervous" diseases formed a large group, and they ranged from so-called functional or general neuroses (epilepsy, hysteria, and neurasthenia, the organic origin of which was assumed but not identified) to the symptoms of "overwork," such as mental fatigue or nervousness. At the beginning of the twentieth century, physicians in Russia, as elsewhere, believed that "only a rare person among us can boast of not having suffered from one or another neurosis. Each of us may one day develop a number of either neurasthenic or hysteric symptoms, as well as high sensitivity, fatigue, headaches, and so on and so forth."[90] The clientele of nervous clinics and sanatoria varied widely and included persons recovering from psychic or somatic diseases, some cases of incomplete recovery, persons with periodic psychoses, general neuroses, and psychopathic constitutions, drug addicts, and "mentally exhausted" and "nervous" patients. The insane were not usually accepted in nervous clinics; if they were, it was advised to have a separate building or at least a separate entrance for these patients.[91] Nervous clinics were therefore less terrifying than the infamous "yellow houses," the usual color of madhouses in Russia. Patients in clinics benefited from a freer regime, which enabled them to develop normal interests. Nervous clinics and sanatoria offered a wide range of physiotherapeutic procedures: electrotherapy, baths, massage, sea-bathing (in M. Ia. Droznes's sanatorium in Odessa), mineral waters, sour clotted milk, grape juice, and even sour horse milk (*kumys*). But the main treatment addressed the mind. Physicians who worked in the clinics mainly had a psychiatric education or at least some experience of work in asylums and mental hospitals. They emphasized the value of a special way of life and an atmosphere that resembled close family relationships.[92] Thus, the old methods of moral treatment were modified by less restrictive conditions.

The philosophy of "moral treatment" was developed a century earlier in England by the founders of the York Retreat, who, as Anne Digby has shown, believed that a "proper regulation of the mind is essentially connected with the prevention of the disease." Lockean educational ideals inspired an analogy between the patients in the retreat and children. John Locke stated that "the great secret of education lies in finding the way to keep the child's spirit easy, active and free; and yet, at the same time, to restrict him from many things he has a mind to."[93] The Moscow psychiatrist Korsakov expanded this analogy further: as in a family, where "concern and thoughts for other persons . . . do not let the soul feel emptiness," close and friendly relationships between patients and staff in the clinic filled the time and stimulated "healthy" emotions. The founders of the York Retreat saw the superintendent as the "master of the family"; the marriage of its first superintendent to its matron seemed to confirm this ideal. By the same token, Korsakov claimed that a woman's presence was important for establishing close relationships: looking after the patients, she entered into small details of their life and created an intimate and caring atmosphere. The doctor "simply does not have time for this." But he also should not be accessible: if he had the image of a distanced and authoritative patriarch, the patients and staff would value every small sign of his attention and immediately obey his orders.[94]

One more parallel between the York Retreat and other private madhouses, also usually called "retreats" or "refuges,"[95] and the institutions for the nervously ill was the importance of the countryside location. Korsakov believed that life in a rural clinic would allow patients to become hardened by walking barefoot and partaking of fresh air, sunbathing, and healthy food. The clinic's influence was moral as well as physical. A simply designed countryside medical institution prevented "unnatural" and "unhealthy" living. Korsakov recommended the accommodation of patients in wooden huts, typical houses of Russian peasants. He did not encourage the noisy entertainment characteristic of city life, such as picnics, amateur theatricals, and promenades in a carriage. The idea that a simple life, in peace with nature and people, would sober the mind and cure the soul echoed religious ideals shared by such different people in different times as the founders of the York Retreat at the end of the eighteenth century and Tolstoy more than a hundred years later.

Although compromised in the nineteenth century, when asylums often degenerated into custodial institutions, the idea of moral treatment still appealed to psychiatrists. Alongside other aspects of moral treatment, the eclectic approach adopted by the keepers of the York Retreat ("if one remedy failed, then another was tried")[96] was given new life by the pragmatic therapists of institutions for the nervously ill. A new generation of psychiatrists used Korsakov's name as well as his legacy. In fact, Korsakov headed both the Moscow University Psychiatric Clinic and a private institution, where Nikolai Osipov also began to work soon after he graduated from the university. The latter was the oldest private clinic for the mentally ill in Moscow, founded in 1830 by a physician in state service, F. I. Gertsog (1785–1853). As the clinic was designed for wealthy patients, it was more comfortable than public asylums, and the founder set out to make the regimen looser and more humane. As in the York Retreat, window bars were hidden behind wooden frames, restrictive measures were considerably diminished, and patients were treated as mildly as possible. Patients could play games, read, and attend church; they were not disturbed by the public—in contrast to the asylums where people came to watch the insane for entertainment. The regimen introduced by Gertsog was continued by his successors, the psychiatrists V. F. Sabler (director, 1831–71) and Korsakov (director, 1879–97). Korsakov went further than anybody else in Moscow in introducing nonrestraint, and he removed the bars and abolished straitjackets and isolation cells. Bazhenov, Korsakov's pupil and admirer, although a busy director of the Moscow City Psychiatric Hospital and a professor of the Higher Women's Courses, maintained the same atmosphere in the clinic when he became director in 1905. Osipov joined the clinic in 1906 and worked there for about a year, until he was invited to run another private clinic. He returned to Bazhenov's clinic in 1910 and became responsible for it when both Bazhenov and the head physician left for the army in 1914.[97]

Like their predecessors, the new generation of physicians were attracted by a utopian image of the mental institution as a place, isolated from the external world, where the way of life and relationships between patients and staff would have great therapeutic value. The atmosphere of a nervous clinic or sanatorium equally benefited staff and patients: it satisfied the clients' needs for autonomy, self-respect, and a choice of treatment and the physicians' professional interest in criticizing existing theories and experimenting with new methods of treatment. Korsakov, who had an opportunity to work in both an asylum and a private clinic, noticed that, in contrast to the mental hospitals, which allowed general studies, small institutions had better conditions for case studies, for detailed observation in a variety of situations. These "lay monasteries" provided "splendid isolation" for both the patients—from their domestic environment—and for practitioners—from the pressure of work in huge hospitals.[98] The conditions in nervous clinics and sanatoria encouraged physicians to pursue the attitude celebrated by Osipov in his article on Tolstoy and psychotherapy: to heal by the way of life, by the intimate and supportive psychological atmosphere, and by the physician's "personality" and to develop a "personal philosophy" rather than rely on any given theory.

Purification of the Soul

Not by chance, the article in which Nikolai Osipov introduced the idea of the physician-healer was titled "Psychotherapy in Tolstoy's Literary Works."[99] In this article Osipov spoke for a nascent psychotherapy and defined its possibilities, advantages, and differences from hospital psychiatry. Psychotherapy, when it was introduced in psychiatric hospitals at the beginning of the twentieth century, was a radical change, a turn away from the custodial care typical of mid-nineteenth-century asylums to a more promising way of treatment. The very project of psychotherapy was directed against the "therapeutic nihilism" of an official medicine that ignored the patient's inner world and denied the efficacy of psychological treatment. The generation of practitioners who called themselves psychotherapists sought a new professional image that would help establish the difference between their occupation and hospital psychiatry and other medical specialties. The Tolstoy-inspired image of the physician who was "more than a professional"—a healer or a philosopher—perfectly served this purpose. Tolstoy's idea of the importance of "natural wit and wisdom" provided words with which to oppose traditional theories. For Osipov, this language was not just rhetoric intended to encourage his colleagues to advance beyond conventional psychiatric knowledge. He was deeply convinced that Tolstoy was an intuitive psychologist and that his novels contained excellent descriptions of psychological problems and their "psychotherapeutic" cure.

Osipov gradually entered into an imaginary dialogue with the writer, gaining more psychotherapeutic inspiration from Tolstoy than from his own medical and scientific background. In both of Tolstoy's major novels—*War and*

Peace and *Anna Karenina* (1875–76)—he found illustrations of "natural" psychotherapy: the heroines Natasha and Kitti are much more intuitive than their doctors and understand better the remedy needed for their recovery. Kitti (in *Anna Karenina*) is skeptical about her treatment: "Her whole illness and the treatment appeared to her stupid and even ridiculous. Her treatment seemed to her as absurd as piecing together the bits of a smashed vase. Her heart was broken. Why did they want to dose her with pills and powder?"[100] Natasha (in *War and Peace*) recovers in spite of her treatment, not because of it: "In spite of the vast number of little pills Natasha swallowed, and all the drops and powders out of the little bottles and boxes, of which Madame Schoss, who had a passion for such things, made a large collection, and in spite of being deprived of the country life to which she was accustomed, youth prevailed: Natasha's grief began to be overlaid by the impressions and incidents of everyday life, and ceased to press so painfully on her heart. The ache gradually faded into the past, and little by little her physical health improved."[101] Yet, albeit unconsciously, the physicians did help in Natasha's case:

[The doctors'] help did not depend on making the patient swallow substances, for the most part harmful (the harm was scarcely appreciable because they were administrated in such small doses), but they were useful, necessary and indispensable because they satisfied a moral need of the sick girl and those who loved her—and that is why there are and always will be pseudo-healers, wise women and homeopaths. They satisfied the eternal human need for hope of relief, for sympathetic action, which is felt in the presence of suffering, the need that is seen in its most elementary form in the child which must have the bruised place rubbed to make it better . . . The doctors in Natasha's case were of service because they kissed and rubbed the bad place, assuring her that the trouble would soon be over if the coachman drove down to the chemist's in Abatsky square and got a powder and some pills in a pretty box for a rouble and seventy kopeks, and if she took those powders in boiled water at intervals of precisely two hours, neither more or less.[102]

The moral Osipov drew from these examples was that illness with spiritual roots needed an appropriate treatment, just as Tolstoy directed his young heroines into religion, prayer, and contemplation about the meaning of their lives. In the therapy-informed language of today, Kitti and Natasha "do not need a medical doctor to address their illnesses, but rather a counselor or psychologist to deal with their spiritual problems."[103] Osipov modeled at least one of his cases after Tolstoy's ideas: the case of a young woman whose condition had been diagnosed as "degenerative psychosis" but which he rediagnosed as a much milder neurotic disease. He reported that he cured her through a series of conversations, in the course of which she finally found new prospects in life; she then began training to become a teacher for peasant children.[104]

"Ethical," or "rational," therapy was probably most similar to this kind of spiritual treatment, and for a period it was a widely adopted form of therapy in Russia as well as in the West. The Swiss physician Paul-Charles Dubois (1848–1918), who suggested the doctor should "sit down beside his patient and listen to his plaints with the greatest patience," as Edward Shorter emphasizes, laid the basis of a "psychological paradigm" for treating nervous disorders. For a while, his "method" was equated with psychological therapy per se. When, for instance, the director of a nervous sanatorium near Moscow announced that his patients were offered, besides hypnosis, suggestion and psychoanalysis, "psychotherapy in its proper sense," he meant rational therapy.[105] Dubois taught patients to adopt a dignified life, and not to deny their responsibility for illness, as a way to physical health. As a Russian psychiatrist formulated the essence of rational psychotherapy, its goal was "to foster man's spiritual renewal, to restore what is the most elevated and precious—his personality."[106] Osipov, who visited Dubois in 1910, was struck by the similarity of Dubois's and Tolstoy's messages: "Do not fear illness, fear the treatment, and the treatment not in the sense of taking harmful medicines, but, mainly, the treatment in the sense of recognizing yourself ill and therefore liberated from moral demands on yourself."[107] As Osipov interpreted it, Dubois's creed gave direct response to Tolstoy's moral demand of medicine: "The physician should not tell a neurasthenic anything which he himself does not believe, which he could not tell his ill colleague, and which he would not tell himself if he were ill."[108]

The first decade of the twentieth century was a period when European psychotherapy, developing rapidly, differentiated into a number of competing theories. During the nineteenth century psychotherapy had existed in two major forms. The first was "suggestion under hypnotic sleep," which stemmed from the work of early magnetizers and was encouraged by J.-M. Charcot's experiments with hysterics. The French physicians A.-A. Liébeault and Hippolyte Bernheim introduced the second form, "suggestion in a waking state" (*suggestion à la veille*). Other versions of "psychological therapy" soon appeared, from Josef Breuer's and Freud's "cathartic treatment" of hysteria to Dubois's "rational therapy." The pioneers of psychotherapy regarded the newcomers as potential rivals. In 1904, at the peak of Dubois's fame, Bernheim complained that the Swiss physician had "annexed" psychotherapy, just as Germany had annexed his native Alsace a few decades earlier.[109] In the first decades of the century Pierre Janet began to vie with Freud for priority over the cathartic method and contraposed his *analyse psychologique* to Freud's psychoanalysis. Dubois, supported by the Russian-Swiss neurologist Constantin von Monakow, criticized Freud's method in about 1910, and a prominent Berlin neurologist, Hermann Oppenheim, announced a war against psychoanalysis. In the course of these discussions psychotherapy was no longer understood as a single "method" of treatment or even a single theory and came to include a variety of "psychotherapies," competing ways to conceptualize and treat neuroses.

The physicians in Russia, living far from these theoretical quarrels, regarded the proliferating psychotherapies as compatible rather than contradictory.[110] The Russian physician B. S. Greidenberg quoted his German colleague Oscar Vogt: "one should not make separate therapeutic domains out of hypnosis, suggestion, persuasion, and psychoanalysis; they are but different sides of the single method of treatment—psychotherapy, or, more precisely, nervous and psychic therapy; they are different ways that lead to a single goal."[111]

The Russian physicians consciously chose the position of students, and indeed many young psychiatrists completed their education with the stars of European psychiatry. In the late nineteenth century they studied with Charcot, Kraepelin, Valentin Magnan, Paul Flechsig, and Theodor Meynert, and at the beginning of the century they were attracted by Bernheim, Dubois, Freud, and Carl Jung. Those who visited European celebrities often informed their compatriots about what they had learned in reports that resembled travelers' stories. The authors, like travelers to distant countries, wrote about Western "discoveries" in psychiatry as something exotic that should be adjusted to Russian conditions before being adopted. They judged foreign theories as outsiders, cautiously tried them on like new clothes that might not fit, and did not hurry to assimilate the latest fashions. The claims for theoretical novelty did not touch these "provincials," who preferred methods of proved efficacy to new and questionable theories. Osipov remarked that "the psychotherapist should be armed with the knowledge of the psychotherapeutic stars, with the spirit of their doctrines, and fight illness using, at one time, one method, at another time, another method, and not to forget about physiotherapy and even about pharmaceutical therapy."[112] The method should be carefully and thoughtfully chosen to relate to the individual case, and a psychotherapist should not, like a salesman in a shop, offer clients a choice of alternatives—"hypnosis, Dubois, Freud, Oppenheim?" I. B. Fel'tsman, Osipov's colleague and coeditor of the series *The Psychotherapeutic Li-*

brary, reported on his visit to Bernheim: "In what I have seen, I did not find a big difference between Bernheim's persuasion and Dubois' *traitement moral.*" Personally, however, Fel'tsman preferred Dubois, on the ground that the latter "took from Liébeault the soundest ideas about the psychogenesis of the neuroses and the necessity of reeducation." Rational therapy was preferred on the basis that it was, as Fel'tsman expressed it, "at least harmless."[113]

Like many of his colleagues, Osipov found warm psychological contact with the patient, "emotional therapy," the most important treatment. In a book written by Bazhenov and Osipov and published in France—one of the first systematic presentations of the different methods of psychotherapy—Osipov's contribution consisted of a description of the case of Natasha in *War and Peace.* Osipov believed her recovery, due to emotional support from her close family and a rediscovered ability to love, was an example of genuine psychotherapy. The words did not worry Osipov, and he used the terms *rational, emotional,* and *ethico-philosophical* therapy interchangeably, for, he thought, they all conveyed more or less the same idea. By the same token, he once classified psychoanalysis under the rubric of "ethico-philosophical therapy" and defined it as one more technique for achieving psychological cure through intimate emotional and intellectual contact with the patient.[114]

In 1910 a group of young psychiatrists, including Osipov, started the journal *Psychotherapy (Psikhoterapiia)*, which was the first to propagate new methods of treatment and to acquaint Russian physicians as well as a general audience with Western works on the topic. This journal opened its first issue with the article "Psychotherapeutic Views of S. S. Korsakov," in order to demonstrate the journal's continuity with the humanitarian traditions of Russian psychiatry. The article, as well as the earlier work by its author, N. A. Vyrubov, the director of a nervous sanatorium, updated Korsakov's views in the light of the concept of psychoneurosis. Vyrubov did not reinvent the wheel, and in a book published in the same year he recommended traditional treatments: isolation of patients from an everyday environment, special regimens, "friendly and informal relationships among the staff and patients, as well as a range of psychological treatments, which combined '*suggestion à la veille*' and suggestion in hypnotic sleep, the method of Breuer and Freud, and the method of Dubois and their modifications."[115] He thought keeping to a single method was as difficult as it was unnecessary, and he accused those who sought methodological purity of being "pedants." In his sanatorium, Kriukovo, near Moscow, well known among Moscow intellectuals, Vyrubov combined psychoanalysis with rational therapy and the fashionable anthroposophy of Rudolf Steiner.[116]

Psychoanalysis in a Literary Form

The acceptance of psychoanalysis in Russia, as well as in the West, occurred through a loose and liberal understanding of what it was all about, as Edward Shorter has demonstrated. Many observers thought psychoanalysis did not diverge sharply from other views within the psychological paradigm, or, in Dubois's words, from other methods of "psychological treatment for psychological illness."[117] Russian therapists continued to combine the methods of Freud and Dubois longer than did their Western colleagues, even after Dubois, with the help of von Monakow, had begun publicly to oppose psychoanalysis.[118] During the summer of 1910, Osipov visited Freud in Vienna, Eugen Bleuler and Jung in Zurich, and Dubois in Bern.[119] For him, psychoanalysis and rational therapy were complementary forms present in any psychotherapy. He compared them with analysis and reeducation, which, he argued, could not be reduced to Freud's and Dubois's methods: "The term 'psychoanalysis' is much broader than Freud's psychotherapy, as the term 'reeducation' is broader than Dubois'."[120] The first issue of Osipov and Fel'tsman's *Psychotherapeutic Library* was Freud's *On Psychoanalysis* (1911); the second was Dubois's *On Psychotherapy* (1911).

In 1911 the staff of the Moscow University Psychiatric Clinic resigned in protest against the rector's conservative policy in the Kasso affair. After being replaced by their more stiff-necked colleagues, they devoted more time to psychotherapy. Even Serbskii, a psychiatrist of the old school, translated a book by the French physicians J.-J. Déjerine and E. Gauckler on the psychotherapy of neuroses.[121] Osipov was one of the first in Russia to write on psychoanalysis; two of his papers on the topic appeared in 1908 in the *Journal of Neuropathology and Psychiatry* (*Zhurnal nevropatologii i psikhiatrii*).[122] As a result, Freud received "two thick off-prints, in one of which the tangle of Cyrillic signs is interrupted every two lines by the name *Freud* (also *Freudy* and *Freuda*) in European print, while the other makes the same use of the name Jung." During his visit to Freud in 1910, Osipov made a favorable impression on him as a "clear head and convinced follower" and "magnificent fellow."[123]

Although interpreted loosely as a method of psychological treatment, psychoanalysis, unlike rational therapy, still had to confront moral objections. Like many of their foreign colleagues, Russian psychiatrists had difficulties in accepting it.[124] There were very few adventurous psychotherapists—one exception was Vyrubov, who practiced and taught psychoanalysis as early as 1909—and most did not feel the time to promote psychoanalysis had arrived.

Vyrubov could only ask his colleagues not to criticize psychoanalysis while the theory was still developing, hoping that the future would clarify its possibilities and limits.[125] In the beginning, Osipov shared the reservations about the wide application of psychoanalysis. He wrote, for example, that the free-association test "would be very close to moral torture" if it were used by detectives. Like many of his colleagues, Osipov believed that psychoanalysis unnecessarily stressed sex. Later, however, he changed his view, arguing that psychoanalysis had nothing in common with a call for sexual liberation and that "it was completely wrong to conclude that Freud prescribed coitus as a treatment for neurosis."[126] He recalled his argument with Serbskii, who, although he spoke foreign languages well, pronounced Freud's name in two syllables, *Fre-ud,* with an accent on the last syllable. In ancient usage, the Russian word *ud* meant the male or female sexual organ; in Serbskii's time one could still find it in medical books. In response to this, Osipov, who wanted to show his sympathies with Freud's theory, pronounced the name *Freund,* "a friend."[127] In 1911, in front of a large audience—the First Congress of the Russian Union of Psychiatrists and Neuropathologists—he courageously defended psychoanalysis from the accusation of "pansexualism."[128]

Osipov's way to reconcile general audiences with psychoanalysis was to stress its moral engagement. It is significant that Osipov, who rarely quoted other psychiatrists directly, repeated Freud's statement that "man is not only much more immoral, but also *much more moral* than he knows about himself" (emphasis added by Osipov).[129] In his attempts to overcome reservations about psychoanalysis, Osipov once again turned to Tolstoy for help. He borrowed an illustration from Tolstoy's novel *Resurrection,* the main character of which, Prince Nekhliudov, at times expresses a need to purify himself from his "animal being" in order to maintain his "spiritual being." This was, Osipov commented, precisely the division of labor between the two main psychotherapies: rational therapy aimed to maintain the "spiritual self," whereas psychoanalysis helped fight "the beast" by learning more about it. Even if the originators of these therapies disagreed with each other, the therapies were complementary: rational therapy lacked analysis, which Freud's method provided. Osipov argued that "different methods of psychotherapy do not contradict each other, and all are directed towards the same aim: to strengthen the spiritual self in a man."[130] Psychotherapists from Dubois to Freud, he stated, all addressed the soul and propagated the maxim "Know thyself"; they called patients to reason and self-responsibility, and all had a common slogan, "Do not extinguish the spirit!"[131]

Osipov saw a particular closeness between Tolstoy and Freud: "the comparison between Freud's scientific psychology and Tolstoy's fictional psychology reveals many similar insights." Both authors rejected the crude materialism of official medicine, adopted broad philosophical views on human nature, and analyzed "small details and minor movements" as things with deep meaning.[132] Osipov drew a parallel between Tolstoy's and Freud's psychological intuitions in his book-length study of Tolstoy's trilogy *Childhood, Boyhood*, and *Youth* (1856), which he admired as a brilliant examination of a child's psychology. He called the novels "a psychoanalysis in literary form," and subtitled an early version of his book, "Introduction to Psychoanalysis, Introduction to Psychotherapy" (Osipov's study was never published in Russian).[133] He argued that psychoanalysis alone could rival great intuitive psychologists such as Tolstoy, whereas academic psychology usually failed when it attempted to translate literary insights into scientific language. How, Osipov asked in despair, could one conceptualize in scientific terms, for instance, the opening scene of *Childhood*, in which a little boy awakens overwhelmed by contradictory feelings: "If we now cut [Tolstoy's] picture in pieces, we will have to translate into [psychological] states a tenderness that is expressed through caress, touch, kisses, delight, the single feeling of love to God and mother, light and easy joy, pity, the readiness to sacrifice oneself, faith, hope, admiration. Indeed, what a joyless view is our class of states!"[134]

The language of academic psychology was too abstract and general, so any of the fine movements of a child's soul, so artfully described by Tolstoy in *Childhood*, would become meaningless if translated into the language of stimuli, motives, and reactions. The only psychologist who could conceptualize subjective experiences was Freud, he "transcribes the symptoms of neurotics that we do not understand into an understandable language." Osipov argued that Tolstoy and Freud, in literary and in scholarly form respectively, used the individualizing method proper to the human (idiographic) sciences, though he made clear that Tolstoy's "psychoanalysis in a literary form" remained the most perfect method of knowing personality.[135]

There could hardly have been a better way to facilitate the reception of psychoanalysis in Russia than to link it with Tolstoy's writings. In the light of Russian literature, psychoanalysis began to acquire a Russian accent, and it resembled Tolstoy's life philosophy more than a theoretical doctrine. Nevertheless, the translation of psychoanalysis into the language of Russian culture guaranteed its successful reception. The majority of Russian psychiatrists became familiar with psychoanalysis and many practiced it among other methods of psychotherapy, and even patriarchs such as Serbskii admitted the "significant and often striking" therapeutic success of psychoanalysis.[136] In

1910 the Moscow Society of Psychiatrists and Neuropathologists announced a new topic, "Psychoanalysis (Freud and Others) in Diseases of the Nervous System," for an annual competition. Osipov intended to compete for the prize.[137]

Psychotherapy in Emigration: A Nostalgia for Love

The First World War stopped the growth of psychotherapy in Russia. All the editors of *Psychotherapy* except Osipov went into the army, and the journal ceased publication. Osipov was exempt from military service because he was the only support for his mother (his father had died). His coeditor of the *Psychotherapeutic Library,* Fel'tsman, was also in the army, and the series stopped at the fourteenth issue. One consequence was that, as noted above, Osipov's "Analysis of Lev Tolstoy's *Childhood, Boyhood, Youth*" never appeared in Russian. He continued to lecture at the Higher Women's Courses and to work as the chief physician for the Rukavishnikov Shelter for Delinquent Children, as well as acting as consultant in Bazhenov's private clinic and seeing his own private patients. The Provisional Government, which came to power after the abdication of the tsar, in Osipov's words, "dressed him in a military uniform."[138]

The Bolsheviks, who replaced the Provisional Government after the October Revolution, were in Osipov's opinion absolutely unacceptable. In 1918 he left Moscow together with his friends and, like thousands of Russians who followed the White Army to the Crimea, traveled south hoping to reach Europe by sea.

Osipov was forced to share the misery of many Russian civilians who were not taken by the British and French ships and instead fled to Istanbul. With money and luck, some émigrés were able to buy visas and tickets in Turkey and leave for Europe. Osipov was unsuccessful and had to return to Russia. In 1920 he tried to emigrate again, in the third wave of emigration, which probably had the hardest experience of all. Another émigré of that time described in *An Unsentimental Journey* how starving travelers from Russia were locked on ships for many days before they were allowed to disembark on the Turkish coast. The refugees were then sent to the White Army camps, where endless military drills, lack of food, and epidemics killed many of them. The author, a former law student, succeeded in escaping from the military camps, but life in the camps for civilian refugees was hardly better. In Istanbul he tried all kinds of jobs: he was a clown, palmist, dishwasher, and street salesman, and he worked in a photographic atelier and a laundry. Finally, he succeeded in reaching Europe and settled in Prague, where the Czechoslovak government offered stipends and an opportunity for former Russian students to continue their education.[139] Osipov also arrived in Prague in 1921, after crossing the Black Sea and passing through Belgrade and Budapest.

The Czechoslovak government offered Russian émigrés accommodation and financial assistance; former university professors were promised life-long stipends. The initiator of the "Russian action," President T. G. Masaryk (1850–1937), was a philosopher with scholarly interests in Russian culture and literature, interest that had taken him twice to Yasnaya Polyana among other places in Russia. He had definite negative views about the October Revolution. There were expectations that the Bolshevik regime would soon be replaced by a more liberal one and that the new Russia would need specialists, especially lawyers, and in 1922 a Russian department of law was founded in Prague to train lawyers.[140] By the end of 1924, the financial help given by the Czechoslovak government exceeded the total sum spent on Russian refugees by all other European governments.

In spite of this support, the life of Russian émigrés involved an intense struggle fighting against depression and hunting for new sources of subsistence. The refugees were not allowed to take positions in state enterprises, but they could work in the private economy. Faced with the task of creating employment for themselves, the Russians opened small enterprises as well as schools and colleges. The latter served the interests of both teachers, who obtained jobs, and students, who received professional training that increased their chances in competing for vacancies in the private economy. The needs of the Russian community stimulated the rapid growth of voluntary associations: there were more than 140 political parties and public and professional societies. The most important organization to mediate relations between the Russian community and Czechoslovak officials was the Association of Russian Town and Country Self-governing Authorities in Prague, which united former *zemstvo* and municipal workers. In addition, there were numerous organizations for Russian youths, students, women, engineers, physicians, chauffeurs, and local communities of Siberian people, Cossacks, religious groups, and many others.

Yet practical necessity was not the only motif of the émigrés' activity. They also sought to preserve their sense of identity, and many of them believed they would be able to return to their country and contribute to its cultural life. For the émigrés, nostalgic about Russia, the work in voluntary associations and cultural institutions gave purpose and hope. A number of cultural and academic institutions were established: the Russian Historical Archive

Abroad kept records of the history of the emigration, and the Russian People's University, modeled after the Shaniavskii People's University in Moscow, offered primary school education for the working class, popular lectures for the general public, and research seminars, such as the seminar for lovers of the Russian language.[141] The last elected rector of Moscow University (as opposed to those appointed by the Soviet government), the zoologist M. M. Novikov, who was expelled from Soviet Russia with a large group of intellectuals in 1922, became rector of the People's University in Prague.[142] The philosophers N. A. Berdiaev, V. V. Zen'kovskii, I. I. Lapshin, and N. O. Lossky and the historians A. A. Kizevetter, S. I. Gessen, and E. F. Shmurlo carried on their academic work in Prague. The linguist Roman Jakobson led a group of Russian and Czech scholars, which became known as the Prague Linguistic Circle. Tolstoy's former secretary V. F. Bulgakov founded the Russian Cultural and Historical Museum in Zbroslav.[143] Alongside the academic institutions were numerous associations of men of letters, Russian publishing houses, theaters, ateliers, and clubs with weekly teas, soirées, and charity performances. Émigré publishing houses continued to publish Russian classics and contemporary fiction; the largest Russian publishing house in Prague, Plamia, published more than thirty titles a year and a "thick" literary journal, *Russia's Will* (*Volia Rossii*). Russian intellectuals animated Prague's cultural life, and the city became known in the 1920s as the "Slavic Athens."[144]

Despite the difficulties of the exile, Osipov, with the temperament of a leader, felt very much at home in the Russian community. After arriving in Czechoslovakia, he was offered a position as chief physician in the psychiatric clinic of the new Masaryk University in Brno, but he declined the offer, partly because he was conscious of the difficulties of running an institution in a foreign country, partly because the majority of his friends were settling in Prague.[145] He started working instead at the Charles University in Prague, in the period before the government began to regulate refugees' employment, and he was one of the few Russians allowed to obtain a position of *Dozent*. He had the opportunity to open an outpatient psychiatric service in the University Polyclinic and continue the work with neurotics that he had begun in the outpatient department of the Moscow University Psychiatric Clinic. He learned the Czech language, acquired a private practice in the city, and published widely in the Czech, German, and Russian languages. A sociable and likable person (his friends affectionately nicknamed him "Little Ship," perhaps because he was rather short and thickset and swayed as he walked), he quickly became a well-known figure in émigré and Czech intellectual circles. He frequented all sorts of academic gatherings, from the meetings of the

Society of Russian Physicians in Czechoslovakia to philosophical seminars. In 1925 he started his own seminar in psychiatry, which eventually moved to his home. Russian and Czech students who attended the seminar reported that Osipov was an excellent teacher.[146] He also taught in the Russian People's University and often gave popular lectures around the country on psychiatry, psychology, and literature.

The life of the émigrés, though, was far from peaceful and untroubled. In the mid-1920s, the political situation in the Soviet Union stabilized and prospects for a quick return to Russia began to vanish. Czechoslovakia's establishment of diplomatic relations with the Soviet Union slowed down the "Russian action": stipends for professors were gradually reduced, and student stipends stopped completely in 1931. In 1928 the Czechoslovak government issued a law that protected the national labor market, and the refugees either had to adopt Czechoslovak citizenship and compete for jobs or leave the country. Some émigrés moved to other countries; others returned to the Soviet Union in response to the Soviet repatriation campaign. For those who stayed, it became even more difficult to preserve their "Russianness." There were different ways: some, like a character in one of Vladimir Nabokov's novels, kept her Russia with her by taking into exile her shawls, wooden dolls, and Russian-made jewelry. Some, like the poet Marina Tsvetaeva, "carried Russia within herself" and would "lose her only with life." For some, the status of refugee acquired symbolic meaning as the only connection with their country. "Remember that you are a refugee," the editorial of an émigré newspaper reminded its readers in 1933, "be patient, hope, work, go to charity performances and to clubs, talk, dance, be charitable, but do not forget that you are a Russian. And do not have any citizenship other than the Russian one."[147]

A particular feature of émigré public life was frequent celebrations of anniversaries of famous public figures, from tsars and emperors to scientists and writers. In 1928 the Russian community celebrated Tolstoy's centenary; in 1931, the half-centenary of Dostoevsky's death; and in 1937, the centenary of Pushkin's death. Between these major occasions, the jubilees of V. M. Garshin, Goncharov, Turgenev, and other nineteenth-century writers provided social occasions. Congresses of the Union of Russian Academic Associations Abroad usually culminated in a closing session centered on a classic writer: the Fourth Congress in 1928 celebrated Tolstoy, the Fifth celebrated Turgenev. Several permanent seminars of the Russian People's University were devoted to literary topics: Bem's seminar on Dostoevsky, E. A. Liatskii's seminar on Tolstoy, and S. V. Zavadskii's seminars for lovers of the Russian language. Contributions to seminars on philosophy and even natural sciences often contained discussions of writers and their works. Literature, which was as much a public as an individual matter, united the politically, economically, and socially divided Russian community and sustained its sense of national identity. Not by chance, the books most often borrowed from the Russian libraries were the novels of Dostoevsky and Tolstoy.[148]

Physicians were as nostalgic as other émigré intellectuals. M. P. Polosin, a physician and the former head of Orenburg City Council, settled in Prague with the Czechoslovak Legion in 1918. He was appointed director of a Russian tuberculosis sanatorium. When not engaged in his medical work, he wrote the autobiographical *Childhood* and *1918* and a piece of literary criticism, *Pushkin's Mistakes*.[149] The psychiatrist G. Ia Troshin, who had led the attempt to "democratize" the St. Nicholas Hospital in Petersburg in 1906 (see Chapter 1), as an émigré wrote extensively about literature and music and published several works on Pushkin. Of seventy public lectures and talks given by Osipov between 1922 and 1931, more than a dozen were on literature and the writers Turgenev, Goncharov, Dostoevsky, Tolstoy, I. A. Krylov, A. S. Griboedov, and M. E. Saltykov. He lectured to the Society of Russian Students, Society of Russian Physicians, and audiences at a poet's club, the Russian Library, and elsewhere.[150] Osipov was regarded as an expert on Russian literature, so his presence on the organizing committee of the Tolstoy centenary celebration was thought to be "absolutely necessary."[151] Osipov treated these occasions seriously and prepared academic talks for each of them. When asked to give a talk on Dostoevsky, Osipov noted, "It is necessary to re-read all Dostoevsky! I do not want to get away with general ideas."[152] He also continued the analysis of Tolstoy's works from psychiatric and especially psychoanalytic perspectives that he had begun in Russia.

Psychoanalysis continued to occupy a significant place in Osipov's psychotherapeutic work as well as in his teaching: he was invited to lecture on psychoanalysis at the Charles University (which, as the historian of psychoanalysis in Central Europe remarked, was second only to the University of Budapest in introducing psychoanalysis into the curriculum). One member of Osipov's psychiatric seminar, the psychiatrist and neurologist F. N. Dosuzhkov (1899–1982), later became a founder (in 1936) of the Czechoslovak Society for the Study of Psychoanalysis and a training analyst for several generations of Czechoslovak psychoanalysts.[153] Osipov's talks and lectures about the psychological interpretation of famous writers and their characters were followed by discussions in the intimate atmosphere of Russian gatherings, with the inevitable tea from a samovar, and they were an effective vehicle for dissemination of psychotherapy and Freudian ideas. His listeners were excited to learn that one could interpret Gogol's and Dostoevsky's phantasmagoric stories as dreams and find a key to their irrationality. Osipov argued that "no matter how phantasmagoric the work is—it is phantasmagoric by content only, whereas its constitutive idea is real and alive."[154] He discovered illustrations of the Oedipus complex in Dostoevsky's *The Landlady* and *Eternal Husband* (1870), analyzed the psychological origin of jealousy in Tolstoy's *Anna Karenina,* explained the pathological laziness of Goncharov's title character in *Oblomov* (1859) by neurotic complexes, and traced the adventures of libido in Turgenev's novel *First Love* (1860).

Osipov found an attentive and grateful audience among both literary critics and dilettante lovers of Russian literature. His friend E. A. Liatskii (1868–1942), the historian and literary critic, confessed in a letter to Osipov, "At your suggestion, I studied Freud and, in many respects, clarified your point of view for myself."[155] Dostoevsky scholar A. L. Bem followed Osipov's lead in interpreting Dostoevsky's writings as a product of dreamlike activity. He found that "the composition, style, and manner" of Dostoevsky's short story *Eternal Husband* was similar to the "psychology of dreams" and that its phantasmagoric character had its roots in the writer's personality. Under Osipov's influence, Bem came to the conclusion that creative writing eased Dostoevsky's inner tension and rescued him from mental illness. In his turn, Osipov celebrated a "new approach to Dostoevsky," which did not explain his writings by biographical details but instead tried to "recreate his life through the study of his creative writings." He agreed that "Bem's statement that Dostoevsky's writings are dreams is correct and very successful—all Dostoevsky's style is a style of daydreams, dreams, and delusions, processed by consciousness."[156]

Both Bem and Osipov thought they were using a radically new method—the analysis of "small details" in order to reveal the author's conscious or unconscious intentions. Bem wrote that his article on Griboedov, an early-nineteenth-century Russian playwright, was "further approval that the very method of work is correct": "For myself, I call my method of work the method of 'small observations.' Everybody who carefully reads my last work will understand clearly that, although Freud is not mentioned, and moreover there is nothing 'sexual' in it, in essence Freud's method played a great role. This method is exactly the same as that which Freud understood as the analysis of 'everyday life,' that is, of the writer's small errors and mistakes, which completely reveal his creative impulses . . . I would like to try sometime to give a theoretical basis to the 'differential' method in literature, to show what fruitful results it may bring when skillfully used."[157]

It was a major change in the Russian tradition of literary criticism. The critics were brought up in the tradition of realism, which, since V. G. Belinsky's time, judged literature and writers according to their contribution to public life and social movements. Now they found much in common between the analysis of literature and art and the analysis of the unconscious. To use Carlo Ginzburg's phrase, they united psychoanalysis and art criticism in a single paradigm—the analysis of "tiny details" to reveal important characteristics of the author's style and motives.[158]

Though many Western scholars responded to the disasters at the beginning of the century with Stoic and existential philosophy, the Russian thinkers who fled from the Bolshevik regime turned towards a philosophy of love as an absolute value and a source of redemption.[159] Tolstoy's version of Christianity, ridiculed by the generation of the 1860s, now appealed to émigré Russians as the only antidote to the destructive and disastrous epoch. The religious renaissance of the late nineteenth century, started by Dostoevsky, Tolstoy, and Vladimir Solov'ev, culminated in the foundation of the Religious and Philosophical Meetings, where intellectuals mixed with Orthodox priests. It received a new impulse from the catastrophe of 1917. Religious philosophy had no possibility of surviving in the Soviet Union, but in compensation it formed a main strand of Russian thought abroad, where almost all the prominent religious thinkers, including Merezhkovskii, Berdiaev, and Lev Shestov, found themselves after the Revolution. Some other philosophers, previously little concerned with such issues, turned towards moral and religious problems. For instance, Osipov's friend and fellow émigré E. V. Spektorskii (1875–1951), in his *Christianity and Culture,* published in Prague in 1925, articulated the role of religion for all spheres of spiritual, social, and even material culture—for philosophy, science, and art, for the development of the idea of personality, of legal justice, and the state. I. I. Lapshin (1870–1950), in *La phénoménologie de la conscience religieuse dans la littérature russe,* showed that even the most fanatical "nihilists" from the 1860s, Chernyshevsky, N. A. Dobroliubov, and D. I. Pisarev, were deeply religious in their youth.[160]

Psychoanalysis, as one more theory of love, was obviously discussed in this milieu, but the response was ambivalent. Many thought it concentrated on the dark sides of human nature. As the philosopher Lossky, another émigré to Prague, emphasized, "the terrible discoveries made by Freud and his school may prove fatal to man unless ways are pointed out for transfiguring the low instincts lurking in the realm of the subconscious." His colleague V. V. Zen'kovskii argued against Freud's and Emile Durkheim's attempts to explain religious experiences as derivative of other experiences. On the other hand, Freud's notion of libido was perceived to have some connections with the Platonic Eros. It gave another émigré philosopher, B. P. Vysheslavtsev, the opportunity to reinterpret Christian love as a product of the sublimation of Eros and God as the most meritorious object of love, the source of this sublimation. In Lossky's words, Vyshelavtsev argued that "the training of imagination, feeling and will in the spirit of Christianity . . . through connecting our imagination and will with the concrete goodness of the Absolute, the living personality of the God-man and the saints . . . is the only way to attain the fullness of perfect life." His followers praised "new arguments to prove that Christianity can only serve this purpose if it is interpreted as truly the religion of love and freedom, as the good news of the kingdom of grace, and not distorted by legalism or fanatical intolerance."[161]

The position that Osipov, an expert on psychoanalysis, took in the discussion was important for these circles. It was known that Osipov had gained Freud's sympathy during his visit to Vienna in 1910 and had remained in friendly correspondence.[162] (Devoted to Freud personally, Osipov, together with the Czech psychoanalysts Jaroslav Stuchlík and Emanuel Windholz, suggested putting a plaque on the house where Freud was born in Příbor (Freiberg, Moravia) in commemoration of his seventy-fifth birthday.)[163] The émigré intellectuals believed, however, that Osipov's views were broader than psychoanalysis, and they emphasized that he "cured not by hypnosis or psychoanalysis, but by psychotherapy in the whole, by completeness and by the astonishing harmony of his own personality."[164] His friend Lapshin described Osipov as a master of "intuitive" diagnostics.[165]

Lossky recalled that he once asked Osipov why he did not read on the tram: "On the tram I never read: everybody who gets in is more interesting and valuable than any book," was the answer.[166] Lossky believed that Osipov not only was an original "intuitive" psychologist but also had recast Freud's psychological theories in the spirit of modern religious philosophy, including Lossky's own personalist metaphysics. He quoted from Osipov: "The empirical value of Freud's research will not be affected if the central place is ascribed not to physiological attraction, but to Love in the eidetic sense as an absolute value. In our spatio-temporal world Love is embodied in varying degrees, beginning with the very lowest, that of identification (I love this apple and, in virtue of that love, eat it, i.e., destroy it). Then love expresses itself in sensuality—genital and extra-genital—and tenderness. Finally it finds expression in special experiences of intimacy between people—the highest form of Love's manifestation in the human world." Lossky ascribed to Osipov the view that love was a basic factor in cosmic life, far earlier than sexual passion and not reducible to mere physiological attraction. He regretted that illness and death prevented Osipov from developing in detail his theory of love, "which was to explain the connections between persons in a way different from that of the Freudians with their tendency to pansexualism."[167]

Dividing his sympathies between Tolstoy and Freud, Osipov once commented that he valued psychoanalysis because it came as close as possible to Tolstoy's "intuitions" into human psychology and had the same goal—"purification of the soul." He was convinced that psychoanalysis was not the only cure for neurosis and that reading Gogol's short stories, which "overcome fears by acceptance of absolute values," could help as well. Ten years after the Bolshevik Revolution, Osipov wrote an article titled "Revolution and Dream," which he intended to send to Freud. In this interpretation of phantasmagoric revolutionary reality, he mixed Freud and Tolstoy and regarded revolutions as a regression of Eros to the lowest stages, to narcissism, and then to death—an absolute absence of love.[168] As an émigré he resumed work on his unfinished manuscript "Organic Natural Philosophy in Contemporary Russian Science" and prepared for publication a book chapter, "Life and Death," a biologist's reflections on Tolstoy's "eternal questions." When, in the early 1890s, Tolstoy was in the process of writing an essay he had titled "On Life and Death," he decided to omit "Death": "this word lost completely the meaning which it had in the title. God allow that [the essay] will act in the same way at least on some readers." Osipov retained "Death" in the title of his own essay, but he asserted with the same pathos as Tolstoy that life has an absolute value.[169]

Decadents, Revolutionaries, and the Nation's Mental Health

One can, of course, blame neither Pushkin nor Dostoevsky for what is going on now in Russian literature and
Russian reality. Yet there must be some connection
between the last half-century of our literature and our
reality, between the grandeur of our reflection and the
misery of our action. It appears sometimes that Russian
literature has completely exhausted Russian reality; like a
giant single blossom of *Victoria Regia,* Russian reality
produced Russian literature and is now unable to produce anything else. In dreams we were gods, in the waking state we have not yet become humans.

—D. S. Merezhkovskii

Equally cold-hearted and wicked, the Mephisto of artists,
the Demon of poets, and the Degenerate of psychiatrists,
all of them mirror . . . the real "Demon" of humankind,
a genuine pathological evil worse than death itself—it is
dying, decline, the decay of life and of the psyche.

—I. A. Sikorskii

Was There Decadence in Russia?

"Although the degenerates multiply in periods of decadence, it is also
through them that States are established," Emile Durkheim wrote in *Suicide*
(1897), and he illustrated this conclusion by a comparison of French and
Russian literature: "The sympathy accorded to the [Russian literature] in

France shows that it does not lack affinity with our own. In the writers of both nations, in fact, one perceives a morbid delicacy of the nervous system, a certain lack of mental and moral equilibrium. But what different social consequences flow from these identical conditions, at once biological and psychological! Whereas Russian literature is excessively idealistic, whereas its peculiar melancholy originating in active pity for human suffering is the healthy sort of sadness which excites faith and provokes action, ours prides itself on expressing nothing but deep despair and reflects a disquieting state of depression." For Durkheim, it was ideals and values that manifested a society's stage of development. In contrast to "an ancient and disoriented society," in which "disgust with life and inert melancholy . . . readily germinate, . . . in a youthful society an ardent idealism, a generous proselytism and active devotion are more likely to develop." Though the Russians, like the French, exhibited psychological weariness and "lack of equilibrium," they had preserved, at least in art, their ideals and values and remained therefore a youthful nation. By contrast, he thought, the old European civilization had entered a period of *anomie* and was in danger of dying.[1] Disappointed in the Old World, fin de siècle Europeans saw in "colossal, youthful and barbaric" Russia "a promising dawn" of the new civilization.[2]

The Russian intellectuals, however, did not nourish such hopes about their own country. Unlike their neighbors in the West, they saw Russia in the light of sunset and discussed it as also having entered a state of *anomie*. In the words of I. A. Sikorskii, a professor of psychiatry at the St. Vladimir University in Kiev, at the turn of the century Russia was experiencing the "decline of idealism and lofty motifs in society, weakening educational influence of the older on the younger, of fathers on children, [and] an increasing number of crimes and suicides." Like Durkheim, Sikorskii based his diagnosis on literature. He compared two short stories with similar plots but separated by several decades. In a contemporary short story by Anton Chekhov, *Heartache* (1886), a cab driver, Iona, longs to tell somebody that he has recently lost his son. But neither his passengers nor other drivers listen to him, as they are preoccupied with their own petty thoughts, and Iona ends by telling his sorrow to his horse. Sikorskii recalled an earlier story, Ivan Turgenev's "poem in prose," *Masha* (1878; written circa 1875), in which a cab driver has just buried his wife. But, in contrast to the Chekhov story, his concerned passenger "noticed immediately a sad, gloomy expression on the driver's face, noticed sorrow in his voice and first started speaking to him."[3]

Nineteenth-century Russians, brought up on the romantic idea that the nation's spiritual life reached its apogee in art, believed the quality of literature was a sensitive indicator of society's moral state. They would have agreed that the literature of the 1860s and 1870s reflected the brightest period of Russian history and, moreover, that Turgenev, Tolstoy, and Dostoevsky contributed to raising up the nation by preaching the values of freedom, democracy, enlightenment, and humanism. It was the period of political thaw, emancipation of serfs, and progressive reforms in government. Populism—the belief that Russia had its own noncapitalist path into the future based on the structure of rural society—inspired the Russian intelligentsia to "go to the people," endeavoring to satisfy the peasants' educational and medical needs and to raise their political consciousness. The hopeful atmosphere changed completely in the 1880s: the murder of Alexander II by a terrorist organization in 1881 led to a period of reaction, with the autocracy firmly in control, severe censorship, constraints on education and public life, and arrests and executions of political prisoners. In the words of a historian, "the buoyant optimism of the Russian intelligentsia in the 1860s and the heroic, apocalyptic mood of the 1870s now gave way to the ideology of the so-called 'little deeds' advocating social conformism and a sober and prosaic attitude to life."[4]

The heyday of the Russian novel was also over by the 1880s: Dostoevsky died in 1881, Turgenev two years later, and Tolstoy, after his spiritual crisis in the late 1870s, abandoned fiction for moral philosophizing. By contrast, turn-of-the-century writers appeared weak and insignificant, preoccupied by an aesthetic rather than a moral quest. The new movements in art, decadence and symbolism, brought about fears that literature had lost its guiding role in society. Though in fact the philosophical issues remained of paramount importance even for the most "aesthetic" artists of that period,[5] the general public saw decadent and symbolist art as "devoid of idea, an art that was left to its own devices, an expenditure of technical energy without an accepted philosophical intent." As the literary historian John E. Bowlt comments, in spite of the symbolists' claim that their art was intimately linked to "the most passionate idealist impulses of the spirit," they were castigated for the betrayal of the "grand idealism" cultivated by the preceding generation of writers.[6] A critic writing for a popular magazine complained that, though previously life had been difficult for young Russians, they had had the comfort of Ivan Turgenev, Nikolai Chernyshevsky, and Nikolai Mikhailovsky and an ideal to which they could devote themselves. Now Russian youth had "instead of Turgenev, Artsybashev [a decadent writer]; instead of Insarov [a noble character in a Turgenev novel], Sanin [the hero of an erotic novel], instead of Mikhailovsky [a journalist and ideologist of Populism], Solomin, with a cry of 'Down with shame and purity.'"[7]

Literary critics took the word *decadence* from late Roman history to characterize the literary manner of Théophile Gautier and Charles Baudelaire. At first, the poets willingly accepted the name, which accentuated their belief that they were strangers in a mundane world. Decadence, however, was soon held responsible for the decline of morality and distortion of classical art forms. As in the West, the terms *decadent* and *symbolist* were used in Russia for the artists who portrayed eroticism, ecstasy, frenzy, and decline. In the early to mid-1890s, both trends became familiar to the public when the journal *Northern Herald* (*Severnyi vestnik*) began to publish poetry, prose, and manifestos of mainly Western decadents, and when the almanac *Russian Symbolists* (*Russkie simvolisty*) featured young native authors. The almanac had a *succès de scandale* with a notorious "poem," "Oh, Cover Your Pale Legs," published in the 1895 issue, the author of which, Valery Briusov, chose Verlaine as his guide and employed such images as "violet hands," "translucent kiosks," and "nude crescent moon."[8] The new art soon became a part of everyday life in Russia. At the turn of the century, there was not only a "Moscow [Aubrey] Beardsley" (Nikolai Feofilaktov, who portrayed half-dressed women), but also "Russian Oscar Wildes" whose extravagances challenged the bourgeois way of life. In a turn-of-the-century story, *Decadent,* two merchants' daughters chat on a train. One is unfortunately married to a poet calling himself "Oskar Wildovich," and the disenchanted women conclude that decadents are good-for-nothings who seek the favor of the middle class for their money.[9]

Decadent writers were held in contempt not only by the editors of popular self-education magazines and by the merchant class; some physicians added their authority to these critical voices. In 1901 Sikorskii diagnosed a new clinical form—*idiophrenia paranoides*—in the works of poets and writers who identified themselves with the decadent and symbolist movements. Fearful that the "degenerate trend in literature . . . is able to spoil and pervert the reader's tastes," Sikorskii suggested psychiatrists should unite their efforts with "scientifically educated *littérateurs*" to protect literature. F. E. Rybakov (1868–1920), a psychiatrist at the Moscow University Psychiatric Clinic, argued that modern literature was dominated by "petty plots" and preoccupied with the "little nothings of life": "Literature has never presented such a mass of pathological types—degenerates, neurasthenics, psychopaths—as it does now . . . All of them are types whose place is not at the feast of life but in a sanatorium or psychiatric clinic; they are degenerates, morally insane, impulsants, they are all slaves of their instincts and passions." Rybakov preferred Dostoevsky's "mentally ill" characters to the degenerates or the decadent writers: the mentally ill were at least "alive, acting, having sometimes deep ideas," whereas the hero of modern fiction was a "dead, ruined person." He worried that the "absence of ideals" would inhibit the readers' moral search and concluded that, though "an ill, disbalanced, nervous soul may reach great ecstasies, . . . it will never have produced firm social ideals or solid principles of world culture."[10]

Like their Western colleagues, Russian psychiatrists characterized the decline of modern art by drawing a comparison between the works of professional artists and the art of the insane. Many of them, like Cesare Lombroso, collected items of art and writing by their patients. Rybakov referred to a "small collection of the works by my patients written even before the so-called new wave in literature [in which] one can find motifs not completely alien to the modern forms of fiction." The Moscow neurologist G. I. Rossolimo, who also collected works by the mentally ill, observed in 1901, "When fifteen years ago, I happened to look at the drawings and to read verses of the mentally ill, I was deeply impressed by their ugliness and fantastic content—they were so different from what art and poetry produced at that time. Only fifteen years later, this infinite difference almost disappeared—so similar have the works of some sane and insane artists become." Following Lombroso, Russian psychiatrists sought for common features in the works of the insane and in modern art, such as abuse of symbols and allegories, fanciful and fantastic metaphors, synesthesias such as colored perception of sounds. Rybakov, for instance, quoted K. Bal'mont's poem, in which "the sun smells herbs and fresh flowers, lights with bell ringing," as a symptom of "confused thinking."[11]

Like Max Nordau, who feared decadent artists would exercise an almost hypnotic suggestion on the public,[12] Rossolimo warned that lowering artistic standards could bring about an "epidemic of art." "Show me a middle-class family where the music—piano, violin, or singing—would not be heard," he asked rhetorically, and answered, "If you point me out such a family, I would show you in response such houses where the musical instrument is taken by force, especially if there are more women in the family. Go for a walk in the countryside of a big city in spring, summer, or autumn, and you would not find any spot where one or several producers of oil etudes would not be sitting in front of a village house or a grove; in winter they all are waiting for any exhibition to open, longing to tickle their artistic fancy and communicate their impressions from the manner, background, atmosphere, and nuance."[13] He thought psychiatric control of aesthetic education was needed because modern art reinforced nervousness in society: certain kinds of painting, sculpture, and especially poetry, as well as theater performances and amateur theatricals, because they might be harmful to a young person, should be excluded, and musical education in secondary school should be limited to choral singing.

Rossolimo's talk at the annual meeting of the Moscow Society of Psychiatrists and Neuropathologists in 1901—one of the earliest manifestations of a nascent mental hygiene movement—made an ambivalent impression on his colleagues. Some of them shared his fears that the new artists, whose vulnerable minds were dominated by "psychological automatism," could provoke a psychic epidemic. Others protested against this extreme position. Many psychiatrists disagreed with Rybakov and Rossolimo that modern art was the product of diseased artists. They sought for social rather than psychological causes of the decline of art and attributed both the state of art and the artists' mood to unfavorable conditions in tsarist Russia. Psychiatrists agreed with the point made by radical critics that art was now dominated by mediocrity and invaded by mentally disturbed decadents only because everything free-spirited, bright, and forceful had been censured and oppressed. The Moscow psychiatrist M. O. Shaikevich, criticizing Rossolimo's extreme views, wrote that his "severe and categorical diagnosis" did not take into account the "social-psychological and social-pathological influences on artists that distort their art." The "depressing conditions of the day," Rossolimo continued, produce a "sensual tone of disappointment, dissatisfaction, and tiredness, . . . reinforce egocentric feelings, . . . increase the feeling of weakness in oneself, and create the need to find a ground in something, even in mysticism."[14]

Psychiatrists like Shaikevich emphasized that artists describe only what they see and cannot be held responsible for the corruption of morals. Psychopathology portrayed in art is neither the artists' invention nor the result of their immoral preoccupations: "pathological" characters in literature are "primarily a reflection of well-known social conditions."[15] Sikorskii argued that by portraying degeneration and moral decline, the "young writers of the realist school"—Anton Chekhov, Maxim Gorky, Vikentii Veresaev, Leonid Andreev, and Alexander Kuprin—aimed to illustrate the social and psychological tendencies of the epoch. The youngest of the group, Leonid Andreev, made his name as a writer who described strong feelings and extreme situations. Like many of his young contemporaries, Andreev spent his youth in a search for a palpable expression of the Demon, the abstract notion of evil, which he sought to personify in his drawings and writings. He succeeded especially, Sikorskii claimed, in portraying the dark sides of degeneration—people guided by their instincts rather than by moral choices and rational decisions.[16]

Chekhov, Sikorskii argued, was the first to describe how the "old evil which has been temporarily suppressed by the reforms of Alexander II, is reappearing in new forms." He portrayed "vulgar" (*poshlye*) and dull people devoid of ideals, who passively submitted themselves to the flow of life: his "miserable, half-alive [characters], resembling progressive paralytics" were the product of the dark times. Another physician, M. P. Nikinin, also praised Chekhov for revealing "social ulcers." When Chekhov portrayed "neurasthenic" characters, he pointed to the causes of neurasthenia in society, "to the same social ailments as we psychiatrists point to." Psychiatrists, Nikinin thought, shared with Chekhov the hope that, "with the improvement of social conditions, the number of neurasthenics will decrease and the number of active society members will increase." Even Rossolimo, though he found Chekhov's portrayal of neurasthenics unconvincing, finally agreed that the "neuroses" of his characters resulted from the harsh requirements of life and work in a modern society and especially from "our Russian conditions."[17]

With the exception of Rybakov and a few others, psychiatrists disagreed with the view that modern artists were "debauched degenerates" who appealed to a small audience determined to satisfy its dirty instincts. On the contrary, Sikorskii argued, their art served moral purposes: it warned of the dangers of immoral life and degeneration and reminded the audience that "only well-developed ideals can protect man from moral failure." Speaking about modern painting, Sikorskii mentioned one tableau—a group portrait of the members of the State Council by Il'ia Repin—as providing remarkable evidence of hypocrisy and pomposity in the higher bureaucracy in Russia. All the contemporary arts, in his opinion, conveyed the same message: there was something wrong with Russian life, a life that could no longer continue in the same way.[18]

"We can no longer live like this," declared the headline of a liberal newspaper in the spring of 1905, and soon everyone was repeating the phrase. Surrounding events added fuel to these feelings. A political crisis developed after the disastrous defeat in the Russo-Japanese war. Tsar Nicholas's inauguration of moderate reforms in mid-1904 unleashed a wave of opposition. The assassination of the conservative Minister of the Interior, V. K. Pleve, opened the way for a war against the autocracy. The main wave of strikes began after Bloody Sunday (January 9, 1905), and the revolution entered a violent stage.[19] A few years earlier, a young psychiatrist, V. V. Vorob'ev (1865–1905), argued that "degenerate talents, cumulatively, can produce abnormal trends in art, like decadence, ultra-impressionism, ultra-symbolism, etc."[20] In December 1905, during one of the clashes with the troops in Moscow, Vorob'ev was fatally wounded by a policeman while delivering medical assistance to rebels on the barricades.[21] Contrary to the imagined threat of decadence and degeneration, everyday life had proved to be a real danger.

Russian Hamlets

In 1905 the medical profession was quickly moving towards political opposition. The tradition of relating the growth in incidence of mental diseases to political and social conditions in Russia, however, had emerged long before.[22] Russian physicians were persuaded that social and political changes were necessary to make the country healthy. Though physicians of all political attitudes mentioned the lamentable state of public health, the liberal and socialist-oriented among them linked any improvement in the health care system to wide-scale reforms. The historian John Hutchinson has demonstrated that the slogan of the leaders of community medicine, "healthification" (*ozdorovlenie*), had much resonance. It implied the delegation of more responsibilities to the local self-governments (*zemstva*) in charge of public health in the provinces and the liberation of the professional intelligentsia employed there from bureaucratic control. To "make the country healthy" gradually became a synonym, at least for the radical part of the medical profession, for democratic reforms. In the words of physician and writer Vikentii Veresaev (pseudonym of V. V. Smidovich, 1867–1945), "a physician—if he wishes to be a physician and not a bureaucrat—must before everything fight for the removal of the conditions which make his work senseless and fruitless."[23]

Not all physicians, however, had the stamina to respond to this ardent call, putting their careers at risk. The main character of Veresaev's novel *Notes of a Physician* (1901) did not fit the image of a vigorous and heroic figure; this sincere and sensitive young *zemstvo* doctor faces all kinds of difficulties working in a remote "deaf" province, and he sometimes surrenders to them. Some physicians perceived Veresaev's weak hero as a slander on *zemstvo* physicians and the medical profession in general.[24] N. A. Vel'iaminov, president of the St. Petersburg Medical-Surgical Society and a professor of the Military-Medical Academy, characterized the book as "unhealthy" and the author as an ambitious and selfish neurasthenic. During the months after publication, physicians' responses pro and con filled the pages of medical, literary, and popular journals. Sikorskii was among the sympathizers, believing in the goodness of Veresaev's fictional character and interpreting his weaknesses as the reverse side of his longing for a moral life, his search for ideals. "Everything that the people of the 1880s lacked," Sikorskii argued, "conscientiousness, sense of guilt, constant need of moral self-improvement—all this one can see in Veresaev's characters." The psychiatrist criticized those who were unable to draw a distinction between the hero's and the author's views and emphasized that a novel is the product of creative writing and should not be taken for a pamphlet or a medical treatise. Yet Sikorskii agreed that Veresaev's doctor lacked some essential features of the perfect positive hero: intelligent, endowed by refined sensitivity, but by no means a fighter, he remains passive when he should act. Sikorskii suggested that Veresaev's weak-willed hero, with his "incomplete" character, was a typical but undesirable figure in an atmosphere where great changes were anticipated. He should gain the attention of physicians and psychologists as a type with an "underdeveloped will."[25]

At the turn of the century, doctors, politicians, and social thinkers equally used the concept of will. They thought of weak will mainly as a symptom of social inferiority, an organic property of "the other"—a child, a woman, a madman; or a Jew, a Negro, a Slav, a "primitive"—of anybody different from the white European rational male.[26] A white educated male was allowed to have weak will only in cases of neurasthenia or "nervous exhaustion," the illness that the physician George M. Beard diagnosed in middle-class American businessmen at the time of rising industrial society. In the 1880s and 1890s, the "malady of the century" took over the European continent. The historian Robert A. Nye mentions, for example, that at the time of heightened concern about national decline in France, studies of national character became a veritable industry. French authors compared strength of will and entrepreneurial spirit in different nations: whereas some were anglophile, others preferred the vigorous American character or made reference to Germany, whose younger generation manifested "the spirit of endurance and perseverance" that characterized their ancient ancestors.[27] In contrast to the individual treatment provided for neurasthenia—which, as the American neurologist S. Weir Mitchell suggested, consisted of rest cures and mild attitudes towards the patient—treatment on the national scale involved "education of will" and hardening of the younger generation. Durkheim, in his recommendations for moral education, stressed that "an inability to restrict one's self within determinate limits is a sign of disease" and suggested that practice in self-control and self-discipline should be part of the education of the will. The nationalists proposed the "cult of fatherland" and military training as the means to strengthen the national character and "pour steel" into the hearts of French youth.[28]

Among other nations, the Russians, or the Slavs in general, were held to

be a notoriously apathetic, weak-willed, and indolent people, their "melancholic" temperament caused by a cold and dark climate. In his comparison
of different European nations, Henry Havelock Ellis remarked that "indolence, apathy, resignation, mystic fatalism, are noted by all as the weakness of
the Russians."[29] The Russians would have agreed that their national character was, in the words of a French author, "more passive than active, more resis-
tant than entrepreneurial, more obstinate than having a will of its own, more
meek than rebelling, more showing respect for power than strong and dom-
ineering."[30] In Russia, however, the language of will, which often went together with the rhetoric of neurasthenia and degeneration, had political rather
than biological connotations. Complaints about the weakness of national
character and degeneration among Russians increased during the periods of
political reaction, in the 1880s and after the defeat of the 1905 revolution.

In the late 1880s, the Khar'kov psychiatrist N. I. Mukhin called degeneration "a bizarre and unfair fate" for the Russians, "both a reward for their
labors and a punishment for their sins." He thought that, though there were
still "places and happy corners where life is so peaceful and circumstances are
so beneficial that one can find strong people with solid nervous systems," the
bulk of the population was degenerating. "Overwhelmed by civilization,
working feverishly, suffering from all kind of shortages, receiving insults from
everywhere, and drinking in order to forget the unfortunate life or out of
idleness and boredom, this mass could not preserve a strong nervous system."
He referred to the neurasthenic character of the Russians, this "pathological
ground where the flowers of degeneration develop," as a product of "shortages" and "insults," of poverty and an oppressive regime, rather than an accumulation of inherited illnesses. In the aftermath of the 1905 revolution, psychiatrists overtly interpreted unfavorable political conditions as the cause of
degeneration. At the meeting held in 1908 in memory of B.-A. Morel, the
French psychiatrist who coined the term *degeneration*, V. M. Bekhterev, the
leader of St. Petersburg psychiatrists, pronounced capitalism the main cause
of degeneration. He gave a Marxist twist to the discussion, identifying the
evils of degeneration with the problems brought about by capitalism, which
increased the divide between the rich and the poor and spread an exhaust-
ing competitiveness.[31]

Observers generally sought the origins of neurasthenia in the speeded-up,
stressful life of modern society. In addition, Russian psychiatrists emphasized
political causes. Under an oppressive regime, they argued, people were especially prone to neurasthenia because their energy and best intentions could
not find an opening. The Moscow psychiatrist M. Iu. Lakhtin wrote that

"Russian historic conditions" are responsible for the appearance of "broken" individuals (*stradaiushchie ot nadryva*), those severe, reserved, nonsociable people who are especially susceptible to a mental disturbance. Political conditions transformed individuals "full of noble intentions but unable to engage in social action" into psychasthenics, and their altruism became pathological. P. P. Tutyshkin (1868–1937), a psychiatrist-Bolshevik, openly identified the cause of the weakening energy and will of the nation as political reaction after the 1905 revolution. He cited as evidence the rising rate of hysteria and neurasthenia and the decreasing resistance to authority. At the national meeting of psychiatrists in 1911, the Khar'kov physician B. S. Greidenberg argued, with reference to conditions in Russia, that the increasing rate of neuroses and the predominance of an "incomplete psychological type" were symptoms of a "transitional historical epoch," great social cataclysms, and political revolutions.[32]

As earlier, psychiatrists turned to literature to express their concern with ticklish political questions. While writing about the supposed mental illness of one of Andreev's literary characters, Amenitskii interpreted it as a problem common to a time of political reaction, when "unstable individuals of borderline degenerate constitutions . . . [are] the first victims . . . of the struggle with the oppressive social moods." A physician known only as "Dr. V. M. B–r," also illustrated the increase in weak-willed individuals under the oppressive regime with examples from the literary world: "When the brain exhausts all its powers and other organs become atrophied, the will weakens as a result. Someone, who loses his will, loses also life force and becomes a victim of pessimism; the wave of pessimism took over writers like Nadson [a decadent poet], V. Garshin, who has the whole gallery of 'little Hamlets,' and others. Moreover, do not some of Lev Tolstoy's main ideas bear traces of deep disappointment with science, civilization, and the success of the educated part of humanity?"[33]

By mentioning Hamlet in this context, Dr. B–r continued a discussion that had been going on in psychiatry for several decades. The historians William Bynum and Michael Neve have observed that for the High Victorians, Hamlet was insane because of his inability to act and the disjunction between his desire and his will. Henry Maudsley mentioned Hamlet's lack of action in his *Physiology and Pathology of the Mind* (1867). After translation of the book into Russian in 1871, the Russian audience could read that "men of great reasoning powers . . . are notoriously not infrequently incapacitated thereby from energetic action, they balance reasons so nicely that no one of them outweighs another, and they can come to no decision: with them, as with Hamlet, meditation paralyses action." Later British psychiatrists considered Hamlet insane for different reasons, finding Shakespeare's character "sympathetic and moving only if mad."[34]

This was the opposite of Russian psychiatrists' perception; they refused to recognize Hamlet's insanity precisely because they sympathized with him. As the physician A. N. Kremlev wrote, if we accept that "everything that Hamlet does during the first three acts he does in a state bordering on madness, then all the deep meaning of his words, all his wit, all his disclosures and revelations . . . lose any sense." In Russia Hamlet was emblematic not only of a reflective, inactive type of person but also of resistance to the authorities. As Ellis commented in relation to Hamlet's popularity in Russia, "Acute yet not massive in intellect, finely receptive, nobly ideal, infirm of purpose and will, struggling impotently in a political world that was, as he said, 'a prison,' and throughout all a temperamental artist, every Russian of the nineteenth century who sought to stand upright and be himself felt that he was a Hamlet confronting a Hamlet's fate." Dr. B–r argued that Hamlet is neurasthenic, not mad or degenerate; because neurasthenia (he might have been familiar with Durkheim's definition) is a social characteristic, a state of society rather than a disease: Hamlet is a social type, not a medical patient. In the contemporary as well as Shakespearean epoch, "people were kicked out of routine life, some were depressed by doubts, disappointment in the old religion, way of life, morals; some were excited by new prospects—in brief, their spiritual sphere was in an extraordinary, abnormal state." A social abnormality does not necessarily lead to clinical insanity. An "incomplete psychological type," a "type of transitional epochs," to which both Hamlet and his Russian doubles belonged, had different prospects. The type, Dr. B–r wrote, will move "towards degeneration, if unfavorable external conditions continue to oppress the light sides of a personality, or towards a critically thinking and acting person, if the conservative, repressive atmosphere ceases to act."[35]

Lacking vigorous characters, turn-of-the-century Russian novels were peopled by "little Hamlets." Sikorskii found the number of characters with "underdeveloped will" in Russian literature frightening, but he thought he well understood the cause: "Because weak will is a national feature of the Russians, as well as other Slavic peoples, it is portrayed in abundance by literature. Oblomov became a common name for an inactive person; many Russian educated men are contemplative to the degree that they have Hamlet's inhibitions, indecisiveness, and inability to act. Chekhov and Veresaev give the brightest examples of when, *faced by the prospect of acting, a person is impotent and is himself aware of it.*"[36] Sikorskii mentioned the title character of

I. A. Goncharov's novel *Oblomov,* a good-hearted but apathetic and idle Russian aristocrat whose name had for a long time been synonymous with laziness and weak will. The influential critic N. A. Dobroliubov, suggesting that Oblomov's "indolence and apathy are the result of upbringing and environment," transformed Goncharov's hero into an all-Russian phenomenon, "Oblomovitism."[37] In the critic's opinion, Oblomov was a direct descendant of the "superfluous people" who had often appeared in Russian literature—the Byronic young men of noble origin, endowed with every talent and enjoying every pleasure of social life, who nonetheless suffered from spleen and lack of purpose, not knowing where to apply their energy in the suffocating conditions of tsarist Russia.[38] In characterizing Oblomovitism, radical critics condemned a regime based on serfdom and the absence of political freedoms, circumstances that, they believed, inevitably produced idle and unworthy individuals. Oblomov, generalized into a social type, also gave psychologists the material with which to analyze the development of laziness in children; it set up a negative model showing how not to bring up children if the nation wanted to be vigorous and strong.[39]

In a country peopled with Hamlets and Oblomovs, strong and active characters were exceptions. The strong-willed characters, such as the heroes of Chernyshevsky's novel *What Is to Be Done?* (1863), were rare and exotic and caused a sensation in the reading audience. In his essay "Hamlet and Don Quixote" (1860), Turgenev lamented that though everyone belonged to one of these types, in his own times there were disproportionately more Hamlets than Don Quixotes.[40] Yet, as if it were a miracle, at the height of reaction in the 1880s, a Russian Don Quixote appeared; like Cervantes' character, he seemed to be a madman.[41]

In Search of the Positive Hero

As Don Quixote seeks to do good by tilting at windmills, so the main character of Vsevolod Garshin's story *The Red Flower* (1883) does so by battling with a flower, as the historian Peter Henry has observed.[42] *The Red Flower* is the story of a mental patient who is gripped by the obsession that a dahlia in the hospital grounds harbors Cosmic Evil. He engages in "spectral" battles with it, but the hospital staff does everything to prevent him from achieving his mission of destroying evil and saving humankind. Yet he wins his last "illusory" battle and dies, holding the red flower in his stiffened fingers. As Henry comments, *The Red Flower* could have been perceived as a call for the humane treatment of mental patients. But in Russia, where the connection between "madness" and outspoken criticism of society had a long history, the audience willingly read a political message into the story. At the height of reaction, when "normal" philistines carried on with their lives, a really bright character, a rebel, had to be a madman, a person driven by an "abnormally" developed will. In an essay written after Garshin's death, the writer Gleb Uspenskii stressed that in appalling and hopeless social conditions only the insane could think of improving life. The critic Mikhailovsky, comparing Chekhov's *Ward No. 6* (1892) and Garshin's *The Red Flower*, preferred the latter: unlike Chekhov's "apathetic" and "indifferent" hero, Garshin's madman showed all the essential virtues of a noble and self-sacrificing hero.[43]

Psychiatrists also found *The Red Flower* remarkable. Ellis regarded it as "the most perfect story of madness."[44] Sikorskii appreciated the masterful descriptions of "symptoms" that usually only psychiatrists knew about, such as manic exaltation, the period of transition from a lucid interval to a frenzied condition, the coexistence of normal and pathological states, and peculiar associations of ideas and their transformation into obsessions. But he especially valued the idea, clearly expressed in the story, that "mental illness does not eliminate the higher characteristics in the mentally ill—intelligence and dignity." Referring to the last episode of *The Red Flower*, he wrote, "When the sick man who had exhausted all his energy under the influence of a noble but mad delusional idea was found dead, he had a calm, peaceful expression on his face; his tired features expressed a kind of proud happiness . . . Psychiatrists a long time ago knew that even in a very heavy illness like progressive paralysis, which gives the person an extreme madness and almost wipes out all human features, the patient's feeling and thought may still sparkle brightly either under the influence of sympathy or in some other circumstances."[45]

The main promoter of mental hygiene in Russia and a specialist in child psychology and psychiatry, Sikorskii graduated from the Medical-Surgical Academy in 1876, then worked at the Academy and later at the St. Nicholas Hospital in Petersburg. Sikorskii met Garshin soon after *The Red Flower* was published. The psychiatrist and the writer formed a friendly relationship. After their first meeting in 1883, Garshin remarked that "great psychiatrists (so far there have been almost none) will be given great power, and power for good, for a great psychiatrist cannot be a brute." During their subsequent meetings Sikorskii remained, Garshin recalled, "as usual, warm-hearted [*dobrodushen*], serious, and bright." Garshin became interested in the psychiatrist's work, and Sikorskii offered him his recently published book on education. Garshin wrote to his mother in 1884 that Sikorskii's review of *The Red Flower* fully rewarded him for the odd and hostile reviews of other critics.[46] The relationship, however, did not last long: in 1888, supposedly in a fit of his periodic illness, Garshin killed himself, throwing himself down a stairwell.

In spite of his recurrent mental illness, Garshin was much loved during his life and admired after his death. His close friend V. A. Fausek wrote, "I frequently thought that if one could imagine a fully harmonious state of the world, it would be when everybody had acquired the same character as Vsevolod Mikhailovich. His main feature was an extraordinary respect for the rights and feelings of others, an ability to recognize dignity in every person, not a rational, reflective ability, but an unconscious, instinctive one, inherent in his nature." Like Tolstoy, Garshin wrote to Alexander III begging him to forgive the terrorists who killed the previous tsar (Alexander's father). He also pleaded with Count Loris-Melikov, a Petersburg high official who was attacked by a Polish Jewish student, to spare the young man from the death sentence. After his visit to Loris-Melikov, Garshin went to see Tolstoy in Yasnaya Polyana. Soon thereafter he had a breakdown, and his illness was diagnosed as "cyclic psychosis." In a later psychiatric account of this story, Garshin and Tolstoy "discussed all night how to bring happiness to humankind, and [Garshin] left totally convinced of his mission. On his way from Tolstoy, he bought a horse and, like Don Quixote, traveled around Tula region preaching the elimination of world evil. Finally, he was sent to a psychiatric hospital where he spent a few months."[47]

Though aware of Garshin's illness, psychiatrists were so impressed by the man and his literature that they accepted that in exceptional circumstances, as in the case of Garshin himself, the impact of illness should be neglected. Several psychiatrists, led by their professional curiosity, attempted to examine the evidence of Garshin's manic-depressive psychosis. All the same, they willingly recognized that the writer's noble nature was preserved throughout his illness. In his essay about the writer's illness, N. N. Bazhenov wrote, "The uninitiated person thinks that mental illness completely distorts the human cast of mind. For many cases, especially for those where the intellect is not damaged, this is definitely wrong; even when the disease is at its height, one can still find cardinal determining features of the person. The very content of delirium is borrowed from the person's normal psychology. In that sense Garshin's delirium was very typical. During the attacks, as well as in his normal state, Garshin remains the same hater of evil, full of active love for people, ready to sacrifice himself for their sake."[48] Bazhenov titled his essay "Garshin's Spiritual Drama," as opposed to "Garshin's Illness."

During the first Russian revolution (1905–7), psychiatrists found "Garshin's type" among their patients. Lakhtin reported the case of a patient in a state of hallucinatory confusion, who, like the character in *The Red Flower,* believed that the struggle between dark and light forces had become concentrated in himself and that he had to sacrifice his life in order to stop bloodshed, eliminate the world's evil, and save those who were perishing. In addition, Lakhtin observed several patients whose illness he diagnosed as psychasthenia; he explained that their disease originated in an inability to express their noble intentions and feelings. The psychiatrist termed this category of patients "pathological altruists," implying that in the oppressive atmosphere after the defeat of the 1905 revolution, their unwanted altruism took distorted, pathological shape. His description of altruism as "pathological" was not dismissive; it by no means diminished the value of altruism, just as "the value of a pearl is not diminished by the fact that it is a pathological formation of a shellfish." Pathological altruists could also be found in the past—Lakhtin mentioned Socrates, Mohammed, Jeanne d'Arc, Auguste Comte, and a literary character, Don Quixote.[49]

To be a pathological altruist was not a male prerogative; Lakhtin found a female version of this condition in so-called "fiancée's fear"—the anxiety that young women supposedly experienced before marriage because they doubted the strength of their feelings and feared they did not deserve their husbands.[50] Women had even fewer opportunities than men to fulfill their altruistic feelings; they did not have any other outlet than marriage, and the best chance for them was to marry a noble man. Turgenev's novel *On the Eve* (1860) provided a cultural model for female self-sacrificial behavior: the heroine, Elena, fulfills her noble intentions by marrying a Bulgarian nationalist and in this way sacrifices herself to the revolutionary movement.[51] Lakhtin understood fiancée's fear in this way, as a particular anxiety of young noble women that their "sacrifice" in marriage would not be great enough.

With the coming of the first revolution, psychiatrists no longer considered Don Quixote a madman. Though one of them diagnosed paranoia in Cervantes' hero, he admitted that Don Quixote's illness did not pass into the stage of psychic weakness and that he ended in a lucid state.[52] Following this precedent, psychiatrists reclassified as sane other supposedly pathological but progressive literary characters. This was the case, for instance, with Maxim Gorky's characters. Gorky's prose, drama, and poetry, which welcomed the revolution and glorified "the madness of the brave," brought him immense popularity in the first few years of the twentieth century.[53] Though earlier, discussing Gorky, some psychiatrists had doubted the sanity of his characters—considering, for instance, the title character of his novel *Foma Gordeev* (1899) "a typical neurasthenic or psychasthenic"—now they hastened to give them a clean bill of health. Foma Gordeev, an intellectual with a higher cause, finally kills himself, supposedly in a bout of illness. Psychiatrists, however, decided that this end was "inappropriate for [him] as a literary type." In his article "Pathological Features of Gorky's Characters" (1904), Shaikevich argued that though Foma is "more a man of emotions than reason, . . . there is nothing pathological in him." Having not found any "organic predisposition for a psychosis," Shaikevich had every reason to claim that Foma's "search for a pure life . . . does not originate in illness."[54]

Compared with an apathetic individual or a philistine fearful of social change, even a paranoiac seemed an improvement. N. Vavulin, author of *Madness: Its Meaning and Value,* became persuaded through his own experience that "madmen" are in fact the most normal people. During the 1905 revolution, Vavulin was imprisoned for several months and, though previously a healthy man, had hallucinations in his solitary confinement. This caused him to reflect on mental illness, and he concluded by suggesting that in some historical epochs a "paranoiac" had advantages over a "normal" member of the established order. With a touch of irony, Vavulin wrote, "A paranoiac in general is the most harmonious phenomenon in human nature. He does not know conflict, contradictions, reproaches of conscience and those accursed questions that poison the existence of others. A paranoiac is always convinced that he is destined for great events."[55]

Revolutionary ferment transformed Russian society, which now emphasized activity, heroism, and self-sacrifice as its main values. It inspired many psychiatrists to reassess the meaning of mental illness and their understanding of the normal and abnormal. The Moscow psychiatrist and psychotherapist Iu. V. Kannabikh (1872–1939), in an essay on the notion of normality, paraphrased Nietzsche: "the one who is ethically normal is not an average man but a man who has achieved the highest completeness and amplitude of life." He implied that the conditions for this kind of normality could be achieved only with the political liberation of Russia. Similarly, the influential Moscow psychiatrist A. A. Tokarskii, in a public lecture about the fear of death, claimed that human life is measured by intensity not by duration: "The really intense life begins for a person with the moment when he for the first time goes beyond his personal existence and gives his life to others."

Indeed, A. I. Iarotskii (1866–1944), a psychiatrist from Dorpat, stated that the length of one's life depended on the amount of one's idealism. On the eve of the 1905 revolution Iarotskii was arrested for participation in a Marxist reading group and exiled. He spent some years in Paris working with Elya Mechnikov, the famous immunologist who studied the positive impact on overall health of the bacterial flora of the gut. Iarotskii came to believe the significance of gut bacteria was grossly exaggerated: "In my view, one cannot agree with Mechnikov when he claims that the bacteria of the large intestine play the dominant role [in maintaining the healthy condition of the organism] in old age. It is impossible to rely on Mechnikov's sour milk only . . . By contrast, Tolstoy's teaching appears much more appropriate, as [he] explains premature aging in our generation by the conflict between moral requirements and the constraints of the political regime." In his book *Idealism as a Physiological Factor* (1908), Iarotskii wrote that striving for ideals is the only means to preserve sanity in Russia, which after the failure of the revolution more than ever resembled a prison.[56]

Neurasthenia and Its Radical Cure

Historians emphasize that, like ideas of weak will and degeneration, the concept of neurasthenia was value-laden. In the United States in the nineteenth century, as Joan Burbick remarks, neurasthenia was considered a disease that was specific to the refined and civilized and united Americans with their English or European predecessors.[57] In Russia, this concept also had political uses. It supported the arguments of professionals in charge of the nation's mental health who wanted to intervene in the public debate on political and social issues, such as reforms of local government, school education, and new trends in art. Like their Western counterparts, Russian psychiatrists believed the "brainworker" was especially prone to nervous diseases.[58] Yet, unlike the neurasthenic businessman exhausted by "cruel competition for the dollar" but spoiled by the easily available pleasures of life, as described by George M. Beard and S. W. Mitchell,[59] the Russian neurasthenic was an altruist who rarely gained any material privileges from his labor. The Russian neurasthenic did not have the advantages of his Western counterpart, who, once receiving the diagnosis, was then allowed to "move in neurasthenic circles."[60]

The archetypal Russian neurasthenic was a hard-working, intelligent, often poor and physically unfit person, oppressed by a lack of freedom and suffering from unfulfilled desires to serve the people. He was seen as needing psychiatric help. It was because he treated this kind of patient that the Moscow psychiatrist S. S. Korsakov gained fame as an "honored physician in service to the Russian mental worker."[61] Korsakov was himself an example of an overworked intellectual, and he died of a heart attack in his early forties. A few years after Korsakov's death, his student and friend N. N. Bazhenov contemplated the idea of a special clinic for the neurasthenic intelligentsia. In a speech at the opening of a private hospital for mentally ill soldiers and officers from the Russo-Japanese front, he expressed a wish that after the war the hospital could be transformed into "a permanent clinic for the laborers on another battlefield, where no fewer victims fall, that is, a clinic for those professionals who could not afford other private clinics." The members of the intelligentsia, Bazhenov stressed, had an indisputable right to treatment in better conditions than those offered in public hospitals.[62]

Participants at the conference of the Pirogov Society of Russian Physicians in 1904 discussed the question of providing special institutions for "individuals with shattered, weak nervous systems, exhausted, nervous, neurasthenics, hysterics, hypochondriacs." The psychiatrist S. S. Stupin raised the issue of "nervous sanatoria" for those who, having sacrificed their health for the good of society, could not afford private clinics and sanatoria. He argued that subsidized institutions on the German model of "people's sanatoria" should be made available to those with nervous illness.[63] The majority of psychiatrists at the conference, however, found the idea of sanatoria *pium desiderium,* desirable but not obligatory, and suggested they would be of little help in current social and political conditions.[64] A much more efficient method to fight neurasthenia and degeneration, they argued, would be to eliminate the causes of nervous illnesses found in malnutrition and unsanitary living conditions, which could be achieved only through social reforms.

A year later, the Moscow professor of neurology V. K. Rot (1848–1916) proposed the establishment of the All-Russian Society for Struggle with Nervous Diseases to propagate mental hygiene and organize sanatoria for nervous and overworked patients with low income. Once again, his colleagues rejected the idea. M. Ia. Droznes (1847–1912), director of a nervous sanatorium, agreed that sanatoria were important, but he concluded a talk with what he believed was a better suggestion: to eliminate as quickly as possible "the etiological factor that is conducive to the spreading of nervous and mental diseases in the population—an extremely oppressive, bureaucratic regime that restricts the personality." A psychiatrist-Bolshevik, S. I. Mitskevich, compared prophylactic measures such as sanatoria with "pathetic palliatives," and he called for the radical cure of the "fundamental evil of our era," capitalism. To propagate sanatoria was, in his opinion, "to foster bourgeois Pharisee attitudes that the social evil is being treated, while in fact the money would be thrown into a bottomless barrel."[65] Tutyshkin, also a Bolshevik, argued that "degeneration is caused by such scourges of humanity as alcohol, syphilis, TB," which could be fought only with the "general measures that would change the social and political regime."[66] Trying to defend his position in the continuing debate, Rot argued that he did not deny the necessity of reforms but feared they might come too late. He quoted a Russian proverb: "before the sun rises, the dew will have eaten the eyes out." He emphasized the need for urgent measures to help neurotic members of "the working intelligentsia"—teachers, physicians, writers—who were "not so numerous that one could watch calmly how they perish." Rot referred to the "well-known examples of writers prematurely dead from alcoholism, who could have been saved if treated properly."[67] Yet the majority agreed with the radical opinion that sanatoria would not be needed if conditions changed.

The country was indeed on the move. The 1904 meeting of the Pirogov Society had adopted as its final document a demand for representative government, and its last session had been interrupted by a military orchestra, the noise of which, the police hoped, would prevent voting on the final resolution. The next year was decked in revolutionary colors. *Zemstvo* radicals organized themselves into a coalition and called a number of congresses, which were dominated by the professional intelligentsia. They demanded changes in the government, an amnesty for political prisoners, and a declaration of civil rights and freedoms. Towards the end of the summer, the government sought to deflate growing opposition by establishing a consultative national assembly and signing a peace treaty with Japan. Yet the law that established a national assembly based the franchise on property ownership, and it reaffirmed the autocracy and failed to secure freedoms and civil rights. In response, a new national *zemstvo* congress was called in mid-September 1905 with the purpose of selecting a slate of constitutionalist candidates and actively campaigning for them in the coming elections.[68]

A few days prior to the *zemstvo* congress, psychiatrists held their second national meeting in Kiev, organized by Sikorskii and others. It began with an emotional speech by Bekhterev, in which he argued that the absence of civil liberties endangered mental health and was responsible for the "lack of vital capacities" in people. He explicitly blamed the regime as an obstacle preventing the free development of personality, and he ended his speech quoting a line of poetry: "Open my gaol, give me brightness of the day." The electrified audience carried the speaker out of the room on their shoulders.[69]

The sponsors of the meeting, the wealthy Kiev bourgeois, were scandalized, and the police closed the congress until Sikorskii obtained an authorization to continue.

It was Sikorskii's irreproachable reputation during his twenty-year professorship at the St. Vladimir University in Kiev that gave him enough standing to organize a psychiatric meeting in the agitated year of 1905. Sikorskii's career began in Petersburg, and he was appointed to the chair in Kiev in 1885. There he founded the psychiatric journal *Questions of Nervous and Mental Medicine* (*Voprosy nervno-psikhicheskoi meditsiny,* 1895–1905) and published extensively on child psychiatry, psychology, and mental hygiene. In his understanding, mental hygiene embraced a wide range of topics, from children's education to degeneration, psychic epidemics, and religious cults[70] A connoisseur of the arts, he was convinced that the psychiatrist should use literature as the most precise indicator of society's health: "the highest ideal life of Russian people is manifested in creative work, and the psychiatrist, without doubt, should know this higher life as closely as the ill, declining, decadent life. They are two poles of spiritual existence, and one should know them better in order to understand the large area between. This intermediate area forms a wide arena in which the psychiatrist applies the foundations of psychic diagnostics and the principles of nervous and mental prophylactics and health care."[71]

Despite Sikorskii's excellent standing, long before the day of the psychiatric conference, in a special letter to the organizers, the Ministry of the Interior warned that psychiatrists should not discuss any issues beyond their professional competence.[72] Sikorskii attempted to cool down the atmosphere by avoiding any reference to politics in his talk. In his address to the conference, he spoke on the "psychological foundations of education" and the civilizing role of literature.

Sikorskii's political sympathies were not with the radicals, especially after the government had announced the program of reforms and addressed the opposition's most urgent demands. Like Hippolyte Taine, who in his history of the French Revolution characterized the Jacobean leaders as pathological fanatics,[73] Sikorskii saw revolution in general as a triumph of crude force. During revolutions, the weak will of the Russian people could be a real danger: "that is why any fanatic can lead us easily, and that is why we fail to defend our personalities in a struggle with ourselves or with others whose will is stronger." Instead of throwing themselves into revolutionary activity, Sikorskii argued, his compatriots should have strengthened their will. He challenged the radicals with words he attributed to modern writers: "you are too self-confident pronouncing loud words, operating with high principles, hoping to transform society without having done the most important thing, without transforming your own soul!"[74]

While the radicals at the 1905 psychiatric meeting attacked the government's policies, Sikorskii focused his criticism on the school system, which in his opinion concentrated on the education of intellect at the expense of feelings and will. Education should strengthen will, he argued, but strong will by itself could be destructive and should therefore be kept in balance with feelings and intellect. Gorky's characters, for instance, were uneducated; they were strong but lacked purpose: "they were too long in unnatural conditions of life . . . so their souls became distorted." Their prospects, however, were better than those of the weak characters in Veresaev's novels, because, "if only given education, . . . these people [portrayed by Gorky] are able to elevate themselves to a broader, philosophical understanding of life." Educated feelings and strong will were the keys to morality, continued Sikorskii, so the role of literature in the education of feelings was hard to overestimate. The best mentors of feelings and will, the mother tongue and national literature, should not have a place inferior to Latin and Greek in school programs: "education should not be replaced by philology!"[75]

Sikorskii's efforts notwithstanding, the conference adopted a politically extreme resolution that announced the crucial role of government repression in the etiology of nervous and mental diseases and demanded that the government cease violence, liberate political prisoners, and introduce the principal human rights and freedoms.

With the later course of the revolution, however, the radical voices sounded less confident. In the autumn of 1905, the peasants, encouraged by the political discussions about expropriation of land, burned estates of the gentry in the hope that terrified landlords would leave the land to them. In December Moscow witnessed an unrest in which people died on both sides of the barricades. After that, as the historian Roberta Manning comments, "the mainstream of gentry opinion . . . sought to enhance government authority in order to combat revolution, even at the expense of a traditional *zemstvo* concern, the protection of the civil liberties of citizens." *Zemstvo* congresses, the former driving force behind the opposition movement, now condemned terrorism and welcomed government repression; at one congress the physicians even offered toasts to the armed forces as "the firm support of the fatherland and order."[76]

Alarmed by the growing violence, as the historian Laura Engelstein remarks, more and more psychiatrists interpreted the revolution as a social pathology that threatened civilization and progress. Like Sikorskii, they invested their hopes in the elevating influence of culture and education. Bazhenov, at that time the president of the Society of Moscow Physicians and a member of the liberal Constitutional Democratic Party, expressed his concern for the peaceful development of revolution. In the pamphlet *Psychology and Politics* (1906), he warned about the danger of the Bolsheviks' call to unleash a mass uprising. He feared the masses were prone to suggestion and unable to act constructively, and he reminded the revolutionaries that psychology teaches that crowds have their own laws, which would interfere with Bolshevik plans to control and direct mass activity: "brain, nerves, and anthropological characteristics of the citizens, not historical antecedents or economical interests lie at the foundation of any social or political regime." For an illustration of where the revolution went wrong, Bazhenov referred to the attempts to "democratize" psychiatric hospitals and establish "dictatorship of the revolutionary people." Bazhenov, who acted as a peacemaker in two such cases, saw them as barbaric violations of hospital regimes that had interrupted the normal conditions of work and adversely affected the patients. The only way to improve life, he suggested, lay in "very slow and piecemeal changes of the soul" through education and culture.[77]

The Palliative of Mental Hygiene

The defeat of the revolution in 1906 hit the medical profession perhaps more than any other. The radical physicians employed in *zemstva* were sacked or forced to retire. In 1907, the journal of the Pirogov Society mentioned the names of 1,324 physicians in the martyrology of the repression.[78] As at the beginning of the revolution, psychiatrists were again alarmed by the "uncontrolled violence" of the government, blamed the regime for producing "broken" individuals, and welcomed social changes as their best cure. The *zemstvo* psychiatrist V. I. Iakovenko (1857–1923) argued that the government's violent actions created an atmosphere of lawlessness and fear and contributed to an "epidemic of mental diseases." By contrast, the revolution was "healthy and progressive" for the intelligent but mentally unstable individuals to whom it gave an opportunity to act, providing an outlet for their energy and relieving tension. Another psychiatrist, M. Zhukovskii, wrote that during revolutions "disbalanced, hypochondriac, and apathetic individuals recover, revive, and become useful members of society."[79]

In 1911, at the first meeting of the newly founded Russian Union of Psychiatrists and Neuropathologists, its president, Serbskii, called on physicians to show courage, reminding them about their duty to protect national health in the oppressive political atmosphere. Alluding to the poet Konstantin Bal'- mont's well-known lines "I wish to be proud, I wish to be brave," Serbskii said, "While poets only wish to be proud and brave, we representatives of science must be. Guided by her light we must declare openly and loudly that it is wrong to make people go mad, to drive them to suicide and mental illness."[80] The police used Serbskii's speech as a pretext to close the meeting. As discussed in Chapter 3, only a few months before the congress, Serbskii had resigned his professorship at Moscow University, together with more than a hundred of his colleagues, in protest against the reactionary policy of the Minister of Education, L. A. Kasso. The staff of the Moscow University Psychiatric Clinic (University Clinic), which Serbskii headed for a decade, had joined the director shortly thereafter.[81] In his speech to the psychiatric congress in 1911, Serbskii used Kasso's name in a *jeu de mot,* saying that all these *cas sots* ("silly cases") would pass after a while.[82] Yet the situation at the university appeared to stabilize, and Serbskii was replaced by Rybakov, a former assistant at the University Clinic who had not resigned together with his colleagues.

Rybakov was from the *meshchane,* that is, he was probably the son of a small tradesman or artisan. He had to climb the ladder of state employment from the very bottom before receiving his first promotion together with his doctor's degree. At the age of thirty-one, he was finally appointed as an assistant in the University Clinic and married the daughter of a high-ranking civil servant. In 1911, when he was made director of the emptied institution, Serbskii's spirit was still in the air, so Rybakov had a difficult time trying to "tame" the clinic. On one occasion, when he tried to use a patient for a demonstration during his lecture, the physician who treated this patient refused to help him, saying it would be "as the comrades decide."[83] Serbskii himself had not encouraged the use of patients in the lecture room. Rybakov, who believed Serbskii still had an influence on the staff, wrote to him demanding the "establishment of a *modus vivendi* which would protect senior physicians from the despotic influence" of yesterday's students.[84]

Moscow academics boycotted Kasso's appointees, and the University Clinic ceased to be a center for Moscow psychiatrists. Its biweekly conferences, Little Fridays, attended by physicians from many hospitals, found another host institution, and both the First Congress of the Russian Union of Psychiatrists and Neuropathologists and the International Congress for Mental Care in 1913 ignored the University Clinic.[85]

Rybakov's scientific interests had always gravitated towards hypnosis and psychotherapy. He contributed to the temperance movement in Russia, organizing the first outpatient service for alcoholics at the University Clinic in 1896, where he treated patients by hypnosis. At the meeting of the Moscow Society of Psychiatrists and Neuropathologists in 1899, he argued that "the mentally ill and drunkards are blood brothers" but that drunkenness was a social rather than an individual illness. This statement notwithstanding, he continued to see alcoholics as medical patients and to apply to them every method of treatment. In 1904 he reported to the Pirogov Society congress positive results with the hypnotic treatment of alcoholics, and his recommendations to establish outpatient services for alcoholics and to use hypnosis were included in the final resolution of the congress, though only with the qualification that the real cure of alcoholism lay in reforms rather than in medical treatment.[86] Indeed, while his radical colleagues continued to demand social changes, Rybakov voted for mental hygiene; when they argued that the state's uncontrolled violence had a pathogenic effect on the population, he cautiously mentioned that it influenced only predisposed, fragile individuals. At the Second Congress of Psychiatrists and Neuropathologists in 1905, in the debate on Rybakov's talk about outpatient services for alcoholics, a colleague criticized the proposed local measures and called for major changes:

We [physicians who can treat alcoholism] are few, and against us is the whole way of life with its rituals and habits, against us is society, finally against us is the government which receives one-fourth of its billion-ruble budget from selling alcohol . . . Our work is difficult, it is a Sisyphean labor, and its results in the social sense are scant. That is why in this case as in others the focus should be made not on treatment but on prevention of diseases. Taking this into account, I absolutely disagree with the ninth point of Dr. Rybakov, "The ideal organization of treatment, etc." God forbid! Our ideal is completely different. The ideal of our struggle is the Russia in which economic and social reforms will foster the sober way of life of the entire population.[87]

Rybakov's interest in such treatments as hypnosis and suggestion led him into experimental psychology. After the death of Tokarskii, who headed the experimental psychology laboratory in the University Clinic and taught the course to medical students at Moscow University, Rybakov replaced him and continued these experimental activities. In addition to psychophysics and Wundtian experiments, he used tests designed by Francis Galton, Hugo Münsterberg, Benjamin Bourdon, Hermann Ebbinghaus, Emil Kraepelin, and Alfred Binet and Victor Henri, as well as by his compatriots and colleagues A. N. Bernstein and A. P. Nechaev (1870–1948). He also constructed his own devices and in 1910 composed an "atlas for studying personality by means of experimental psychology, adapted for pedagogical and medico-diagnostic purposes."[88]

Together with Bernstein and Rossolimo, Rybakov organized the Society of Experimental Psychology (1910), "an association of those who are interested in medical and psychological aspects of education."[89] One of the society's self-appointed tasks was to promote testing in mental hospitals and schools. Bernstein, a leading supporter of Kraepelin in Russia, propagated the idea of an "objective" approach to the patient's consciousness, independent of its content and based on formal signs of disease. The best-known Russian test was Rossolimo's "psychological profiles," which consisted of a diagram ("individual profile") plotted using the results of eleven separate measurements of such things as attention, perception, memory, and fatigue.[90]

Psychiatrists of the old school argued that if tests were applied widely, half of the population would be found insane.[91] The mental hygienists, however, silently accepted this conclusion. They drew a permeable boundary between normality and insanity in terms of performance rather than biological defect. Rybakov formed his own criterion of insanity based on a person's "working capacity" and "ability to act according to his will." Understood like that, illness became a threat to anybody. The only protection from all-permeating insanity, in his view, was mental hygiene in the form of "sensible continuous exercise of mental capacities and rationally organized work." Culture and education, he firmly believed, should fight the irrational in the human mind: "reason, this pilot of personality, is born from great culture. The history of humanity demonstrates: the lower man's place is on the staircase of cultural development, the less he is able to suppress his beast within; the more civilized he is, the easier and freer he controls it." A staunch supporter of Nordau, Rybakov feared the corrupting influence of lower standards in art and blamed the decadent cult of insanity for placing "talent and illness on the same pedestal."[92]

While the conservative Rybakov held optimistic views about the possibility of treating and preventing insanity, radical psychiatrists continued to assume that an oppressed nation could never be healthy. Thus, in the summer of 1909, a young Moscow psychiatrist interested in psychoanalysis, M. M. Asatiani (1881–1938), went to Zurich to see C. G. Jung. He had high expectations from the meeting with the rising star of psychoanalysis, with whom he wanted to discuss the problems of Russian practitioners in general and analysts in particular.[93] As Jung reported in a letter to Freud, Asatiani "complained about the lack of therapeutic results" of what he called "resistance therapy." Jung explained Asatiani's situation by "the imperfection of his art," but also thought "the trouble lies with the Russian material, where the individual is as ill-differentiated as a fish in a shoal." Freud wrote back suggesting another, no more flattering reason: "Your Russian [Asatiani was in fact Georgian] probably has some utopian dream of a world-saving therapy and feels that the work isn't getting on fast enough. The Russians, I believe, are especially deficient in the art of painstaking work."[94]

Asatiani's own perception of this meeting was entirely different. Though a young man, he had already had a rich political experience. During the 1905 revolution he worked in the Moscow University Clinic and witnessed the courage with which the director, Serbskii, shut the doors against the police who were seeking out revolutionaries. Asatiani's understanding of his conversation with Jung was colored by political overtones. He wanted to communicate a political message—that psychoanalysis is inapplicable in Russia because of the country's lack of political freedom, not because of the nature of the "Russian material." When he described his visit to Jung to his Russian colleagues, Asatiani attributed his own understanding to the Swiss maître: "in conclusion, Jung remarked that psychoanalysis requires particular social conditions, which are not in contradiction with individuals and provide for free personal development. In Russia, where the peculiar social regime [*osobyi obshchestvennyi stroi*] hardly fosters free personal development and obstructs the independence of individuals, psychoanalysis must meet great difficulties and is therefore problematic to conduct."[95]

The political troubles of the day, which caused this gap in understanding between Russian psychiatrists and their colleagues abroad, also created a divide between two groups of psychiatrists within the country. Physicians on the left and on the right of the political spectrum interpreted in different ways the causes and cures of neurasthenia, weak will, and degeneration. Radical psychiatrists argued that neurasthenia originated in external political circumstances, which caused an inner tension in potentially active individuals and made it impossible for them to find an outlet for their altruistic intentions. They saw reform and revolution, which would provide the political conditions for individual freedom, as the only means to cure mental diseases. By contrast, conservative psychiatrists believed neurasthenia was a product of local causes—overwork, malnutrition, and ignorance—and should be given local treatment, which they found in education and mental hygiene.

Both groups, however, identified in literature an index of mental health, a representation of what was healthy and what was harmful for the nation. Literature provided illustrations of decline, degeneration, mental instability, and lack of ideals, but it also inspired hopes for regaining national strength. Though psychiatrists stressed the negative effect of literary decadence on mental health, they found much of contemporary art inspiring rather than degrading. Once again, psychiatrists shared an expectation so widespread in Russia: that literature should provide guidance for society, especially during critical periods when the country's future was in the balance.

FIVE

The Institute of Genius

Psychiatry in the Early Soviet Years

Social construction and psycho-physical self-education
will become two aspects of one and the same process. All
the arts—literature, drama, painting, music and architecture will lend this process beautiful form . . . Man will
become immeasurably stronger, wiser and subtler; his
body will become more harmonized, his movements
more rhythmic, his voice more musical . . . The average
human type will rise to the heights of an Aristotle, a
Goethe, or a Marx.
                                              —Leon Trotsky

Under the influence of mental illness, unexpected abilities can emerge from within the human organism.
                                              —P. I. Karpov

Historians have often described revolutionary Russia as a laboratory for utopian projects inspired by Romanticism and the Enlightenment. As Richard
Stites remarks in *Revolutionary Dreams: Utopian Vision and Experimental Life in
the Russian Revolution,* the post-revolutionary period "was one of those rare
moments in history when a large number of people actually tried to break
the mold of social thinking that sets limits to mankind's aspirations, that defines 'human nature' in a certain unchangeable way, that speaks in realistic,
prudent and ultimately pessimistic tones."[1] The post-revolutionary epoch
was conducive to dreams of reshaping human nature, and many dreams were
put into practice. The Moscow Institute of Brain, the Central Institute of
Labor, and the Psychoanalytic Institute were all founded in the first decade

after the 1917 Revolution, under state sponsorship.[2] Compared with these projects, the Institute of Genius, however bewildering it may appear today, was no more utopian.

The idea to study and "protect" geniuses in a special institution may be seen as a caricature of psychiatrists' aspiration to share the political culture of the arts, or even as the quintessence of their desire to control culture. This idea argued for a state institution in which artists, scientists, and other "geniuses" would become subjects of medical and psychological studies. Though grim sounding, this project was inspired by the Enlightenment vision of genius as an ideal of humankind as much as by the notion of genius as illness. The Institute of Genius contained in a nutshell a pre-revolutionary dreamlike project, the realization of which had suddenly become possible. The authors of the project wanted, as a start, to create a central institution in the context of state-regulated public health. Their ideal, however, was a healthily organized society that would automatically prevent illnesses and abuses of talented people and would integrate art into everyday life. The adventures of this project are revealing about what happened to psychiatrists' attitudes towards literature and art and to the genre of pathographies in the vibrant post-revolutionary decade.

Psychiatry in Disarray: 1917–23

Within a year after Russia entered the First World War it became clear that the psychiatric service, despite the experience of the Russo-Japanese war, was as unprepared as the army itself. The psychiatric service was under the overlapping jurisdictions of the Red Cross, the Ministry of the Interior, and the Ministry of Defense. Poor coordination between these administrations added to difficulties caused by lack of transportation, medicaments, nursing staff, and physicians. With the beginning of the Revolution, the situation in the army became even more chaotic. Less than a week after the abdication of Nicholas II in March 1917, the Petrograd Soviet of Workers' and Soldiers' Deputies decreed that soldiers were "to enjoy all the rights of a citizen," could form associations and unions, and could not be punished or prosecuted without a trial.[3] As the historian W. Bruce Lincoln comments, soldiers formed groups to discuss anything from war and peace to "insulting remarks" made about the Revolution by their officers and to elect their own committees.[4] For a period, these committees coexisted with the old structure, adding to the chaos in the army.

The army physicians suffered from the loss of control. As during the 1905 revolution, when under the slogan of "democratization" nurses and junior staff forced head physicians to retire and elected their own administration, in the spring of 1917 psychiatric nurses, many of whom were former soldiers, turned against their seniors. Ironically, one episode involved the same physician, N. N. Reformatskii, who in 1906 had suffered the humiliation of being carried out in a wheelbarrow by the rebellious staff of the St. Nicholas Hospital in Petersburg. In March 1917, Reformatskii, a head of the West Front psychiatric division of the Red Cross, gave an order to transfer some psychiatric nurses to other locations without their consent. As a result, a group of nurses broke into Reformatskii's apartment at midnight and required him to "abdicate." The group's leader, a female physician recently elected to the soldiers' soviet, reassured him that this act would save him from "rougher treatment" by the crowd of soldiers.[5]

To add to the disarray in army psychiatry, the mental hospitals countrywide were under a threat of liquidation. In April 1917, the Russian Union of Psychiatrists and Neuropathologists called an extraordinary meeting in Moscow to discuss both urgent action and the future of psychiatry under the new regime. Threatened by the growing anarchy, psychiatrists longed for central control, "a single central administration, either under *zemstvo* or military jurisdiction, to which everything should be submitted."[6] But, though willing to accept centralization as a way to deal with the emergency, the meeting participants still wanted to see a more democratic organization of psychiatry in the future, with psychiatric associations, university psychiatry, and the public equally represented.[7] The most radical participants wanted to decentralize psychiatric care and organize a network of local facilities under the supervision of the local authorities, instead of a few centrally controlled large hospitals. Some psychiatrists raised the question of collegiality in hospital administration, arguing that hospitals should be directed by elected councils with the participation of nurses and the public. In the unpredictable political situation, however, the ideal of democratization remained a distant goal. More sober participants warned their optimistic colleagues that "the new owners of the cherry orchard"—the revolutionary soviets—might have their own views on what to do with psychiatry.[8] One observer remarked that, in order to establish effective mental health care, psychiatrists now had to direct their propaganda to a different audience and to ally with new authorities.[9]

As opposed to those colleagues who welcomed decentralization of mental health care, the Moscow psychiatrist L. M. Rozenshtein (1884–1934) argued that Russian psychiatry was not equipped to take this decisive step and to refuse central funding. In Russia, unlike Scotland and other countries with well-developed philanthropic support for mental institutions, mental health had always been a state concern. Rozenshtein believed that in Russia, where nonpsychiatric physicians had little interest in mental health care, society was almost certainly unprepared to take the care of the mentally ill into its own hands. Even before the war, he had become persuaded of the advantages of centralized psychiatry, and he had found a precedent in the mental hygiene movement organized in the United States by Adolf Meyer.[10] Inspired by the tradition of Russian community medicine, Rozenshtein argued that psychiatry should be centralized by a welfare state, and he was prepared to negotiate his project with "the new owners of the cherry orchard," whoever they might be. Soon thereafter he discovered that a socialist government was more sympathetic than others to the goals of preventive medicine. Eventually, Rozenshtein became the most active proponent of mental hygiene and designer of preventive psychiatry in the Soviet Union.

Though the intelligentsia welcomed the February Revolution of 1917 and supported the Provisional Government, whose main task was to organize the transition to a representative political system, it was alarmed by the Bolsheviks' seizure of power in the autumn of 1917.[11] Many professionals left the country; those who stayed witnessed an even worse destruction of social order, but they also saw more signs that the new government was concerned with public issues. Russian community physicians had struggled for decades to obtain state support and to demonstrate to the authorities that public health begins with social reforms. The most active physicians therefore invested their hopes in the Revolution.[12] Their most daring wishes came true when the new government proclaimed that medical services would be free of charge and directed towards the prevention of diseases and when it established a ministry of public health headed by a physician.[13]

Founded early in 1918, the government's Council of Medical Collegia was later reorganized in a ministry, Narkomzdrav (People's Commissariat of Public Health).[14] Following Lenin's call to use "bourgeois specialists," though under proper supervision, in Soviet organs, the council approached the Russian Union of Psychiatrists and asked it to delegate three physicians "competent in organizational matters" who would be willing to work in its Psychiatric Commission. In spite of heavy losses during the First World War and the Revolution, the union replied promptly and constructively. The members were convinced that central control alone could both save psychiatry from final destruction and help numerous "victims of the war and revolution." In a letter to the council, the leaders of the union argued that "mental health care is the state's duty [and should be] sustained through state agencies with strict control and subordination of local organizations to central ones."[15] The union's recently elected president, P. P. Kashchenko (1859–1920), the secretary, L. A. Prozorov, and a member, I. I. Zakharov, volunteered to work on the Psychiatric Commission. At the first joint meeting, the commission drafted a plan of urgent measures to evacuate the mentally ill from the front line and to aid hospitals on the edge of survival. The commission intended to fund these actions from the budgets of organizations that had had psychiatric departments and now, like the Red Cross, were to be abolished.

The first concern of the Psychiatric Commission was to preserve mental hospitals, many of which had not received fuel, food, and drug supplies for months.[16] In some of them patients had either died or been let out; in others, patients and staff had starved. The total number of patients in Russian and Ukrainian mental hospitals shrank to a quarter of that in the prewar years (12,950 in 1923 versus 42,229 in 1912).[17] During the Civil War, the death rate in hospitals reached 40 percent; in the Tver' Psychiatric Colony, 378 patients died in 1917, 467 during the first eight months of 1918, and 138 in August 1918 alone.[18] Though the commission created an emergency fund to aid the hospitals, it could provide no more than one-tenth of the prewar level of funding. As shown in a 1920 survey, only one of forty-eight hospitals had a sufficient food supply, fourteen reported that it was only "satisfactory," and others were heavily undersupplied. The following year was marked by a famine that reduced official food quotas in hospitals to a thousand to twelve hundred calories per person per day. The temperature in wards was below freezing point, though trees in hospital parks and gardens were cut down for fuel. Without hot water, drugs, and sanitary equipment, hospitals were overrun by tuberculosis, typhus, and cholera.[19] Violence in overcrowded wards increased, and restrictive measures were introduced—which in some hospitals went as far as armed guards—where nonrestraint had been the rule.[20] Kashchenko, head of the Psychiatric Commission and an experienced *zemstvo* psychiatrist, reported to Narkomzdrav that Russian psychiatry had never been in such a critical state.[21]

Lev Markovich Rozenshtein and the Soviet Conception of Public Health

In the years preceding the First World War, the majority of psychiatrists shared the view that the betterment of the nation's mental health would come from improved social conditions. They argued that in a well-designed or "healthy" society, psychiatry would not be needed and would be replaced by prophylactics such as mental hygiene. The most radical of them demanded global social changes and rejected any local solution to the mental health problem as a cowardly compromise. After the Revolution they were able to test their theories. Socialist Russia was building the very society that would, in principle, create a hygienic environment that eliminated the social and economic causes of mental illness. The radicals argued that psychiatrists should reconsider the place of their profession in society, reorient it towards the prophylaxis of mental disease, and restructure the psychiatric service according to the agenda of mental hygiene. Yet in 1918, when the country was lying in ruins, it appeared too early to test the impact of any changes or to go ahead with the project of preventive psychiatry. More than ever, the current situation required rescue actions, implying there was still a long way to go before psychiatry became redundant. Very few psychiatrists could think adventurously about the reconstruction, which would inevitably divert resources so much needed for the hospitals. Rozenshtein was one of the dreamers.

Rozenshtein joined Narkomzdrav during its first months and soon thereafter played an important role in the Psychiatric Commission. A combination of personal features helped his advancement to the leadership of Soviet psychiatry.[22] He had worked for a number of years with V. P. Serbskii and N. N. Bazhenov and he considered them his teachers. Thus, though he was an ardent supporter of the new conception of psychiatry, which he believed was the most appropriate for the socialist state, he never failed to emphasize continuity between Soviet and pre-revolutionary psychiatry. His successors, Soviet psychiatrists, regarded Rozenshtein as a link between the past, which now appeared heroic and glorious, and their own generation.[23] On the one hand, Rozenshtein contributed to the legend of "the Moscow school of psychiatry" when he traced the genealogy of Moscow psychiatrists from S. S. Korsakov to its current leader, P. B. Gannushkin.[24] On the other hand, his radical socialist past made him acceptable to the new authorities. In 1906, when Rozenshtein was a graduate student at the Novorossiiskii University in Odessa, he had been arrested for his revolutionary activity and, after seven months in prison, exiled from his hometown. He then found his way to Moscow University, where, after graduation, he gained an appointment at the University Psychiatric Clinic.

The Moscow University Psychiatric Clinic was in its liveliest period at the end of that first decade of the new century and, as Rozenshtein later remembered with nostalgia, resembled the renowned Burghölzli hospital in Zurich. Like their Swiss colleagues, Moscow psychiatrists sought to escape the dead-end of custodial psychiatry and became interested in psychotherapy.[25] Excited about new possibilities of psychological cure, young psychiatrists from the University Clinic traveled to the sources of psychotherapeutic wisdom in Bern, Vienna, and Zurich and held lively discussions on a wide range of topics.[26] The years that Rozenshtein spent at the clinic were a formative experience for him. In 1911 it was a matter of honor for Rozenshtein to follow Serbskii when he resigned as a result of the conflict between the faculty and the conservative administration.[27] Like some other young psychiatrists who left the clinic with Serbskii, Rozenshtein was employed by Bazhenov, and he became his assistant at the Higher Women's Courses. Alongside his work in the clinic and his teaching, Rozenshtein attended to private patients, discovering in his practice "so-called neurotics and nervous and psychological symptoms in sane people that were unfamiliar to physicians."[28]

Rozenshtein was also interested in the recent developments in psychology and conducted at least one piece of experimental research, on memory in alcoholics.[29] An interest in the problem of alcoholism led Rozenshtein to formulate his idea of "neuropsychiatric dispensaries," which he later implemented on a large scale. In Russia as elsewhere, the last decades of the nineteenth century witnessed the rise of antialcohol movements in which psychiatrists played an important part. Psychiatrists took the initiative to organize outpatient services for alcoholics, in which they used hypnosis and psychotherapy. Rybakov organized such a service in the Moscow University Clinic. The efficiency of outpatient services remained questionable, especially given that the state received nearly one-third of its budget from its monopoly on spirits and did nothing to support the efforts of the antialcohol movement. Yet Russian psychiatrists actively discussed the possibilities for a better institutional setting for the treatment of alcoholic patients. In 1907 S. S. Stupin proposed using the dispensary model, which had already been tried in Germany. He suggested that institutions for alcoholics, closely connected with temperance societies, should combine "an outpatient service, a clinic for acute cases, a hospital and a colony for the chronically ill, and special supervision for the alcoholics in care." Rozenshtein supported this project.[30] At the same time, Russian psychiatrists discussed the suggestion put forward by their Western colleagues of combining in the same institutions the treatment of alcoholics and patients with minor mental disorders.

Dispensaries as such were new in Russia, though in England and Ireland they had traditionally provided general outpatient services to the poor. Dispensaries for the tubercular began to develop early in the twentieth century, first in Germany, France, and Britain. Unlike general dispensaries, they did not provide treatment but rather were centers of community work. Cases of tuberculosis were diagnosed and patients received cod-liver oil and advice about home hygiene and, in "early" cases, were referred to sanatoria. In Germany, tuberculosis dispensaries, called Information and Welfare Clinics, provided a model of organization adopted by Russia's antialcohol, infant care, cancer, and anti–venereal disease campaigns.[31] Activists in community medicine appreciated the advantages of dispensaries as centers of community care. Tuberculosis dispensaries, at least, were conceived as a "sorting, isolating mechanism rather than a curative resource." Their aim was to process "all the tuberculosis material of the district," keep records, sort out patients "for appropriate treatment," and follow up on cases afterwards.[32]

The idea of using the dispensary as a model for the combined institutional care of alcoholic and nervously ill patients was realized for the first time in Russia by Rozenshtein. The integration of mental health service in the community was a sensitive issue in Russian psychiatry. At different periods, Rozenshtein's colleagues tried out such forms of welfare psychiatry as family care, countryside colonies, sanatoria with beds for poor patients, and outpatient departments in mental hospitals. In 1913, with a group of his compatriots, Rozenshtein went to inspect the organization of psychiatric services in a number of European countries. At the end of their trip they visited the much admired charity hospitals in Scotland and attended the International Congress of Medicine in London.[33] In one session of this meeting, Rozenshtein heard a talk by the Swiss–American psychiatrist Adolf Meyer, "The Aims of a Psychiatric Clinic."

Just a year earlier, Meyer had founded the National Committee for Mental Hygiene, and now he triumphantly summarized his and his colleagues' approach to mental health. In this approach, psychiatrists cooperated with social workers in the community, acting upon the social causes of mental illnesses and directing efforts towards their prevention. A psychiatric institution of a new type, Meyer argued, would include an outpatient department and dispensary, and it would "work in a close harmony with the larger suburban asylum or hospital." In contrast to the hospital, the new institutions would be oriented towards the community, and the psychiatry practiced in them would become a part of social medicine. "We have come to recognize," Meyer declared, "the need of the study of each patient . . . from the point of view of his being or trying to be a member of a community."[34] Rozenshtein became so persuaded of the advantages of Meyer's approach that, eighteen years later, he enthused about it at the First International Congress of Mental Hygiene.[35] After returning from his trip in 1913, he set up an outpatient service for alcoholic and nervously ill workers as the equivalent of a community center, in a factory village near Moscow.

The war interrupted this experiment and called Rozenshtein to the front, where he spent three years as a psychiatrist in the army. By that time he was already a convinced follower of the psychological theory of the neuroses, and from this standpoint he contributed to the discussion of shell shock, a hot issue in psychiatry during the First World War in Russia as elsewhere.[36] In Russian psychiatry the notion of war neurosis dated back to the Russo-Japanese war, when the army first introduced a psychiatric service. Alongside cases diagnosed as psychoses and epilepsy, army psychiatrists came across unusual symptoms that they related to hysteria or neurasthenia. At the time, practitioners often dismissed such complaints as pretended or faked, but some of them believed in the reality of these symptoms. A physician at the Kharbin army hospital in the Far East, P. M. Avtokratov (1857–1915), in his reports published in Russian and German journals in 1906, described the disturbances as acute and neurasthenic psychoses of depressive character related to war conditions.[37] In the subsequent discussions psychiatrists agreed that widespread alcoholism and the unpopularity of the war might have been responsible for the rise of mental diseases in the army. By contrast, at the outbreak of the First World War there was supposedly less alcoholism as a result of the abolition of the much criticized state monopoly for alcohol. This war was also considered more popular than the war with Japan. Yet the army had many cases of both psychoses and neuroses, and the issue of war psychoses remained obscure. According to a physician's report, nobody in the front line or in military hospitals knew what to do with the "nervously ill," and army officers and psychiatrists alike tried to pass them along to someone else.[38]

The question of war neuroses divided psychiatrists into two camps: those willing to recognize them as a separate group and those who, not finding any place for them in Emil Kraepelin's classification, did not want to admit their existence. Psychiatrists who recognized the reality of war neuroses tended to be familiar with recent developments in psychotherapy.[39] The main bulk of psychiatrists, however, sought the causes of shell shock in organic injury, ignoring the fact that the folk name for such "contused" soldiers was *skonfuzhennye* (confused), hinting at the psychological nature of the trauma. Following the discussion in foreign medical journals, the psychiatrist T. E. Segalov suggested that traumatic neurosis might result from three types of causes: psychological trauma, namely fear experienced during artillery battle; physical damage to peripheral nerves, similar to that caused by a hit; and damage

to the central nervous system caused by a quick change of air pressure, resulting from the firing of a gun (an effect similar to a sudden change of altitude).
It was thought that the physical trauma might cause other neurological diseases besides neuroses and psychoses. Segalov therefore calculated a safe tra-
jectory for firing, high enough to protect those on the ground from what he
called "decompression."[40] Though the psychiatrists who searched for organic
explanations of traumatic neurosis willingly accepted Segalov's version, a few
psychotherapeutically oriented physicians argued that "it is too early yet to
lock psychological causes away . . . in the archives."[41] Rozenshtein thought
the role of the physical trauma, the actual "contusion," was grossly exaggerated. In his view, the combat and the shooting were nothing but the last drop
that caused the previous traumatic influences to overflow. These "latent traumatic reactions," he said, were "emotional," that is, psychological in origin.
The article in which he presented these observations, "On Psychopathology
of the Contused," was severely cut by an army censor.[42]

The horrible sequence of wars and revolutions made Russian psychiatrists
receptive to the notion of psychological trauma. The term "victims of war
and revolution" began to appear both in psychiatrists' publications and in
minutes of their meetings with state officials. (With time, the "and revolution" was dropped out of loyalty to the regime that emerged from the 1917
Revolution.) Rozenshtein, among others, warned about an "increasing nervousness" in the population "worn out by two wars, famine, and the Revolution." Historically, the notion of nervous exhaustion prepared the ground
for the idea of mental hygiene, and Rozenshtein's rhetoric about nervousness had the same effect. He contemplated a project of "neuropsychiatry," a
"new psychiatric synthesis" in which "psychiatrists and mental hygienists
[would] go hand-in-hand with materialistically thinking psychotherapists,
who accept in part the theories of Freud and Adler." Neuropsychiatry, or
"active psychiatry," would, he argued, develop methods for the early detec-
tion and diagnosis of mental illnesses and would contribute to their prevention; social psychiatry, mental hygiene, and psychotherapy were all "further
advancements towards more active psychiatric practices."[43] As a major stage
in the transition from custodial to preventive psychiatry, Rozenshtein envisaged the differentiation of a new area of psychiatry. As opposed to "major"
psychiatry, which dealt with acute diseases, mainly psychoses, a new, "minor"
psychiatry would recognize and treat so-called soft diseases—psychoneu-
roses and other minor disorders. He thought this group of tractable "soft"
diseases would become the main focus of a psychiatry able to prevent more
serious and incurable mental illnesses.

Like preventive medicine in general, preventive psychiatry assumed disease had social causes that a rationally organized society would eliminate. Rozenshtein stressed that in Russia "the old community medicine," traditionally concerned with social causes of disease, provided a better foundation for preventive psychiatry than did medicine in the West. He also credited the new regime with "exceptional opportunities for a new theoretical synthesis in psychiatry as well as for its subsequent application to healthification of everyday life and work."[44] In the early 1920s, however, his call for preventive psychiatry appeared unrealistic to the former *zemstvo* psychiatrists who dominated both Narkomzdrav and the Union of Psychiatrists. The first psychiatric meeting after the Revolution urged the restoration of mental hospitals as well as the old psychiatric system. Two years later, the project on mental hygiene still seemed impossible in a country on the edge of survival. During the national famine in 1921, Rozenshtein studied cases of necrophagia and anthropophagia and did not make any plans for mental hygiene.[45]

One argument against mental hygiene, then, was the lack of resources, but another came from clinical psychiatrists who opposed plans to reshape their field. The project of preventive psychiatry, as well as social medicine in general, appeared threatening to conventional medicine, and from the beginning it contained the potential for serious conflict. Yet inside Narkomzdrav the idea of social medicine was very influential and it was promoted in the early 1920s. By 1922 social hygiene was introduced into the university curriculum, and both an institute and a journal of social hygiene were founded.[46]

The first Soviet "commissar" (minister) of public health, N. A. Semashko (1874–1949), following the lead of both German proponents of *soziale Medizin* and Russian community physicians, placed a heavy emphasis on sanitation and improvement of living conditions rather than on treatment. He attempted to fulfill the notion of a sanitary utopia on a scale as yet unseen.[47] As the delegates of the Eighth Party Congress proudly stated in 1919, "the dictatorship of the proletariat has already made possible an entire range of hygienic and curative measures unachievable within the context of bourgeois society."[48] "After we have finished with pandemics of typhus and have freed our hands," Semashko wrote in 1924, "we will elaborate the plan for the general healthification of the country and will gradually fulfill it."[49] Unlike the old medicine, concentrated in hospitals as the centers for traditional treatment and custodial care, the new preventive medicine would be based in a completely different type of institution. The centers of preventive medicine would combine treatment, prophylaxis, and sanitary education and would be modeled after tuberculosis or alcoholic dispensaries. The dispensary for nervous and alcoholic patients, which Rozenshtein had established before the war, was now to become a model for the mainstream institutions of Soviet psychiatry.[50]

Institutionalizing Mental Hygiene

Emphasizing the importance of industrialization for agrarian Russia and celebrating the construction of the first Soviet power station, Lenin uttered a much quoted phrase: "communism equals Soviet power plus the electrification of the entire country." Paraphrasing Lenin, Rozenshtein could have said that communism was Soviet power plus "dispensarization" of the entire country. At the Second All-Russian Conference on the Questions of Psychiatry and Neurology in November 1923, he took the floor and spoke about "the new tasks of Soviet psychiatry." These tasks, as he and his ally, the psychiatrist P. M. Zinov'ev (1883–1965), argued, consisted of developing mental hygiene and organizing neuropsychiatric dispensaries—medical, social, and educational institutions for the mentally and nervously ill. They envisaged dispensaries becoming regional centers for mental health care, regulating admissions to mental hospitals, psychiatric colonies, and sanatoria for neurotics. But dispensaries were also to fulfill functions previously unknown to psychiatry: outpatient counseling services, supervision of patients after discharge from hospitals, and screening of the population's mental health. The dispensary was to be as much a social as a medical institution, an institution to provide those in care with suitable jobs and occupations and healthy entertainment. A heavy emphasis was placed on sanitary education: the best target for preventive medicine was not the insane person but "sane people around him."[51]

Rozenshtein and Zinov'ev suggested that, though the dispensary's clientele would sometimes overlap with the hospital's, preventive psychiatry should address mainly those cases in which "the disease did not yet damage the working capacity of the organism." It was assumed that neurotics would benefit most from the dispensary's help: as weak-willed individuals, they needed "a certain automatic order" in life, and their activity should be regulated. This explained why the methods to be used in dispensaries were "borrowed from psychotherapy" and included "a great deal of mass suggestion." Zinov'ev said that neurotics provided "the best material" for dispensaries. Yet he warned that psychiatrists could not expect neurotics to come to the clinics on their own initiative, because they usually did not identify themselves as ill people and were not aware of the opportunities for treatment. Neurotics should be rescued by specialists in mental hygiene who would "search out the mentally ill and those . . . in danger of mental illness." As part of this task, dispensaries were to train social workers to conduct inspections at workplaces and in residential areas.[52] Unlike individual psychotherapists who indirectly selected their potential clientele by influencing public opinion, dispensaries would be given enough official power to act directly and decisively. Thus the attempt to obtain state support was crucial for the institutionalization of mental hygiene. But this proved to have a negative side: the official status of mental hygiene reinforced its coercive character, which was especially clear in the case of dispensaries.

Clinical psychiatrists dominated the meeting at which this project was presented. They discussed the revival of hospitals and did not mention the dispensary project in their final documents.[53] But by this time Rozenshtein had strengthened his standing in medical as well as political circles, and his opinion could not be ignored. In 1921 he acquired a doctoral degree and started teaching at Moscow University; two years later his first monograph, *Psychic Factors in the Etiology of Mental Illnesses,* appeared.[54] He became a top Narkomzdrav officer and joined pro-Bolshevik professional and political associations. Eventually he concentrated in his hands all the major posts available to psychiatrists. He was president of the Russian (subsequently Soviet) Union of Psychiatrists and Neuropathologists, founded and presided over the Society of Psychoneurologists-Materialists, and edited its journal, *Soviet Psychoneurology (Sovetskaia psikhonevrologiia)*. He was a member of both the Society "Marxism and Leninism in Medicine" and the All-Russian Union of Associations of Scientists and Engineers (VARNITSO). With time, the balance of forces in the Psychiatric Commission also changed, the influence of *zemstvo* psychiatrists faded, and the ideas of preventive psychiatry won out.

In 1924 Rozenshtein succeeded in opening the first department of mental hygiene at the Moscow Psychoneurological Institute, the institute founded in 1920 as a counterpart to V. M. Bekhterev's Psychoneurological Academy in Petrograd. The dispensary was established as a "practical" service attached to the department. After a few months, however, the dispensary had outgrown the institute, which, in any case, was soon to be abolished by Narkomzdrav. The dispensary was given independent status, a new title—the Moscow State Neuropsychiatric Dispensary—and funding from the centralized state budget.[55] The state funding of the dispensary while most medical institutions were locally funded demonstrated the significance the government attached to social medicine.[56] With this back up, Rozenshtein was able to overcome the objections of clinical psychiatrists and accelerate the transformation of mental hygiene into the mainstream of Soviet psychiatry.

The dispensary was located in an eighteenth-century palace in the center of Moscow, with enough room for laboratories of speech therapy, psychotherapy, and psychoanalysis, as well as anthropological, neurological, psychophysiological, and psychotechnical laboratories. Rozenshtein had twenty-four members of staff at his disposal, enough to satisfy his eagerness for large-scale actions. Equipment was purchased abroad. The construction of an inpatient clinic began, to be completed for the tenth anniversary of the October Revolution.[57] The subjects of the dispensary's research included war veterans, prostitutes, students from Middle Asia, members of the party bureaucracy, industrial workers, prisoners, alcoholics, and former patients of mental hospitals. The research aimed at practical recommendations for each group. The staff also carried out hygienic inspections of housing across Moscow. One of the buildings they surveyed, known as the "Drunk House," became a continuously studied model of the conditions harmful for mental health.[58]

In the proletarian state, the workers' preferential access to medical care was confirmed by party decree.[59] The dispensary also gave priority to the examination of industrial workers in the workplace, which resulted in the introduction of "sanitary passports." These detailed reports on individuals' physical and mental state as well as on conditions of life and work would, in Rozenshtein's conception, provide for workers "the best opportunity to adjust to industry and [give] industry an idea of the individual's special abilities and inclinations, as well as his defects."[60] After the first eight months, the dispensary had four thousand records; in 1928, over forty-three thousand people were examined at their workplaces. The majority of them were found in need of some kind of mental health care. The dispensary staff, however, realized that their results were, in a sense, artifacts and depended upon the criteria of mental illness and health that had been adopted. Thus, the researchers remarked that the category of "slightly nervous" (*legko nervnye*), introduced to describe individuals on the boundary of health and illness, was so large because of its loose definition. This category included "workers with some pathological reactions, very little developed pathological symptoms, whose social conditions [*sotsial'no-bytovye usloviia*] were negative and who could have developed worse symptoms in the absence of necessary psychological and sanitary care." All the same, the criteria of neurasthenia stretched from "[traumatic] experience of the Revolution" to a limited personal budget, poor housing, and overwork. In the words of a dispensary inspector, "only those who, besides the absence of explicit features of disease, also had sufficiently healthy everyday conditions could be placed in the category of the sane."[61] It is not surprising therefore that the surveys designed "to detect the deformities of character caused by occupation" found up to 54 percent of factory workers, 71.8 percent of medical workers, 75.9 percent of shop assistants, and 76 percent of school teachers were nervously or mentally ill.[62]

People were processed—"dispensarized"—in different ways. A few were directed to hospitals, some were recommended to take a break in sanatoria and rest houses, others were advised to follow an improved regimen, do physical exercises, or get involved in community work. Prescriptions to the workers—do not work extra hours, do not work at night, change the character of your work or occupation—in fact addressed their employers. Advice to change housing was especially hard to follow. Yet dispensary workers claimed their recommendations did not overburden employers' budgets: "what is required is not as much expensive dietary canteens, sanatoria, and so on, as large-scale social action for the healthification of everyday life [and], first of all, for mental hygiene propaganda."[63] Trusting that the conditions of life and work would gradually improve, Rozenshtein and his colleagues announced the "reeducation of individuals and the masses" as the number one task for preventive psychiatry. A. B. Zalkind, the leader of Soviet pedology—a discipline that in the 1920s covered education, child psychology, school hygiene, and many other allied subjects—argued that mental hygiene was "not only a therapeutic and defensive method, but also an educational method, . . . a combination of hygiene and education."[64]

In Rozenshtein's conception of mental hygiene, two Enlightenment projects—socialism and psychiatry—came together, both marked by the characteristic Enlightenment belief in reason and education. The Revolution and the construction of the socialist state were supposed to follow the "iron logic" of Marxist theory. Psychiatry was equally informed by rationalism and understood as moral management and education. Similarly, psychotherapy emerged as rational persuasion, a treatment that, first and foremost, addressed the patient's reason. Like their colleagues abroad, Russian psychiatrists favored rational therapy long before the Revolution, and Soviet ideologists of mental hygiene inherited their beliefs. Zinov'ev classified education and psychotherapy in the same category, as "factors mitigating harmful psychosocial influences." When "psychotherapeutic individualism" became criticized in the Soviet Union for its supposed contradiction with the collectivist ideology, psychotherapy was transformed into "sanitary education in small collectives of neurotics." Thus identified with education, psychotherapy continued to exist within mental hygiene even in the period of the harshest ideological criticisms.[65]

With the aim of, in the language of the period, "bringing sanitary education to the masses," the dispensary organized lectures for different audiences, many in workers' clubs. It also established departments of mental hygiene (literally, "cabinets" and "corners"—*psikhogigienicheskie kabinety* and *ugolki*) in factories and colleges. The department of mental hygiene at the Communist University of the Workers of the East was the main institution for research in mental fatigue as well as in the harmful effects of various deficiencies in student life.[66] In 1924 the Moscow dispensary began to teach a special course for physicians on social psychiatry and mental hygiene.[67] Between the late 1920s and the early 1930s, this course was introduced in some university curricula, and two chairs of "social psychoneurology with mental hygiene" were established, one in Moscow, the other in Khar'kov.[68] Rozenshtein and his colleagues fought to establish a network of dispensaries across the country, pressuring the government to include them in the state budget. The network gradually expanded to all the regions after the Second World War.[69]

Rozenshtein's project appealed to the top Narkomzdrav officials, because it served as a vehicle for gaining complete control over psychiatry. Very early in the Soviet years, mental health care became a state monopoly. Though some private clinics opened under the New Economic Policy, when it ended in 1928, as an observer commented, "private psychiatric facilities disappeared from the face of the earth."[70] All psychiatric institutions, including hospitals, sanatoria, and colonies, were transferred to Narkomzdrav, with the exception of university clinics and, for a period, railroad hospitals. The mental hygiene project contributed to the homogenization of psychiatry, which became concentrated in two types of institutions: dispensaries and mental hospitals. According to Rozenshtein's plan, the former should control the latter. His plans seemed to have unlimited credit with Narkomzdrav. In 1924 Semashko spoke of specialists in mental hygiene as a leading force in the country's healthification: "We are talking about healthification of labor. But, the first word in the matter should be given to the neuropathologist. The problems of optimization of work, which preoccupy our workers' state so much at the moment, cannot be solved without the neuropathologist and psychiatrist. We are talking about healthification of our archaic, barbarian everyday life, but in this matter as well one should listen to the neuropathologist with special attention. We are talking about proper education of the younger generation. But who is the best pedagogue (now it is more correct to say, pedologist) if not the neuropathologist and psychiatrist!"[71]

All psychiatrists were required to take part in this transformation to social psychiatry. In 1925, one Moscow psychiatrist voiced the expectation that "the entire Moscow health care organization will be gradually transformed into a single multifunctional dispensary, where every part (hospitals, outpatient and emergency services, sanitary education, and statistics and other services) is closely connected with every other."[72] In a society designed to be "healthy," it was assumed that a state-regulated system of mental health care would guarantee the efficiency of the psychiatrists' efforts. In the early 1930s, Frankwood E. Williams, the medical director of the United States National Committee for Mental Hygiene, made several trips to the Soviet Union at Rozenshtein's invitation. His hosts explained to him how the state system of mental hygiene worked, and he was shown dispensaries, sanatoria, and pioneer camps around the country. He left Russia deeply impressed, and he followed up his visit by publishing reports, articles, and a book on what he had seen. The message conveyed to his colleagues was that an efficient system of total mental hygiene, a goal never achieved in his own country, could succeed only under certain social conditions. Only in the hands of a socialist state, genuinely concerned with its citizens' health and able to organize a national campaign, could mental hygiene reach the masses, transform their lives, and improve human nature. It was in Russia, he believed, that a new, better human type was about to be born with the help of mental hygienists.[73]

Mental Hygiene for Geniuses

In Russia at the turn of the century, many people, from psychiatrists to politicians, believed in social engineering, though they envisaged various methods. The reformists invested their hopes in the improvement of social conditions, the radicals in Communist revolution. In contrast, the professionals insisted that not just economic and political changes but special measures were essential to alter human nature. These measures, under the names of eugenics, psychotechnics, and mental hygiene, had already been proposed in the West. After the Revolution, proponents of these measures in Russia had the chance to implement them on a scale as yet unseen.[74] In 1921, when Rozenshtein was contemplating his plans for social medicine and preventive psychiatry, another, similar project appeared: a project to take care of talented people who, as its author claimed, had often been exploited and abused. "Who does not know the sad pages from great people's biographies," he rhetorically asked, and summarized these pages himself:

Complete misunderstanding of new ideas of a talented person by his contemporaries; prosecution of any creative innovation if it contradicts the tastes and wishes of the powerful; incredible exploitation of artists' work by editors, re-sellers, agents of different kinds; abuse of *wunderkinds;* talented people living in poverty and dying early as a result of inability to adapt to social and economic conditions, to be servile and please their patrons, to advertise themselves and sell their souls; their abuse by the corrupt media; or the opposite—when talented people have to serve the vulgar tastes of the petty bourgeoisie, produce pseudo-art, prostitute art, literature, science, theater, when they clown, pose, arrogantly advertise themselves. All this in order not to starve.[75]

Though socialism should eliminate the conditions that made abuse of geniuses possible, the author assumed the situation would not improve automatically. Geniuses, he argued, owing to their individualistic, unsociable tendencies and frequent ailments, found adjustment to any society difficult. Asocial by nature, they easily fell victim to society and perhaps to incarceration in asylums and prisons; but, if cured of their illnesses and socialized on a par with everybody else, they might lose their creative abilities. The author suggested that a special branch of medicine—aesthetic medicine—should protect geniuses from abuse and increase the output of their work.[76]

Only in a socialist society, where protection of the weak is state policy, could aesthetic medicine become a reality. Alongside general departments of social welfare, the state should establish special institutions for geniuses: dispensaries and "departments of social welfare for mad geniuses" (*sobez genial'nogo bezumtsa; sobez* is an accepted abbreviation for a social welfare department). The institutions would assist in protecting talented people from hostile environments and placing them in favorable conditions for the completion of socially valuable work.[77] The new policy towards the so-called bourgeois specialists, a category that included scholars and engineers, encouraged this plan. The government changed from attacking them to "winning them over." Introduction of the New Economic Policy in 1921 eased scholars' conditions, and establishment of the Central Commission on Improving the Life of Scholars promised state support and privileges such as sanatoria.[78]

The "new man" was the announced ultimate objective; preoccupied with counteracting the disastrous consequences for children of wars, famines, and revolutions, the Soviet government worked out a number of educational and care programs.[79] The plan for institutions for geniuses was designed to take care of children—both *wunderkinds* and those who appeared mentally retarded at school but nevertheless grew up as talented people—within this framework. It suggested that children should be either directed to special schools or provided with individual developmental counseling. Apart from these welfare institutions, the author of this plan, G. V. Segalin, proposed a program of research on deceased "geniuses" coordinated by an Institute of Genius. "Since a talented person's brain and body have not yet been objects of systematic study," he wrote, "the Institute is to decree the compulsory dissection of brains of all outstanding people without exception, and, if necessary, also a postmortem on the corpse, which then will be kept in the anatomical theater for subsequent study."[80]

Other tasks assigned to the institute included experimenting with stimulants known to produce creative states of mind and to control artistic production. Segalin warned that in contemporary bourgeois society art was degenerating into "almost hysterical forms" (*pochti sploshnoe klikushestvo; klikushestvo* was considered a particularly Russian form of hysteria that affected peasant women). An objective expertise in art would help museums and galleries distinguish a genuine work of art inspired by a "real creative illness" from a fake produced by a pretended "mad artist." Working in parallel with a forensic psychiatrist, a specialist in "aesthetic medicine" would provide expertise for the courts in questions of pornography and "antisocial" art in general.[81] This was relevant under the freer conditions of the New Economic Policy, when artists' groups and movements proliferated and private publishing houses reappeared. In an attempt to control these groups, the government readjusted its policies towards literature and art and established new institutions of censorship.[82]

The project for aesthetic medicine was strikingly similar to earlier psychiatric ideas on controlling art and aesthetic education formulated by, among others, G. I. Rossolimo, one of the first proponents of mental hygiene in Russia. Rossolimo, who developed these ideas early in the century (see Chapter 4), stayed in Russia after the Revolution, and his work in child neurology, psychiatry, and psychology gained state support. Having recognized his own ideas in the aesthetic medicine project of an unknown psychiatrist from the provinces, Rossolimo helped arrange for the project's presentation in his Institute of Child Neurology in Moscow. He also helped establish a commission that included the painter Vassily Kandinsky, the literary critic Iu. A. Aikhenval'd, the psychologist N. A. Rybnikov, and the psychoanalyst I. D. Ermakov. The commission, however, never functioned. The project for aesthetic medicine was abandoned, and its author, Segalin, disappeared from Moscow.[83]

Progeneration in a New Country

Girsh (Grigorii Vladimirovich) Segalin (1878–1960) was the son of a wealthy Jewish manufacturer from Moscow. For many years, he studied arts and anatomy in Russia and Germany. He had already become an "eternal student"—of the type so well portrayed by Chekhov—when he decided to take a medical degree. He studied at the universities of Jena and Halle (his departure from Russia perhaps stimulated by the growing anti-Jewish mood and the pogroms at the beginning of the century). In the last decades of the nineteenth century Jena gained a reputation as a "citadel of Social Darwinism," owing to Ernst Haeckel and his followers. In 1898 the Jena historian Ottokar Lorenz published a book on genealogy relating his approach to August Weismann's concept of the ancestral germplasm.[84] In 1905, the same year that Segalin arrived in Germany, Haeckel founded his Monist League with the goal to reform life, art, and psychology on a biological basis. Segalin may have been particularly attracted by the correspondences that contemporary artists found between Haeckel's organicist ideas and their own art, such as the natural forms fashionable in art nouveau and in the eurhythmic dances of Isadora Duncan.

In 1904 Jena hosted a competition for the best essay on the application of the laws of evolution to society, which stimulated a variety of sociobiological projects. In the same year, the Jena psychiatrist Wilhelm Strohmeyer launched a research program for psychopathology based on statistical genealogy, an idea soon enthusiastically developed by Ernst Rüdin. The racial hygiene movement established itself a year later. Though Segalin could not sympathize with the project of purifying the Aryan race, he became enthusiastic about another eugenic idea, the cultivation of geniuses. The Nietzschean aphorism that "the way forward led from being a species to a super-species" inspired Alfred Ploetz to write the first monograph on racial hygiene, but it also inspired a cult of geniuses, which penetrated medicine and biology with the help of such authors as Max Nordau and Otto Weininger.[85]

After returning to Russia in 1913, Segalin passed special examinations required to convert his German medical degree into a Russian degree and to qualify for state employment. He was already thirty-seven when he started teaching psychiatry at the University of Kazan', but three years later his career was again interrupted when he was mobilized and worked in a psychoneurological hospital of the Red Cross in Kiev (which from 1915 was headed by V. F. Chizh; see Chapter 1). After the Bolsheviks had taken over the Ukraine, Segalin worked in the Red Army medical commission organized to fight the

typhus epidemic. Demobilized, he settled in a town in the Urals, Ekaterinburg (after 1925, Sverdlovsk), where he helped organize a medical school at
the newly established University of the Urals. He taught psychiatry and neurology at the university and founded a laboratory of psychotechnics at the
Polytechnic College. He was also active in the public sphere as a member of
the local government commission on minor criminals; as an expert in political trials, so common during the Stalin years; and as a consultant to a variety of institutions, from the Institute of Work Hygiene to the opera theater.
Having become part of the Soviet medical establishment, Segalin did not give
up his artistic interests. In the university clinic, using patients as models, he
painted a gigantic tableau, "Madhouse or Victims of the War." During the
Second World War he founded a portrait gallery of local celebrities and veterans for which he painted several portraits. Segalin also wrote journalistic
sketches and was even elected to the National Writers Union, a sign of the
highest official recognition.[86]

In spite of his acquiring local influence, Segalin's main project remained
an unfulfilled dream. The reason did not lie in the project's implausibility,
since it paralleled such developments as the introduction by psychiatrists in
Germany of hereditary-data banks for research on the inheritance of both
negative and positive qualities—mental disease and fitness, leadership, and
genius.[87] Segalin's contemporaries also believed that his idea to collect the
brains of outstanding people anticipated Bekhterev's idea of a "Pantheon of
Brain."[88] But, unlike Bekhterev, Segalin was an eccentric provincial who,
after having spent many years abroad, had not sufficiently established himself
in Russia. Though the presentation of his project in Moscow went well, he
failed to maintain the interest of those physicians who had access to power.
He reoriented his project towards a journal, which he launched in 1925 and
published almost single-handedly.

To his townsmen, Segalin appeared "a mad original, bearing some fantastic ideas," but an observant contemporary found him "though not without
oddities, a most interesting person."[89] Segalin was in correspondence with
Maxim Gorky, who "loved to collect such people," as well as with other
celebrities. He also arranged contributions to the journal from August Forel,
Wilhelm Lange, and Walther Riese.[90] The journal had a long and loud title:
*Clinical Archive of Genius and Talent (of Europathology), Dedicated to the Ques-
tions of Pathology of a Gifted Personality as Well as of Creative Work with Any Psychopathological Bias.*[91] It consisted of two main divisions, a theoretical one,
filled mainly with Segalin's own writings, and a section of pathographies. In
the first theoretical article, Segalin announced the creation of a new acade-

mic discipline, which he termed interchangeably *ingeniology*, the study of creative work of any origin, "healthy" as well as "pathological," and *europathology*, the study of the effect of mental illness on creative work. The latter term was derived in part from the Greek word *heureka*, "I have found it," (from which "heuristic" also originates), but it also resembled such neologisms of the time as "eugenic" and "eurhythmic." Whatever the name, the new discipline was to study creative people, from children to mad geniuses, under a variety of conditions and from normal states to bouts of momentary madness. As one of his purposes, Segalin mentioned the construction of creativity tests, schemes for "practical semiotics and diagnostics," in order to distinguish "the inspirations of an epileptic" from those of a hysterical person. By looking at a person's artistic style, a psychiatrist would be able to diagnose the disease "as easily as a chemist detects the composition of minerals in the sun by its spectrum."[92]

But Segalin's main focus was on mental illness, which, so he firmly believed, could produce and stimulate creative abilities. In Germany he was exposed to the cult of genius and the ideas of racial hygiene. He read authors who elevated the genius above the average healthy person and believed mediocrity rather than disease was the cause of degeneration. These authors thought geniuses, whether ill or healthy, pointed the way to humanity's future and should be worshipped and cultivated.[93] In the same way, the pre-revolutionary pessimistic vision of decline gave way to belief in an unconstrained progressive evolution of the human species. In the 1920s, in the *Soviet Medical Encyclopedia,* the psychologist L. S. Vygotsky (1896–1934) and the psychiatrist Zinov'ev defined *genius*, referring to the work of the Italian psychiatrist Enrico Morselli, as "an evolving, progressive variation of the human type."[94] Segalin suggested that by examining, analyzing, protecting, and stimulating geniuses, the human species could cultivate itself and rise to as yet unknown heights.

The division between the normal and abnormal should be abandoned, Segalin announced, because "nature . . . knows only one division—between repetitive and creative work." The distinction, he argued, should lie not between illness and health but between productive and unproductive illness. Segalin compared creative illness with birth. He had in mind, perhaps, the common image of Russia as a woman giving birth, as the country lay in ruins and awaited regeneration. Many believed that revival was impossible without sacrifices and that the country would have to pay a heavy cost for its Communist rebirth. In 1926 the psychiatrist P. I. Karpov wrote, "In the course of human development some individuals are ahead of others, and because of that they are unstable and vulnerable to mental diseases . . . Humanity makes sacrifices, leaving in its path of development individuals who fall down in a disordered state." The phrase "when you chop wood, chips fly" became proverbial in the language of the day and was often used to justify political repression. Using the same metaphor, Segalin compared human evolution to a gigantic building site where pathologies—"the chips"—were the inevitable cost of progeneration. His own project aimed at minimizing the number of "chips"—the number of geniuses who perished in this process.[95]

Polemics with Eugenics

At the turn of the century genius was treated as a hereditary quality, and as such it interested social hygienists and eugenicists. In 1909 the founders of the International Society of Racial Hygiene made the recently knighted Francis Galton, author of *Hereditary Genius,* its president. In 1923 the German physician Alfred Grotjahn began to lecture on the biology of genius, talent, and feeblemindedness.[96] The Russian Eugenics Society, founded later than its Western counterparts, often followed their lead. At Rüdin's request, Russian eugenicists examined the family tree of the German-born mathematician Leonhard Euler, who lived and worked in Russia. On their own initiative, they traced genealogies of the writers Dostoevsky, Tolstoy, and Mikhail Lermontov, the painter V. A. Serov, the revolutionary Vera Figner, and the composer Alexander Scriabin.[97] The psychiatrists A. G. Galach'ian and T. I. Iudin reconstructed Garshin's family tree and found that many members of his family suffered from manic-depressive psychosis.[98]

Within eugenic circles, belief in the Lombrosian connection between talent and mental illness persisted. Echoing the ancient notion of genius as Demon, Ernst Kretschmer wrote that genius appears when the "Demon" of pathology is added to an excellent hereditary endowment. Segalin sympathetically quoted Kretschmer's aphorism that "a mentally balanced man makes neither wars and revolution nor writes poetry." But, as a degenerationist, Kretschmer believed that though pathology produces a "spark of genius," it also signifies the beginning of a family's decline: "a most favorable situation for the growth of genius is created at the point where . . . old, highly-bred families begin to show symptoms of degeneration."[99] A man of genius was often compared to a reckless person who wasted the family fortune, to "the evening sun rather than the morning dawn."[100] The taint of insanity and the belief that geniuses rarely had gifted progeny and often remained childless caused eugenicists to doubt that geniuses could ever form good human stock.

The leader of Russian eugenicists, N. K. Kol'tsov (1872–1940), made an exception for the breeding of "weak and sometimes even sick geniuses, because one can receive health and strength from average people's progeny, while highly developed abilities are rare." Nevertheless, visibly dissatisfied with Tolstoy's offspring, he wished that Tolstoy had made a eugenic match.[101]

In 1921, however, the geneticist Iu. A. Filipchenko (1882–1930) conducted a survey of scientists and musicians for the recently established Petrograd Bureau of Eugenics. He found that talented individuals had more mentally ill relatives, especially on the maternal side, than did average people.[102] The results reinforced Segalin's belief that "the genesis of a great man is intimately connected to pathology," and he hastened to report on Filipchenko's study in his own journal. He now argued that "genius . . . is the result of cross-breeding between two lines: one carrying potential talent and the other, usually maternal, hereditary psychotism and mental abnormality."[103] The Romantic vision of creative illness was reconceptualized in quasi-genetic terms as a process in which the "gene of insanity releases the gene of creativity," which would otherwise have remained latent in the genius's family.

Belief in the role of mental illness divided europathology from mainstream eugenics. While eugenicists emphasized the importance of eliminating mental illness, even by means of sterilization, Segalin argued vehemently against negative eugenics and especially against sterilization of the mentally ill. Given the tremendous population loss in Russia, sterilization on a mass scale was considered out of the question, and even the most ardent eugenicists referred to sterilization mainly in a critical way, as an imported "Indiana idea."[104] Yet the Russian Eugenics Society discussed sterilization in the early 1920s and did not immediately reject the idea.[105] Kol'tsov remarked that the "sterilization of Cain, from whom, according to the Biblical legend, all townsmen and craftsmen originate, would have been a sign of great shortsightedness." But he assumed it was possible to raise the question of sterilization in the case of Elisaveta Smerdiashchaia, a fictional character in The Brothers Karamazov, a village idiot and mother of an epileptic and murderer.[106] By contrast, Segalin, who believed her illness might have "triggered" talent in her progeny, argued decidedly against her sterilization or that of anyone else. He criticized eugenicists for not being able to identify "progenerative" pathologies, and he saw an unbridgeable gap between "the notion of eugenic value of individuals" and his own notion of "europositive value."[107]

As soon as Segalin started his journal in 1925, eugenicists argued back. In November 1926, during a discussion of europathology at the meeting of the Russian Eugenics Society, N. V. Popov accused Segalin of erroneously identifying eugenics with sterilization, and he criticized the sloppiness of Segalin's research and his use of an outdated method of statistics. Segalin claimed, in effect, that there is a "gene" for creativity and that this gene is in a latent state until released by illness; he called this the "biogenetic law of genius" (so-named by analogy with Haeckel's law, but sharing little in common with it). Popov ridiculed Segalin's biogenetic law, saying that the real genetic mechanism is completely different and that "Mendel knows neither a 'dissociating agent' [which, as Segalin supposed, releases the 'gene' of creativity], nor the appearance of new traits that do not exist in the species." He corrected Segalin's ignorance: "there is nothing but a recombination of genes which produces a phenotype with the traits that were recessive in parental genotypes." Popov attacked Segalin's standing as a scholar and questioned the validity of his references, because Segalin did not cite sources properly. Segalin, in his view, unjustifiably widened the notion of mental illness so that any odd habit and slight deviation became symptoms of disease. This allowed him and his proponents, Popov argued, to speak about even the soundest geniuses—Pushkin, Gorky, Tolstoy—as mentally ill. Popov believed mental illness destroyed rather than stimulated genius. He made his final argument against identifying talent with illness on moral grounds. He claimed that any such attempt gave the reader a "burdening, confused feeling, a taint of dirt . . . not about [the artist in question], but about those people who dig so thoroughly into his misfortunes even for science's sake." Segalin had not yet obtained "any evidence [that would allow him] to dirty the work of our greatest creator, our mother-nature."[108]

Perhaps in response to Segalin's fantasies about the "genetic mechanism" of genius, Kol'tsov claimed that one did not need a hypothesis about mutation to explain genius. In his view, the genotype of genius was nothing but a happy combination of genes "widely spread in the mass of the Russian people." Kol'tsov's article argued not only with Segalin but also with those eugenicists who were worried by the damage done to the Russian population by war and revolution. Some were especially concerned about the loss of "good blood" as a result of the proletarian terror against the upper classes. By contrast, Kol'tsov located the "good genes" in simple folk, and he claimed that the "gene pool" accumulated in the Russian population through the centuries was sufficient to produce many talented people. He took as examples the writers Gorky and Leonid Leonov, the opera artist Fedor Shaliapin, and the university professor N. P. Kravkov, whose modest origins, he believed, would convince everybody of the inextinguishable vitality of the Russian people. Kol'tsov preferred to see genius as robust rather than sickly—"the main qualities of a genius [are] energy, working and entrepreneurial abilities, creativity, and physical health and fitness." Simple folk always have these qualities in abundance, he argued, so all that is needed is to add to this healthy and vigorous stock some "gene-intensifiers" that reinforce "the brain centers of speech and logical thinking." This had often happened in the past, he stated, when the cultured sons of the nobility "sinned" with women from the lower but healthier classes. "Pushkin, Lermontov, [A. I.] Herzen, and Tolstoy must have left many illegitimate children during their stormy youth, when they, in Pushkin's phrase, 'brought sacrifices to Baccus and Venus' chasing pretty actresses and peasant beauties." During the war with Napoleon, the French, with their "highly developed centers of speech," invaded Russia, leaving behind them "gene-intensifiers" to the benefit of the Russian people. Kol'tsov hinted that captured French soldiers lived as far to the East as Nizhnii Novgorod, Gorky's hometown.[109]

Kol'tsov's article had an ideological title, "The Genealogies of Our *Vydvizhentsy.*" In Soviet newspeak, *vydvizhenets* meant someone who was promoted beyond his qualifications because of his political and class background. Implying that people thus promoted could, like the aristocracy, have their own "genealogy," Kol'tsov killed two birds with one stone: he flattered the new bureaucracy and he defended the genealogical project he was developing with other geneticists. Kol'tsov might also have wanted to improve the reputation of eugenics, as a science that is not hostile to social change and social mobility.[110] By referring to writers, artists, and professors as *vydvizhentsy,* Kol'tsov probably also attempted to prove their "genetic" closeness to the masses and therefore to protect the intelligentsia from proletarian attacks.

When Segalin asked August Forel to contribute to his *Clinical Archive,* the Swiss patriarch sent a short note implicitly critical of Segalin's project. Forel wanted to picture geniuses as healthy, and he wrote that "pathological geniuses are not sufficient for us, they should be gradually normalized with the help of eugenics . . . It is necessary to eliminate *Kakogenik* [the spread of bad traits, as opposed to the spread of good ones] which is progressing nowadays."[111] Criticizing Segalin, Soviet eugenicists distanced themselves from the discredited Lombrosian view that genius was pathological. Like their Western counterparts, they believed those who were socially superior should also be biologically superior. They also preferred not to comment on the natural abilities of party *vydvizhentsy.* References to healthy geniuses compromised neither the "greatest creator, nature" nor social creators, the authorities.

A Soviet Genius

In the atmosphere of early Soviet iconoclasm, previously sacred names were reconsidered. The old culture found itself cast into purgatory by proletarian critics. The literary associations, the futurists, and *Proletkult* (the association of workers' cultural organizations; a term derived from "proletarian culture"), who were the first to declare themselves on the side of the new regime, launched a nihilist attack on the past, threatening to "throw Pushkin and Dostoevsky overboard [from] the ship of modernity."[112] As before the Revolution, the new cultural criticism readily found support in psychiatry. Pushkin may have been a model poet for the pre-revolutionary critics and an example of perfect mental health for psychiatrists, but after the Revolution the literary young Turks denounced the classics, and psychiatrists of the younger generation questioned Pushkin's mental health.[113] Zinov'ev wrote that "in order to understand Pushkin . . . correctly, it is necessary to accept that from the psychiatric point of view he was, though a highly valuable person, yet a psychopath." He explained that to call someone "psychopathic" was not a moral judgment and that the word could be freely applied to outstanding people. To exclude any possibility of mental illness in geniuses would be "to justify the Bohemian habits of talented writers and artists as well as their tendency to abuse ordinary people." Geniuses were not an exception to the laws of nature, nor could their arrogant conduct be excused. Similarly, Rozenshtein assumed that Pushkin was a "cycloid," according to Kretschmer's classification of character, and that Pushkin's famous irony resulted from his occasional "hypomaniac states." Another psychiatrist, I. B. Galant, argued from the position of a fashionable endocrinological theory, according to which individual differences were a function of glands. He classified Pushkin as an erotomaniac with hypertrophied gonads and Gogol as a "hypogonadial type" and schizophrenic.[114]

Psychiatrists of the younger generation found "absolutely unjustified" their predecessors' unwillingness, out of respect for writers' suffering, to speak about writers' mental illnesses.[115] In his dreams about the Institute of Genius, Segalin planned for one of its departments to rewrite old-fashioned biographies, which avoided exposing the weaknesses and illnesses of outstanding people. He also encouraged contributors to the *Clinical Archive* to write pathographies of outstanding figures. The psychiatrist N. A. Iurman insisted on a thorough examination of Dostoevsky's "shadowy as well as bright sides." This was soon undertaken by a psychoanalytically oriented author, Tatiana Rozental', who interpreted Dostoevsky's disease as hysterical epilepsy. Segalin agreed with her that Dostoevsky's epilepsy was not genuine but "affective," that is, caused by traumatic influences.[116]

Alongside the ongoing reevaluation of the past, the Revolution initiated extravagant literary experiments, and in the atmosphere of relative political freedom, literary and artistic movements and groups proliferated. The symbolists' successors, the acmeists (a literary movement; a term derived from "acme"), coexisted with the militant futurists, the visionary imaginists, the peasant poets fearful of growing urbanism, and the proletarian writers, who glorified industrialization and argued that the new culture should be based not on art but on science and technology. The Communist Party leaders recognized the existence of nonproletarian writers as "fellow travelers," but they wanted to reform or break "bourgeois" writers such as the poets Alexander Blok, Andrei Bely, and Anna Akhmatova. Not coincidentally, these poets became objects of psychiatric attention. Referring to a literary critic who argued that Blok's poetry was "ill" and his romanticism "unhealthy," the Moscow psychiatrist Ia. V. Mints diagnosed Blok's "condition" as epilepsy.[117]

Mints's colleague from the town of Smolensk, V. S. Grinevich, quoted the pre-revolutionary view, repeated by proletarian critics, that symbolism and decadence were an escape from reality. He stated that so-called peasant poets escaped "from socialism into . . . a fantastic world of *muzhik* [peasant], pious, wooden Russia"; the symbolists and imaginists hid themselves in pre-logical thinking; the acmeists chose mysticism; and the futurists were nothing but Bohemian, déclassé intellectuals with no concern for the Revolution—pretending to be a literary vanguard, they were "anarchists in the worst sense of the word," a criminal crowd dangerous for the new order. Grinevich characterized as a "psychopath" a poet who boasted that he "quarreled with the commissars in the Cheka" ("Extraordinary Commission," security police), and he predicted that one day the poet could be hanged for his "anarchist yeast." (The poet was Nikolai Tikhonov, member of a "fellow travelers" group, the Serapion Brothers.) Grinevich, who presented himself as an "objective psychopathologist," concluded that the unstable, pessimistic, doubting, and schizophrenic "bourgeois" poets should give way to healthy proletarian writers. Unlike the mentally confused "bourgeois" authors, the new Soviet writers were endowed, he stated, with "classic clarity, precision, and simplicity."[118]

The beginning of 1926 was marked by the tragic death of Sergei Esenin. The thirty-year-old poet cut his veins, wrote a farewell poem, and hanged himself in a hotel room. His free spirit and turbulent life made him a target for both Bolshevik criticism and persecution by the GPU ("Principal Political Department," security police). In the language of proletarian critics, "Eseninism" became synonymous with "a dangerous disease undermining the Soviet body politic, a sign of degenerate . . . individualism, incompatible with the prescribed optimistic attitude toward life."[119] His sensational death was thought to have provoked an outbreak of suicides among young people who had become disillusioned with the Revolution. To counteract its destructive influence, the commissar of public health, Semashko, wrote two articles in which he admitted the spread of suicides but warned about exaggerating their danger. He announced that the déclassé Esenin who had taken his life could not be the model for basically healthy Soviet youth.[120]

There was evidence to support Semashko's claim that Esenin was mentally ill and out of touch with reality. Partly to help him recover from his chaotic life and heavy drinking, partly to protect him from rearrest, Esenin had been hospitalized in the Moscow University Psychiatric Clinic a month before his suicide.[121] Like Semashko, some contributors to the *Clinical Archive* perceived Esenin's suicide as proof of his alcoholic psychosis. One of them argued that Esenin buried his talent in a "bestial criminal instinct usual in alcoholics." Esenin, who grew up in a peasant family, often expressed love for nature and animals in his poems; in the psychiatrist's view, these poems reflected his "male zoophilia." Referring to the proletarian critics who found Esenin's poetry incompatible with the vigorous spirit of the time, another psychiatrist claimed that Esenin's decision to kill himself was caused by his "disharmonious conflict with the healthy and lively spirit of his age and his people."[122]

Responding to Segalin's invitation to rewrite biographies as pathographies, a young Moscow psychiatrist, Ia. V. Mints, reassessed even Jesus Christ. Pathographies of religious figures were not a new phenomenon, but psychiatrists felt especially encouraged to write them when atheism became state policy.[123] Mints diagnosed paranoia in Jesus Christ and attributed it to his asthenic constitution. Exercising Marxist analysis, Mints concluded that the founder of Christianity, who originated from a craftsman's family, had a "petty bourgeois" social background. The young atheist then argued that the same was true for Krishna, Buddha, Zarathustra, Mohammed, and Savonarola, and that these prophets had common life histories and common pathologies: "they believe that they are gods destined to save the world, they leave their families relatively late, when they have already grown up, their lives pass in seclusion, solitude, and fasting, they become vagabonds, they hallucinate. The devil tries to seduce them, but is defeated, and then they acquire followers and produce miracles of a similar kind, [for instance,] treating hysterics."[124]

Writers with established reputations were not excused from pathographies. Gorky's mental health was questioned on the ground that the writer made a suicide attempt when he was eighteen.[125] Tolstoy, Dostoevsky, Nietzsche, Byron, N. A. Nekrasov, and Honoré de Balzac underwent the same scrutiny.[126] Segalin diagnosed Tolstoy's "affective epilepsy," discovering traces of the disease in the "epileptic intensity" of his literature as well as in his supposed conservatism. He followed the earlier radical critics who had reproached Tolstoy, writing that in his struggle with tsarism Tolstoy did not go far enough, did not accept the need for revolution. Segalin's article persuaded his colleague from Baku, V. I. Rudnev, who reported that it "clarified for me both Tolstoy's world-view and his sudden change [in the late 1870s] which took all of us by surprise." Rudnev wrote that he found further evidence of Tolstoy's epilepsy in his *Memoirs of a Madman*. This only confirmed Segalin's diagnosis.[127]

It is likely that Segalin's article on Tolstoy finally caused the *Clinical Archive* to be shut down. By the end of the 1920s, the nihilist spirit and wild experiments that followed the Revolution were tamed, and the Soviet literary establishment returned to the classics. Both Tolstoy and Dostoevsky were accepted into the Soviet literary pantheon, though not without reservations. The leading critic of the 1920s, A. K. Voronskii, planned "to limit Dostoevsky's pessimism with Tolstoy and to adjust Tolstoy's optimism with Dostoevsky." He reminded the nihilists that at different times various Marxist thinkers had demonstrated their appreciation of Tolstoy. One of the older Russian Marxists had called Tolstoy "a realist in the genuine sense of the term" because his "work rests on experience, just like scientific investigation."[128] Lenin, though he viciously attacked Tolstoy's philosophy of nonresistance, respected his unique stature in Russian culture and preferred him to the new Soviet writers. He supported the publication of the unprecedented ninety-volume collection of Tolstoy's work. The Tolstoy centenary in 1928 was the first large-scale government-sponsored event celebrating a pre-revolutionary writer. It included a seven-hour celebration at the Bolshoi Theater, with the keynote address by the minister of education, Lunacharskii.[129]

Segalin's article on Tolstoy appeared in 1929 in the fourth year of publication of the *Clinical Archive;* the next issue, though announced, was not published. Following the pattern of Stalinist political campaigns, the journal's end was accompanied by a series of critical articles written not by political leaders but by psychiatrists. A psychiatrist from the provinces, N. I. Balaban, published a critical review of Segalin's article on Tolstoy in the official organ of the Society of Psychoneurologists-Materialists, *Soviet Psychoneurology (Sove-*

tskaia psikhonevrologiia). He argued that Segalin's diagnosis of Tolstoy would confuse the reader familiar with the writer's international reputation. Lenin's and Lunacharskii's view of Tolstoy as a sober realist stood in sharp contrast to Segalin's image of a hallucinating writer. Segalin had argued that Tolstoy, before he was fifty, was at a "manic stage" and that later his "affective epilepsy" switched to a "depressive stage." In Balaban's view, Segalin repeated the outdated cliché about Tolstoy's "sudden crisis" that had already been rejected by literary historians. Balaban insisted that Tolstoy's changes should not be explained by illness, and he criticized Segalin for reproducing suspicious Lombrosian views without enriching medical knowledge.[130]

Balaban's article confirmed the end of Segalin's initiatives. In the late 1920s, Segalin still believed the Institute of Genius stood a chance. His hopes were revived when he heard that "some psychological circles" in Moscow had discussed an idea for a "eurological institute." He also learned about the Academy of Sciences' decision to establish a "central organ" superintending the conditions of scientists' life and work. Further, the success of neuropsychiatric dispensaries encouraged Segalin to raise the question of "special dispensaries for creative people." The ambitions of social hygienists had indeed grown, and they campaigned to place all medical institutions under the control of the "united dispensary."[131] Their objectives were to screen the population, to introduce health passports for every worker, "to calculate the coefficient of work capacity," and to provide "timely prophylactic, curative, sanitary and social aid."[132] In Segalin's mind, dispensaries for geniuses would similarly control "abnormal and asocial art" and stimulate "unproductive euroneurotics" with the help of "eurotherapy."[133] Yet, together with the Institute of Genius and aesthetic medicine, this plan had to be abandoned in circumstances that were becoming unfavorable for mental and social hygiene in general.

By the 1930s, despite its widely publicized strategy for public health that had attracted the attention of socialist-oriented physicians in the West, Narkomzdrav was in crisis.[134] It lacked the funds to cope with the consequences of forced industrialization and collectivization. The welfare services were not able to match the growth of the urban population resulting from famine in the countryside. The gap between the ambition of preventive medicine and the social reality was obvious. In 1931 a government decree indicated the grim situation in the understaffed and undersupplied mental hospitals, where the number of patients many times exceeded the intended population. The decree directed Rozenshtein's Institute of Neuropsychiatric Prophylaxis to coordinate mental care, which diverted the institute from its preventive strategies. The decree also ordered that no other institutions of preventive psychiatry were to be founded.[135] The dispensary campaign slowed down, and its main proponents disappeared from the stage. In 1930 the patron of social hygiene, Semashko, was removed from his post as commissar of public health. The new Narkomzdrav strategy was more class-oriented and concentrated on establishing medical facilities for workers at their workplaces.[136]

Rozenshtein was criticized for an attempt "to expand medical control over all facets of social life and to substitute . . . socialist public health with mental hygiene."[137] Zinov'ev's thoughtless remark that "the dispensary should search for its clients among those who consider themselves healthy" provided an opportunity to turn public opinion against mental hygiene.[138] Hygienists were reproached for broadening the notions of mental illness and occupational trauma to the extent that the whole population was made to appear pathological. Critics stated that an excessively broad concept of mental hygiene granted physician-hygienists unjustified "rights to treat, teach, direct, regulate, and interfere in all the complex relationships of life," including economics and politics.[139] Taken aback, Rozenshtein's colleagues began to claim that many problems with mental health were nonexistent and that "large numbers of people [had] found a tremendous amount of plasticity within themselves, enabling them to adjust to the new conditions." They even announced that the need for state support for "victims of war and revolution" was decreasing significantly.[140] Rozenshtein, who persisted in finding many neurotics in need of mental care, was forced to recant publicly.[141] He died two years later. His Institute of Neuropsychiatric Prophylaxis passed into the hands of clinical psychiatrists who vigorously opposed dispensarization. The new administration renamed the department of mental hygiene the "experimental department" and removed the emphasis on prophylaxis from the title of the institute, which now became the Institute of Psychiatry.[142]

Segalin's marginal position as a provincial psychiatrist protected him from physical repression, but his idea of europathology was destroyed in embryo. Its association with eugenics, which in the West had now acquired racial connotations, made it especially vulnerable. In 1928 both the German Society of Mental Hygiene and the London Eugenic Society initiated a campaign for sterilization as a preventive measure against mental illnesses. Three years later, National Socialists in the Reichstag petitioned for the sterilization of hereditary criminals. The founding father of German racial hygiene, Alfred Ploetz, as the historian Paul Weindling remarks, "metamorphosed from being an admirer of Kautsky to a supporter of Hitler."[143] These developments were completely unacceptable in the Soviet Union and endangered the position of eugenics, notes Mark Adams, historian of Soviet eugenics. In 1930 the Russian Eugenics Society was disbanded and its journal terminated, almost simultaneously with Segalin's journal: "no field that linked the biological and the social survived the Great Break intact"[144] The connection between the social and the biological, a sensitive issue for Marxist philosophy, became the focus of political battles in biology.[145]

Literature was equally politicized. Throughout the 1920s the Communist Party kept a watchful eye on literary struggles. When, by the end of that decade, the most militant proletarian group, RAPP (Russian Association of Proletarian Writers), had strangled all others, a Party resolution abolished all literary associations and established a monopoly of the Union of Soviet Writers, with a Communist faction as its core.[146] Stalin upgraded reformed writers into "engineers of human souls." This phrase, as was said at the union's congress in 1934, meant "breaking away from old-type romanticism, from that romanticism that depicted nonexistent life and nonexistent characters, diverting the reader from the contradictions and oppressions of life into a world of the impossible, a world of Utopia."[147] But the suffocating doctrine of socialist realism, which, as historians have demonstrated, was inaugurated at the 1934 congress, was rooted in pre-revolutionary radical criticism and the idea of the social mission of art.[148]

The sober members of the Writers' Union did not favor the idea that "madmen, hermits, heretics, dreamers, rebels, and skeptics" created literature.[149] Alexander Fadeev, the principal spokesman for socialist realism, once stated that "a new step forward in the development of mankind" would be taken if "socialist ideology" were blended together with "the genius of a true artist." From Fadeev's point of view, however, "the genius of a true artist" was healthy. The Lombrosian idea of ill geniuses became completely unacceptable. The psychiatrists who defended it could not excuse themselves by claiming scientific neutrality. When Cesare Lombroso's contemporaries reproached him for "compromising" genius by his theories, he wrote in his defense, "but has not nature caused to grow from similar germs, and on the same clod of earth, the nettle and the jasmine, the aconite and the rose? The botanist cannot be blamed for these coincidences." In the 1930s it was no longer possible to argue that scientists only revealed the laws of nature; the myth of politically neutral psychiatry ceased to work.[150]

Distancing themselves from the tradition of Lombroso and Paul Julius Möbius, psychiatrists rejected the genre of pathography. Only Zinov'ev still insisted that "everybody is pathological to a certain degree" and claimed that one can write a pathography of any average person. In 1934, however, he also hastened to argue that a "social evaluation of great people's deeds" lay beyond psychiatric competence. Gannushkin, leader of the Moscow psychiatrists, closed the door on the compromised genre. In a book (1933) that became his last message to his confreres, he wrote, "History is interested only in results, and mainly in those elements that have general and eternal, not personal and individual, character. The creative person whose biological value does not have the same significance as his creation, has objectively vanished into the background of history. The debate whether genius is a phenomenon of degeneration or progeneration is fruitless and results from the incorrect confusion of the biological and sociological points of view."[151]

Gannushkin held in suspicion not only pathography but also psychotherapy and psychoanalysis. When, in the early 1920s, E. N. Dovbnia announced a course in psychotherapy, the first at Moscow University, Gannushkin expressed his own opinion in an introductory lecture. He virtually devalued the course, telling the students that psychotherapy in a broad sense was not special, as "at any moment [of contact with a patient] any of us is doing psychotherapy"; psychotherapy proper, by contrast, could be dangerous. Though Gannushkin accepted rational therapy, hypnosis and psychoanalysis made him anxious: "Hypnosis . . . manipulates people into stupid fools . . . Psychoanalysis crudely intervenes in the patient's sexual life, traumatizing his psyche. I have more than once observed that physicians, as in morphine and other drug addictions, may cause the disease. [Similarly], one can speak about patients obsessed by the illness 'Freud.'"[152] Educated in the spirit of conventional French and German psychiatry, Gannushkin saw his patients in terms of inherited constitutions and congenital degeneracy and did not believe they could benefit from psychotherapy. The term *pathography* gradually disappeared. As an alternative, the term *sociography* appeared in literary history to give a name to studies in which a writer's style was analyzed in the light of life history and social milieu.[153] A purely social concept of biography replaced the notion of biological illness as a driving force of creative life, a view that contradicted the officially prescribed optimistic mood.

The other principal promoter of pathographies, I. D. Ermakov (1875–1942), was silenced together with Segalin. Like Segalin, Ermakov was a professional painter, and he was allied with a vanguard group named World of Art (*Mir iskusstva*). After graduating from Moscow University in 1902, he worked in the University Psychiatric Clinic, studied traumatic psychoses during the Russo-Japanese war, and became interested in psychoanalysis. In 1920 he organized a psychoanalytic boarding school for young children, and three years later he cofounded the Psychoanalytic Institute in Moscow.

Contemporaries called his version of psychoanalysis "artistic" or "aesthetic" (*khudozhestvennyi*), because of his interest in works of art and in artists' lives. Between 1923 and 1925 Ermakov published his studies of Gogol and Pushkin and edited the *Psychological and Psychoanalytic Library,* a series of translations and original works. He also wrote pathographies of Dostoevsky and M. A. Vrubel (1856–1901), the painter whom he treated in the Moscow University Clinic.[154] In the early 1920s psychoanalysts hoped they could achieve a synthesis of Freudianism with Marxism, but these debates were abandoned by the end of the decade.[155] Ermakov's Psychoanalytic Institute was closed and the publication of his *Library* stopped. In the 1930s he worked occasionally as a consultant to mental hospitals, until he was arrested on a political charge; he perished in the GULAG in 1942.

In spite of this shadow thrown across the writing of pathographies, their end was not caused solely by the contemporary political events. The criticism of Lombroso's views on genius started in the nineteenth century. Similarly, the question of whether pathography was an appropriate way to treat great men arose long before the 1930s, when Soviet psychiatrists finally dismissed it as a "bourgeois" genre. In other words, even in the Soviet Union, the rejection of pathographies had intellectual as well as ideological grounds. Thus, in 1981, the philosopher E. Iu. Solov'ev criticized pathographies by contrasting the pessimistic view that life is driven by illness, common to psychiatric and psychoanalytic writing, to the brighter outlook expressed in "hermeneutic" or "existential" biographies:

Where a hermeneutic biographer speaks about self-identity, acquisition of selfhood, and sense of mission, a pathographer sees the disintegration of the individual's self and an alien and ill part that was previously integrated. This disintegration is interpreted sometimes as a struggle (S. Zweig), as self-estrangement (K. Jaspers), as a sober irony, which provides adaptive sublimation (S. Freud). The general assumption, however, is that the initial impulse of personal development comes from illness. An endless variety of historical individuals are assembled into a table where in the horizontal boxes there are psychic traumas and anomalies, and in the vertical boxes there are typical ways of reacting to them.[156]

Solov'ev's preference for "hermeneutic biography" was influenced by both the intellectual arguments of existentialism and the ideological arguments asserting social optimism.

The writing of pathographies reappeared with glasnost in the late 1980s. A rehabilitation of the genre came from Segalin's home town, Sverdlovsk (with the end of the Soviet Union, its original name, Ekaterinburg, was restored). Inviting his colleagues to write pathographies, the author attributes their disappearance in the Soviet period to political causes. He calls for the restoration of continuity with pre-revolutionary psychiatry and the revival of projects, such as psychotherapy and the "objective" study of genius, that were interrupted by politicians. Though the Ural psychiatrist, like the members of his profession before him, stresses the "objective" study of genius, his manifesto, written in the style typical of glasnost publications, once again confirms that these studies are firmly anchored in political culture. The rich history of the genre of pathography reflects the rich cultural meaning of psychiatry.[157]

NOTES

Abbreviations

ARAN	Arkhiv Rossiiskoi akademii nauk (Archive of the Russian Academy of Sciences)
Arkhiv psikhiatrii	*Arkhiv psikhiatrii, neirologii i sudebnoi psikhologii*
GARF	Gosudarstvennyi arkhiv Rossiiskoi Federatsii (State Archive of the Russian Federation)
Klinicheskii arkhiv	*Klinicheskii arkhiv genial'nosti i odarennosti* . . . (see Chapter 5, n. 91)
Obozrenie psikhiatrii	*Obozrenie psikhiatrii, nevrologii i eksperimental'noi psikhologii*
TsGALI	Tsentral'nyi gosudarstvennyi arkhiv literatury i iskusstva (Central State Archive of Literature and Arts)
TsGIAM	Tsentral'nyi gosudarstvennyi arkhiv istorii i arkhitektury Moskvy (Central State Archive of the History and Architecture of Moscow)
Vestnik klinicheskoi	*Vestnik klinicheskoi i sudebnoi psikhiatrii i nevropatologii*
Vestnik psikhologii	*Vestnik psikhologii, kriminal'noi antropologii i gipnotizma*
Voprosy filosofii	*Voprosy filosofii i psikhologii*
Zhurnal nevropatologii	*Zhurnal nevropatologii i psikhiatrii imeni S. S. Korsakova*

Archival locations are denoted by f. (*fond*, collection); op. (*opis'*, inventory); d. (*delo*, file); ed. khr. (*edinitsa khraneniia*, storage unit); and l., ll. (*list, listy*, folio, folios).

Introduction

Epigraphs: R. V. Ivanov-Razumnik, *Istoriia russkoi obshchestvennoi mysli: Individualism i meshchanstvo v russkoi literature i zhizni XIX veka,* 3d ed. (St. Petersburg: M. M. Stasiulevich, 1911), 13–14; and I. A. Sikorskii, *Psikhologicheskoe napravlenie khudozhestvennogo tvorchestva Gogolia (Rech' v pamiat' 100-letnei godovshchiny Gogolia, [April 10, 1909])* (Kiev: Universitet Sv. Vladimira, 1911), 11.

1. Paul Julius Möbius, quoted in Francis Schiller, *A Möbius Strip: Fin-de-siècle Neuropsychiatry and Paul Möbius* (Berkeley: Univ. of California Press, 1982), 80.

2. The genre of "pathography" became widespread at the turn of the century, but later was overshadowed by a similar genre, "psychobiography." Though "pathog-

raphy" is again in use, Möbius's authorship is often forgotten and reference is made mainly to Freud. See, e.g., Anne Hawkins, "The Two Pathographies: A Study in Illness and Literature," *Journal of Medicine and Philosophy* 9 (1984): 231–52.

3. For an example of a neurophysiological study, see Loraine K. Obler and Deborah Fein, eds., *The Exceptional Brain: Neurophysiology of Talent and Special Abilities* (New York: Guilford, 1989). Psychological studies usually locate creativity in cognitive processes; see, e.g., Albert Rothenberg, *Creativity and Madness: New Findings and Old Stereotypes* (Baltimore: Johns Hopkins Univ. Press, 1990). Some psychologists relate their work directly to Cesare Lombroso and Max Nordau. Colin Martindale, for instance, argues that the characteristics Lombroso attributed to diseased geniuses could be used to develop a psychology of creative processes. See Colin Martindale, "Degeneration, Disinhibition, and Genius," *Journal of the History of the Behavioral Sciences* 7 (1971): 177–82. For a recent attempt to redefine creativity in psychobiological terms, see Hans Eysenck, *Genius: The Natural History of Creativity* (Cambridge: Cambridge Univ. Press, 1995).

4. Michael Neve, "Medicine and Literature," in *Companion Encyclopedia of the History of Medicine,* ed. W. F. Bynum and Roy Porter (London: Routledge, 1993), 2: 1530.

5. Erving Goffman, *Stigma: Notes on the Management of Spoiled Identity* (Englewood Cliffs, N.J.: Prentice-Hall, 1963); Jack P. Gibbs, *Norms, Deviance, and Social Control* (New York: Elsevier, 1981).

6. See, e.g., Peter Conrad and Joseph W. Schneider, *Deviance and Medicalization: From Badness to Sickness* (St. Louis: C. V. Mosby, 1980). The exploration of madness in terms of control and power was pioneered by such works as Michel Foucault, *Madness and Civilization* (New York: Random House, 1965); Erving Goffman, *Asylums* (New York: Anchor, 1961); David Rothman, *The Discovery of the Asylum* (Boston: Little, Brown, 1971); and Thomas S. Szasz, *The Manufacture of Madness* (New York: Harper & Row, 1970).

7. George Becker, *The Mad Genius Controversy: A Study in the Sociology of Deviance* (Beverly Hills, Calif.: Sage, 1978), 48.

8. Ibid., 28.

9. Mark Micale observes a chronological connection between the emergence of pathographies in France and the medical legitimization of the concept of male hysteria. He also points out that pathography presaged psychobiography and the psychoanalytic criticism of art. See Mark S. Micale, *Approaching Hysteria: Disease and Its Interpretations* (Princeton: Princeton Univ. Press, 1995), 245.

10. On the construction of deviant self-identity by modern American artists, see Ronald J. Silvers, "The Modern Artists' Asociability: Constructing a Situated Moral Revolution," in *Deviance and Respectability: The Social Construction of Moral Meanings,* ed. Jack D. Douglas (New York: Basic Books, 1970), 404–34.

11. George Becker, "The Mad Genius Controversy," in *Genius and Eminence: The Social Psychology of Creativity and Exceptional Achievement,* ed. Robert S. Albert (Oxford:

Pergamon, 1983), 38; R. S. Porter, *A Social History of Madness: Stories of the Insane* (London: Routledge, 1987), 65.

12. Becker, *Mad Genius Controversy,* 48. Sander L. Gilman brings together in his works the issue of medical representations and wider cultural references of racial and gender stigmatization. See, e.g., his *Disease and Representation: Images of Illness from Madness to AIDS* (Ithaca, N.Y.: Cornell Univ. Press, 1988); and *The Case of Sigmund Freud: Medicine and Identity at the Fin de Siècle* (Baltimore: Johns Hopkins Univ. Press, 1993).

13. Schiller, *Möbius Strip,* 81, 79–80.

14. Michael J. Clark, "The Rejection of Psychological Approaches to Mental Disorder in Late Nineteenth-Century British Psychiatry," in *Madhouses, Mad-Doctors, and Madmen: The Social History of Psychiatry in the Victorian Era,* ed. Andrew Scull (London: Athlone, 1981), 292; P. I. Kovalevskii, "Ioann Groznyi i ego dushevnoe sostoianie," in *Psikhiatricheskie eskizy iz istorii,* vol. 2 (Khar'kov: Zil'berberg, 1893).

15. Maudsley quoted in Helen Small, "'In the Guise of Science': Literature and the Rhetoric of Nineteenth-Century English Psychiatry," *History of the Human Sciences,* 1994, no. 1: 44; M. O. Shaikevich, "Psikhologicheskie cherty geroev Maksima Gor'kogo," *Vestnik psikhologii,* 1904, no. 1: 55.

16. Christopher Lawrence, "Incommunicable Knowledge: Science, Technology, and the Clinical Art in Britain," *Journal of Contemporary History* 20 (1985): 503–20; Small, "'In the Guise of Science,'" 47.

17. Chernyshevsky quoted in Richard Pipes, *Russia under the Old Regime* (New York: Charles Scribner's Sons, 1974), 278–79; also quoted by Joseph Frank in *Through the Russian Prism: Essays on Literature and Culture* (Princeton: Princeton Univ. Press, 1990), 154.

18. Pipes, *Russia under the Old Regime,* 279; Victor Terras, *Belinskij and Russian Literary Criticism: The Heritage of Organic Aesthetics* (Madison: Univ. of Wisconsin Press, 1974), 16.

19. R. A. Peace, *Russian Literature and the Fictionalization of Life* (Hull, U.K.: Hull Univ. Press, 1976), 11.

20. Solzhenitsyn quoted in Joe Andrew, *Russian Writers and Society in the Second Half of the Nineteenth Century* (London: Macmillan, 1982), xiv.

21. V. V. Rozanov, "Tri momenta v istorii russkoi kritiki" [1892], in *Sochineniia* (Moscow: Sovetskaia Rossiia, 1990), 156.

22. N. N. Bazhenov, *Psikhiatricheskie besedy na literaturnye i obshchestvennye temy* (Moscow: Mamontov, 1903), 24.

23. I. A. Sikorskii, "Uspekhi russkogo khudozhestvennogo tvorchestva: Rech' v torzhestvennom zasedanii II-go s"ezda otechestvennykh psikhiatrov v Kieve," *Voprosy nervno-psikhicheskoi meditsiny,* 1905, no. 3: 497–504; no. 4: 613.

24. The psychiatrist G. Ia. Troshin, for instance, claimed that Pushkin gave a literary account of schizophrenia in *Queen of Spades* (1834). See G. Ia. Troshin, *Pushkin i psikhologiia tvorchestva* (Prague: Society of Russian Physicians in Czechoslovakia,

1937), 304. Similarly, the psychiatrist N. N. Bazhenov wrote that Dostoevsky "gave exact descriptions of mental illnesses which we did not know until recently." See N. Bajenoff [Bazhenov], *Gui de Maupassant et Dostoïewsky: Etude de psychologie comparée* (Lyon: Stork & Masson, 1904), 24.

25. V. M. Bekhterev, "Dostoevsky i khudozhestvennaia psikhopatologiia," in S. Belov and N. Agitova, "V. M. Bekhterev o Dostoevskom," *Russkaia literatura,* 1962, no. 4: 139.

26. V. F. Chizh, *Turgenev kak psikhopatolog* (Moscow: Kushnerev, 1899), 104.

27. A. O. Kellog (1866), quoted in Ekbert Faas, *Retreat into the Mind: Victorian Poetry and the Rise of Psychiatry* (Princeton: Princeton Univ. Press, 1988), 31.

28. V. F. Chizh, "Pliushkin, kak tip starcheskogo slaboumiia," *Vrachebnaia gazeta,* 1902, no. 10: 217; V. A. Muratov, quoted in T. E. Segalov, "Bolezn' Dostoevskogo" [1907], trans. F. Ge, *Nauchnoe slovo,* 1929, no. 4: 92.

29. The mouthpiece of this approach is the quarterly journal *Literature and Medicine,* published since 1982.

30. Henri Ellenberger, *The Discovery of the Unconscious: The History and Evolution of Dynamic Psychiatry* (London: Allen Lane, 1970), 283: "It has been already pointed out that many of Pinel's case histories seem to be borrowed from Balzac's novels. In the same way, Janet's patients show remarkable similarities with some of Zola's characters . . . However, Hofmannsthal's Elektra resembles Breuer's celebrated Anna O. much more than Euripides' Elektra, and Freud's Dora seems to belong to one of Schnitzler's short stories . . . It was from the same refined and highly eroticized fin-de-siècle milieu that the ones drew their literary characters, the others their patients"; Micale, *Approaching Hysteria,* 245.

31. James L. Rice, *Dostoevsky and the Healing Art: An Essay in Literary and Medical History* (Ann Arbor, Mich.: Ardis, 1985).

32. Bajenoff, *Maupassant et Dostoïewsky,* 36.

33. In 1888 Tolstoy spent a few weeks in Dr. Ogranovich's "sanitary colony for neurotics" near Moscow. See S. A. Tolstaia, *Dnevniki: Part 2: 1891–1897* (Moscow: Sabashnikovy, 1929), 108, 236.

34. Later in the Soviet period, psychiatry was often used as an instrument of political repression. This topic, however, lies outside the boundaries of the present research. There is a large body of literature on the history of psychiatric abuse in the Soviet Union; see, e.g., Sidney Bloch and Peter Reddaway, *Soviet Psychiatric Abuse: The Shadow over World Psychiatry* (London: Victor Gollancz, 1984); Semyon Gruzman, *On Soviet Totalitarian Psychiatry* (Amsterdam: International Association of the Political Use of Psychiatry, 1989); Zh. A. Medvedev and R. A. Medvedev, *A Question of Madness,* trans. Ellen de Kadt (London: Macmillan, 1971); Alexander Podrabinek, *Punitive Medicine,* trans. Alexander Lehrman (Ann Arbor, Mich.: Karoma, 1980); Theresa C. Smith and Thomas A. Oleszczuk, *No Asylum: State Psychiatric Repression in the Former USSR* (New York: New York Univ. Press, 1996); Robert van Voren, ed., *Soviet Psy-*

chiatric Abuse in the Gorbachev Era (Amsterdam: International Association of the Political Use of Psychiatry, 1989).

35. D. D. Fedotov, *Ocherki po istorii otechestvennoi psikhiatrii (vtoraia polovina XVIII veka i pervaia polovina XIX veka)* (Moscow: Institut psikhiatrii, 1957); T. I. Iudin, *Ocherki istorii otechestvennoi psikhiatrii* (Moscow: Medgiz, 1951).

36. Recent Russian-language scholarship is rather scarce and consists mainly of biographical articles scattered in psychiatric journals. The works by A. G. Gerish are the most informative; see his *P. B. Gannushkin* (Moscow: Meditsina, 1975) and *P. P. Kashchenko (1859–1920)* (Moscow: Meditsina, 1980), and references to his works in the chapters that follow.

37. See Julie Vail Brown's "The Professionalization of Russian Psychiatry: 1857–1922" (Ph.D. diss., Univ. of Pennsylvania, 1981); "Heroes and Non-Heroes: Recurring Themes in the Historiography of Russian-Soviet Psychiatry," in *Discovering the History of Psychiatry*, ed. M. S. Micale and Roy Porter (New York: Oxford Univ. Press, 1994), 297–307; "Revolution and Psychosis: The Mixing of Science and Politics in Russian Psychiatric Medicine, 1905–13," *Russian Review* 46 (1987): 283–302; "Professionalization and Radicalization: Russian Psychiatrists Respond to 1905," in *Russia's Missing Middle Class: The Professions in Russian History*, ed. Harley D. Balzer (Armonk, N.Y.: M. E. Sharpe, 1996), 143–67; "Psychiatrists and the State in Tsarist Russia," in *Social Control and the State*, ed. Stanley Cohen and Andrew Scull (New York: M. Robertson, 1983), 267–87; and "Social Influences on Psychiatric Theory and Practice in Late Imperial Russia," in *Health and Society in Revolutionary Russia*, ed. Susan Gross Solomon and John F. Hutchinson (Bloomington: Indiana Univ. Press, 1990), 27–44.

Kenneth Steven Dix, "Madness in Russia, 1775–1864: Official Attitudes and Institutions for Its Care" (Ph.D. diss., Univ. of California, 1977); David Joravsky, *Russian Psychology: A Critical History* (Oxford: Blackwell, 1989).

38. For a good brief English-language presentation of the history of Russian psychiatry prior to the Revolution, see Brown's "Psychiatrists and the State in Tsarist Russia." I draw in part on her account in the following paragraphs.

39. There is a rapidly growing body of scholarship on the history of psychoanalysis in Russia, see, e.g., Alberto Angelini, *La psicanalisi in Russia: dai precursori agli anni trenta* (Naples: Liguori Editore, 1988); Michèle Bertrand, ed., *Psychanalyse en Russie* (Paris: L'Harmattan, 1992); Alexander Etkind, *Eros of the Impossible: The History of Psychoanalysis in Russia,* trans. Noah Rubins and Maria Rubins (Boulder, Colo.: Westview, 1997); James L. Rice, *Freud's Russia: National Identity in the Evolution of Psychoanalysis* (New Brunswick, N.J.: Transaction, 1993); V. M. Leibin, ed., *Zigmund Freid, psikhoanaliz i russkaia mysl'* (Moscow: Respublika, 1994); Magnus Ljunggren, *The Russian Mephisto: A Study of the Life and Work of Emilii Medtner* (Stockholm: Almqvist & Wiksell International, 1994); Martin Miller, *Freud and the Bolsheviks: Psychoanalysis in Imperial Russia and the Soviet Union* (New Haven: Yale Univ. Press, 1998).

One. Gogol, Moralists, and Nineteenth-Century Psychiatry

Epigraphs: Nikolai Gogol, *Diary of a Madman and Other Stories*, trans. Ronald Wilks (London: Penguin Books, 1972), 33–34 (*The Diary of a Madman* first published in 1835); I. D. Ermakov, *Ocherki po analizu tvorchestva Gogolia (Organichnost' proizvedenii Gogolia)* (Moscow: GIZ, 1922), 221.

1. "Your life was an enigma, so is today your death"; P. A. Viazemskii, quoted in Victor Erlich, *Gogol* (New Haven: Yale Univ. Press, 1969), 210.

2. For the English translation see Gogol, *Selected Passages from Correspondence with Friends*, trans. Jesse Zeldin (Nashville: Vanderbilt Univ. Press, 1969).

3. Quoted in Ruth Sobel, *Gogol's Forgotten Book:* Selected Passages *and Its Contemporary Readers* (Washington: Univ. Press of America, 1981), 186.

4. V. G. Belinsky, "Letter to N. V. Gogol" [1847], in *Belinsky, Chernyshevsky, and Dobroliubov: Selected Criticism,* ed. Ralph E. Matlaw (Bloomington: Indiana Univ. Press, 1976), 83.

5. Gogol, *Selected Passages,* 139.

6. Belinsky, "Letter to N. V. Gogol," 85.

7. See, e.g., Victor Terras, *Belinskij and Russian Literary Criticism* (Madison: Univ. of Wisconsin Press, 1974).

8. Isaiah Berlin, *Russian Thinkers,* ed. Henry Hardy and Aileen Kelly (London: Penguin Books, 1994), 116.

9. On the idea of "two Gogols" see Robert A. Maguire, "Introduction," in *Gogol from the Twentieth Century: Eleven Essays,* ed., trans., and intro. Robert A. Maguire (Princeton: Princeton Univ. Press, 1974), 11–13.

10. Gogol quoted in Sobel, *Gogol's Forgotten Book,* 272, 179.

11. Vladimir Nabokov, *Nikolai Gogol* (New York: New Directions, 1961), 129.

12. A. P. Tarasenkov, quoted in V. I. Shenrok, *Materialy dlia biografii N. V. Gogolia* (Moscow: Lissner & Geshel', 1897), 4: 860.

13. Pogodin quoted in Vladimir Voropaev, "Poslednie dni Nikolaia Gogolia," *Literaturnaia ucheba,* 1992, no. 2: 55; N. G. Chernyshevsky, [Review of] "Zapiski o zhizni Nikolaia Vasil'evicha Gogolia, St. Petersburg, 1856" [1856], in *N. V. Gogol' v russkoi kritike,* ed. A. K. Kotov and M. Ia. Poliakov (Moscow: Khudozhestvennaia literatura, 1953), 391–406; I. S. Turgenev, "Gogol" [1869], in *N. V. Gogol v russkoi kritike i vospominaniiakh sovremennikov,* ed. S. Mashinskii (Moscow: GIZ detskoi literatury, 1951), 318 (Turgenev added that after talking to Gogol, his first impression of "fatigue, sickness and nervous restlessness" disappeared); Nikolai M. [P. A. Kulish], *Zapiski o zhizni N. V. Gogolia,* 2 vols. (St. Petersburg, 1856).

14. Shenrok, *Materialy,* 16, 28, 862.

15. Cesare Lombroso, *Genio e follia* [1863], translated into English as *The Man of Genius* (London: Walter Scott, 1891), 98–99.

16. N. N. Bazhenov, "Bolezn' i smert' Gogolia," *Russkaia mysl',* 1902, no. 1: 133–49; no. 2: 52–71. Published also as a book, *Bolezn' i smert' Gogolia* (Moscow, 1902). See

an abridged translation into English, "Dr. N. N. Bazhenov on Gogol," in *The Completion of Russian Literature,* ed. Andrew Field (New York: Atheneum, 1971), 83–99. I quote from the latter edition when possible.

17. "Dr. N. N. Bazhenov," 99.

18. Tarasenkov quoted in Shenrok, *Materialy,* 864.

19. "Dr. N. N. Bazhenov," 85–86.

20. Bazhenov, *Bolezn',* 4.

21. Ibid., 32–33.

22. "Dr. N. N. Bazhenov," 86–91.

23. Chizh's 1902 speech published as V. F. Chizh, *Bolezn' N. V. Gogolia* (Moscow: Kushnerev, 1904), 216.

24. For biographical information on Chizh, see F. S. Tekut'ev, *Istoricheskii ocherk kafedry i kliniki dushevnykh i nervnykh boleznei pri Imperatorskoi Voenno-Meditsinskoi Akademii* (St. Petersburg: Voennaia tipografiia, 1898), 216–20.

25. D. N. Ovsianiko-Kulikovskii, "Iz istorii russkoi intelligentsii: Vospominaniia," in *Literaturno-kriticheskie raboty* (Moscow: Khudozhestvennaia literatura, 1989), 2: 307. Ovsianiko-Kulikovskii intended to give an intimate account of his inner life and even attempted a "psychoanalytic study" of himself.

26. V. F. Chizh, *Kriminal'naia antropologiia* (Odessa: G. Beilenson & I. Iurovskii, 1895), 50.

27. Ovsianiko-Kulikovskii, "Iz istorii," 309.

28. N. N. Bazhenov, "Vtoroi mezhdunarodnyi kongress kriminal'noi antropologii," *Voprosy filosofii,* 1889, no. 2: 17–41.

29. A. K. Vul'fert, "Vozrazheniia na referat d-ra Bazhenova o s"ezde kriminal'noi antropologii," *Voprosy filosofii,* 1889, no. 2: 41–46.

30. V. P. Serbskii, "Prestupnye i chestnye liudi," *Voprosy filosofii,* 1896, no. 5: 669.

31. Stephen Jay Gould, *The Mismeasure of Man* (New York: Norton, 1981), 122.

32. V. F. Chizh, "Obozrenie sochinenii po kriminal'noi antropologii," *Arkhiv psikhiatrii,* 1893, no. 3: 106. On the criticism of Lombroso by Russian psychiatrists see, e.g., P. Tarnovskaia's review of the Russian translation of *The Criminal Man,* in *Vestnik klinicheskoi,* 1885, no. 1: 278–96.

33. V. F. Chizh, "K ucheniiu ob organicheskoi prestupnosti," *Arkhiv psikhiatrii,* 1893, no. 1: 176. A fragment of Prichard's *Treatise on Insanity* (1835), in which the notion of moral insanity was formulated, was first published in Russian as "Nravstvennoe pomeshatel'stvo" in *Arkhiv psikhiatrii,* 1893, no. 3: 53–68, but the treatise was already known to Russian psychiatrists in English or German versions. On the concept of moral insanity, see Eric T. Carlson and Norman Dain, "The Meaning of Moral Insanity," *Bulletin of the History of Medicine,* 1962, no. 1: 130–40.

34. Chizh, *Kriminal'naia,* 46–47, 50.

35. V. F. Chizh, *Dostoevsky kak psikhopatolog* (Moscow: M. Katkov, 1885), 72; Dostoevsky quoted in ibid., 70.

36. Henry Havelock Ellis, *The Criminal,* 3d ed. (London: Walter Scott, 1901), 141.

37. L. V. Blumenau, quoted in T. I. Iudin, *Ocherki istorii otechestvennoi psikhiatrii* (Moscow: Medgiz, 1951), 114. Altogether, twenty-six students obtained their degrees from Merzheevskii's clinic.

38. Tekut'ev, *Istoricheskii,* 216.

39. Joe Sim, *Medical Power in Prisons: The Prison Medical Service in England, 1774–1989* (Milton Keynes, U.K.: Open Univ. Press, 1990), 57.

40. See Paul Nitsche and Karl Willmans, *The History of the Prison Psychoses,* trans. Francis M. Barnes and Bernard Glück (New York: Journal of Nervous and Mental Diseases Publishing Co., 1912).

41. Chizh, *Dostoevsky,* 10–11.

42. V. F. Chizh, *Uchebnik psikhiatrii* (St. Petersburg: Sotrudnik, 1911), 37.

43. V. F. Chizh, "Nravstvennost' dushevno-bol'nykh," *Voprosy filosofii,* 1891, no. 3: 129.

44. On Moreau, see Virginia Berridge and Griffith Edwards, *Opium and the People: Opiate Use in Nineteenth-Century England* (London: Allen Lane/St. Martin, 1981), 68. On Charcot, see Jean Tuillier, *Monsieur Charcot de la Salpêtrière* (Paris: Robert Laffont, 1993), 45.

45. Danillo graduated from the Medical-Surgical Academy in 1874. He was a physician in the army during the Russo–Turkish war (1877–79). Having defended his doctoral dissertation, he studied in France. He returned to Russia in 1884 and, taught at the Military-Medical Academy until his early death. See Tekut'ev, *Istoricheskii,* 197. Besides his work with Richet on coca, Danillo also conducted his own research on the effect of absinthe on animals with one brain hemisphere surgically removed. In 1883 he was elected a member of the Société médico-psychologique, Société anthropologique, and Société anatomique de Paris. Charles Richet reported on this work in *L'Homme et l'intelligence: fragments de physiologie et de psychologie* (Paris: Félix Alcan, 1884).

46. Danillo quoted in Richet, *L'Homme,* 499–500. Danillo and Richet's original reads: "l'ablation du cervaux fait perdre à l'animal opéré le pouvoir d'inhibition; il est devenu farouche, sauvage, tressaillant au moindre de bruit, ne s'arrêtant plus quand il a commencé à fuir." Ibid., 494–95.

47. Andreas-Holger Maehle, "Pharmacological Experimentation with Opium in the Eighteenth Century," in *Drugs and Narcotics in History,* ed. Roy Porter and Mikuláš Teich (Cambridge: Cambridge Univ. Press, 1995), 70.

48. On the double meaning, see Berridge and Edwards, *Opium,* 154–55. On stigmatization of addicts, see Thomas Szasz, *Ceremonial Chemistry: The Ritual Persecution of Drugs, Addicts, and Pushers* (Holmes Beach, Fla.: Learning Publications, 1985); Jordan Goodman, Paul E. Lovejoy, and Andrew Sherratt, eds., *Consuming Habits: Drugs in History and Anthropology* (London: Routledge, 1995); Porter and Teich, *Drugs and Narcotics.*

49. F. E. Anstie, *Stimulants and Narcotics, Their Mutual Relations: With Special Research*

on the Action of Alcohol, Aether, and Chloroform, on the Vital Organism (London: Macmillan, 1864), 246.

50. Roger Smith, *Inhibition: History and Meaning in the Sciences of Mind and Brain* (London: Free Association Books, 1992), 169, 45.

51. Chizh, *Dostoevsky*, 70.

52. E. G. Boring mentioned Chizh, Pflaum, and Geiger as students of Wundt involved in the experiments on attention undertaken from 1885 to 1902. See E. G. Boring, *A History of Experimental Psychology* (New York: Century Co., 1929), 339. Among other Russians who studied or worked with Wundt were V. M. Bekhterev, N. N. Lange, and G. I. Chelpanov.

53. On French experimental tradition, see Jacqueline Carroy and Régine Plas, "The Origins of French Experimental Psychology: Experiment and Experimentalism," *History of the Human Sciences,* 1996, no. 1: 73–84. On the difference between German and French experimental design, see Kurt Danziger, *Constructing the Subject: Historical Origins of Psychological Research* (Cambridge: Cambridge Univ. Press, 1990).

54. G. I. Chelpanov, *Obzor noveishei literatury po psikhologii (1890–1896)* (Kiev: Universitet Sv. Vladimira, 1897), 2.

55. N. N. Lange, "O znachenii eksperimenta v sovremennoi psikhologii," *Voprosy filosofii,* 1894, no. 4: 571.

56. Kurt Danziger, "The History of Introspection Reconsidered," *Journal of the History of the Behavioral Sciences* 16 (1980): 241–57; James McKeen Cattell witnessed that "most of the research work that has been done by me or in my laboratory is nearly as independent of introspection as work in physics or zoology"; quoted in ibid., 244. On the difference between Wundt and Titchener, see also William R. Woodward, "Wundt's Program for the New Psychology: Vicissitudes of Experiment, Theory, and System," in *The Problematic Science: Psychology in Nineteenth-Century Thought,* ed. William R. Woodward and Mitchell G. Ash (New York: Praeger, 1982), 167–97.

57. Mitchell G. Ash, *Gestalt Psychology in German Culture, 1890–1967: Holism and the Quest for Objectivity* (Cambridge: Cambridge Univ. Press, 1995), 24–26.

58. On Cattell in Leipzig, see Michael M. Sokal, "James McKeen Cattell and the Failure of Anthropometric Mental Testing, 1890–1901," in Woodward and Ash, *Problematic Science,* 322–45. Cattell's and Chizh's observations were strikingly different: Chizh stressed the negative effect of narcotics and announced his finding that "moral feelings" are the first to be affected. By contrast, Cattell, who tried hashish in private, was delighted, like "one who first drinks 'the new strong wine of love,'" and reported the absence of a hangover: "Every after-effect was delightful, there has been no reaction!!!" See James McKeen Cattell, *An Education in Psychology: James McKeen Cattell's Journal and Letters from Germany and England, 1880–1888,* select. and ed. Michael M. Sokal (Cambridge: MIT Press, 1981), 50–51.

59. Kraepelin remembered that "as Flechsig had authorized me to organize the equipment for the clinic's psychological laboratory, I had obtained all the necessary

equipment for the measurement of mental reactions and had begun a larger series of tests . . . intended to study the changes in the speed of mental reactions induced by external effects of . . . poisons, . . . ether, . . . chloroform, . . . amyl nitrate, . . . alcohol, paraldehyde, and chloralhydrate and later with morphium, tea, and caffeine." Emil Kraepelin, *Memoirs* (Berlin: Springer-Verlag, 1987), 19–26. For Kraepelin's comments on Wundt, see ibid., 44, 28.

60. See A. H. A. C. van Bakel, "Emil Kraepelin and Wundtian Experimental Psychology," in *Proceedings of the First European Congress on the History of Psychiatry and Mental Health Care,* ed. Leonie de Goei and Joost Vijselaar (Rotterdam: Erasmus, 1993), 115–24.

61. Chizh began these experiments in the summer term in 1884 and continued them through the winter term, 1884–85. See Woldemar von Tchisch, "Über die Zeitverhältnisse der Apperception einfacher und zusammengesetzter Vorstellungen, untersucht mit Hülfe der Complicationsmethode," *Philosophische Studien* 2 (1885): 603–34. The Russian version was published as V. F. Chizh, "Eksperimental'nye issledovaniia po metodu komplikatsii, ob appertseptsii prostykh i slozhnykh predstavlenii (iz laboratorii professora Wundta)," *Vestnik klinicheskoi,* 1885, no. 1: 58–87.

62. V. F. Chizh, "Appertseptivnye protsessy u dushevno-bol'nykh," *Arkhiv psikhiatrii,* 1886, no. 1–2: 32.

63. On Kraepelin's successors, see B. A. Maher and W. B. Maher, "Psychopathology," in *The First Century of Experimental Psychology,* ed. Eliot Hearst (Hillsdale, N.J.: Lawrence Erlbaumm, 1979), 566–67.

64. I. E. Sirotkina, "Psikhologiia v klinike: raboty otechestvennykh psikhiatrov kontsa proshlogo veka," *Voprosy psikhologii,* 1995, no. 6: 79–92.

65. W. H. R. Rivers, "Experimental Psychology in Relation to Insanity," *Journal of Mental Science* 14 (1895): 597: "The simple methods which are found to be suited to children will probably also be suited to the insane, and *vice versa.*" Tokarskii published a description of the experimental design in the psychology laboratory and the results of his experiments in Tokarskii, ed., *Notes of the Psychological Laboratory (Zapiski psikhologicheskoi laboratorii pri psikhiatricheskoi klinike Imperatorskogo Moskovskogo universiteta),* 5 vols. (Moscow: Kushnerev, 1895–1901).

66. Ash, *Gestalt Psychology,* 67.

67. Kraepelin, *Memoirs,* 25.

68. It was a commonplace that drugged and alcoholic states were forms of "temporary insanity." See Maher and Maher, "Psychopathology"; Rivers, "Experimental Psychology." On Kraepelin and *Arbeitswissenschaft,* see Anson Rabinbach, *The Human Motor: Energy, Fatigue, and the Origins of Modernity* (Berkeley: Univ. of California Press, 1992), 189–94. On Kraepelin's notion of "working capacity," see van Bakel, "Emil Kraepelin," 115.

69. See Lise Weinstein, Martin Lemon, and Alison Haskell, "Schizophrenia from Hippocrates to Kraepelin: Intellectual Foundations of Contemporary Research," in

Clinical Psychology: Historical and Research Foundations, ed. C. Eugene Walker (New York: Plenum, 1991), 272.

70. Chizh also combined different techniques using narcotics (amyl hydrate) to hypnotize his patients. See V. F. Chizh, *Turgenev kak psikhopatolog* (Moscow: Kushnerev, 1899), 104.

71. V. F. Chizh, "Izmerenie vremeni elementarnykh psikhicheskikh protsessov u dushevno-bol'nykh (iz kliniki professora Flechsig'a)," *Vestnik klinicheskoi,* 1885, no. 2: 65–66. Chizh reported that Kraepelin contested the results of these experiments and that Wundt thought they needed checking. See V. F. Chizh, "Vremia assotsiatsii u zdorovykh i dushevno-bol'nykh," *Nevrologicheskii vestnik,* 1894, no. 2: 95. Some Russian psychiatrists did repeat these experiments: in Bekhterev's laboratory in Kazan' the psychiatrist M. K. Valitskaia obtained slightly different results for the subjects with progressive paralysis. She found that associations took longer and that the time of reaction to a situation involving choice was shorter than in normal subjects. See E. A. Budilova, "Pervye russkie eksperimental'nye psikhologicheskie laboratorii," in *Iz istorii russkoi psikhologii,* ed. M. V. Sokolov (Moscow: APN RSFSR, 1961), 330. Chizh himself repeated experiments on associations in 1890 and 1891; see his "Vremia assotsiatsii."

72. V. F. Chizh, "Shirota vospriiatiia u dushevno-bol'nykh," *Arkhiv psikhiatrii,* 1890, no. 1–2: 26.

73. On Chizh's self-experiments, see his "Eksperimental'noe issledovanie vnimaniia vo vremia sna," *Obozrenie psikhiatrii,* 1896, no. 9: 674. On his suitability as experimental subject, see his "Pochemu vozzreniia prostranstva i vremeni postoianny i nepremenny?" *Voprosy filosofii,* 1896, no. 3: 245.

74. V. A. Zhuravel', "Psikhologiia v sisteme meditsinskogo obrazovaniia Tartusskogo (Iur'evskogo) universiteta," in *Tartusskii gosudarstvennyi universitet: Istoriia razvitiia, podgotovka kadrov, nauchnye issledovaniia* (Tartu: Tartusskii gosudarstvennyi universitet, 1982), 3: 98.

75. Chizh, "Shirota vospriiatiia," 23.

76. V. F. Chizh, ed., *O razvitii eticheskikh vozzrenii: Iz lektsii Wundt'a* (Moscow: Universitetskaia tipografiia [M. Katkov], 1886).

77. G. Chelpanov, "Izmerenie prosteishikh umstvennykh aktov," *Voprosy filosofii,* 1896, no. 9–10: 19–57.

78. V. F. Chizh, "Prestupnyi chelovek pered sudom vrachebnoi nauki," *Nevrologicheskii vestnik,* 1894, no. 1 (app.): 14.

79. Kraepelin, *Memoirs,* 45.

80. Shmuel Galai, *The Liberation Movement in Russia, 1900–1905* (Cambridge: Cambridge Univ. Press, 1973), 20.

81. Zhuravel', "Psikhologiia," 97.

82. When V. M. Bekhterev was offered a chair of psychiatry in the provincial town of Kazan' in 1885, he accepted it on the condition that the university would open a psychiatric clinic and a psychological laboratory. See V. M. Bekhterev, *Avto-*

biografiia (posmertnaia) (Moscow: Ogonek, 1928). Even earlier, in the 1860s and 1870s, I. M. Balinskii at the Medical-Surgical Academy in St. Petersburg and S. S. Korsakov at Moscow University began to purchase psychometric apparatus, and laboratories were opened there in 1894 and 1895, respectively.

83. Chelpanov, *Obzor noveishei,* 42.

84. "Khronica," *Voprosy filosofii,* 1896, no. 2: 145.

85. V. Serebrianikov, "Eksperimental'naia psikhologiia," in *Entsiklopedicheskii slovar'* (Leipzig: Brockhaus & Efron, 1904), 40: 285.

86. The psychiatrists who attended the defense publicly announced that the priority in experimental psychology was theirs. See "Otchet o dispute N. N. Lange," *Voprosy filosofii,* 1894, no. 4: 564–82. For more about Chizh's protest, see David Joravsky, *Russian Psychology: A Critical History* (Oxford: Blackwell, 1989), 77.

87. N. Girshberg, "O sootnoshenii mezhdu psikhicheskimi sostoianiiami, krovoobrashcheniem i dykhaniem" (M.D. diss., Iur'ev Univ., 1902), quoted in Zhuravel', "Psikhologiia," 100.

88. V. F. Chizh, *Metodologiia diagnoza* (St. Petersburg: Prakticheskaia meditsina, 1913), 40–43.

89. Chizh, *Turgenev,* 104. The work was first published in *Voprosy filosofii,* 1898, no. 4: 624–48; no. 5: 714–93.

90. P. B. Posvianskii, "Chizh, Vladimir Fedorovich," in *Bol'shaia Sovetskaia entsiklopediia* (Moscow: Sovetskaia entsiklopediia, 1977), 27: 978.

91. Chizh's essay was *Pushkin kak ideal dushevnogo zdorov'ia* (Iur'ev: Tipografiia universiteta, 1899). A few years earlier, a philosopher and literary critic, V. V. Rozanov, contrasted Gogol's "dark" and Pushkin's "sunny" genius. He argued that Gogol's "exalted lyrics, a fruit of exhausted imagination," had a destructive influence on readers—"everybody began to love and respect only their dreams"—and that Gogol himself was aware of a strange destructive power in his work. See V. V. Rozanov, "Pushkin i Gogol" [1891], in *Nesovmestimye kontrasty zhitiia: literaturno-esteticheskie raboty raznykh let* (Moscow: Iskusstvo, 1990), 228, 233.

92. Charles Lamb, *On the Sanity of Genius* (1823), quoted in Neil Kessel, "Genius and Mental Disorder: A History of Ideas Concerning Their Conjunction," in *Genius: The History of an Idea,* ed. Penelope Murray (New York: Basil Blackwell, 1989), 198.

93. Chizh, *Pushkin,* 20.

94. Walter E. Houghton, *The Victorian Frame of Mind, 1830–1870* (New Haven: Yale Univ. Press, 1957), 297.

95. Charles Darwin, *The Descent of Man, and Selection in Relation to Sex* [1871], (Princeton: Princeton Univ. Press, 1981), 70, 98.

96. Chizh, "Nravstvennost'," 146–48.

97. V. F. Chizh, "Intellektual'nye chuvstvovaniia u dushevno-bol'nykh," *Nevrologicheskii vestnik,* 1896, no. 1: 27–52; no. 2: 76; no. 3: 1–18.

98. Chizh, *Pushkin,* 18.

99. See Roberta Thompson Manning, *The Crisis of the Old Order in Russia: Gentry and Government* (Princeton: Princeton Univ. Press, 1982).

100. See Nancy Mandelker Frieden, *Russian Physicians in an Era of Reform and Revolution, 1856–1905* (Princeton: Princeton Univ. Press, 1981).

101. See Julie Vail Brown, "The Professionalization of Russian Psychiatry" (Ph.D. diss., Univ. of Pennsylvania, 1981), 350.

102. P. I. Iakobii (1842–1913), as quoted in Julie Vail Brown, "Psychiatrists and the State in Tsarist Russia," in *Social Control and the State: Historical and Comparative Essays,* ed. Stanley Cohen and Andrew Scull (Oxford: Martin Robertson, 1983), 278.

103. V. F. Chizh, "Pis'mo redaktoru," *Nevrologicheskii vestnik,* 1895, no. 3: 174.

104. For Chizh's original article and the beginning of the ensuing debate, see V. F. Chizh, "Pliushkin, kak tip starcheskogo slaboumiia," *Vrachebnaia gazeta,* 1902, no. 10: 217–20; Ia. F. Kaplan, "Pliushkin: Psikhologicheskii razbor ego," *Voprosy filosofii,* 1902, no. 3: 811; V. F. Chizh, "Znachenie bolezni Pliushkina (po povodu stat'i d-ra Ia. Kaplana: 'Pliushkin. Psikhologicheskii razbor ego')," *Voprosy filosofii,* 1902, no. 4: 888.

105. Iulii Portugalov, "Po povodu polemiki prof. V. F. Chizh i d-ra Ia. F. Kaplana (Zametki chitatelia-psikhiatra)," *Voprosy filosofii,* 1903, no. 1: 154. This criticism notwithstanding, Kaplan and Chizh continued their debate over Pliushkin and others of Gogol's characters. See Ia. F. Kaplan, "Pliushkin i Starosvetskie pomeshchiki (po povodu stat'i prof. V. F. Chizha 'Znachenie bolezni Pliushkina,'" *Voprosy filosofii,* 1903, no. 3: 599–645; V. F. Chizh, "Otvet Kaplanu (Po povodu stat'i g. Kaplana 'Pliushkin i Starosvetskie pomeshchiki')," *Voprosy filosofii,* 1903, no. 4: 755–59. See also a review of this debate in V. I. Shenrok, "Itogi gogolevskoi iubileinoi literatury," *Vestnik vospitaniia,* 1902, no. 6: 1–31.

106. I. A. Sikorskii, *Psikhologicheskoe napravlenie khudozhestvennogo tvorchestva Gogolia (Rech v pamiat' 100-letnei godovshchiny Gogolia, [April 10, 1909])* (Kiev: Universitet Sv. Vladimira, 1911), 3.

107. M. O. Shaikevich, *Psikhologiia i literatura* (St. Petersburg: Ts. Kraiz, 1910), 58.

108. See V. F. Chizh's "O bolezni Gogolia: Lektsiia, chitannaia 20 marta 1903 g. v Iur'evskom obshchestve estestvoispytatelei," *Saratovskii listok* 70 (1903), 2; "Bolezn' N. V. Gogolia," *Voprosy filosofii,* 1903, no. 2: 262–313; no. 3: 418–68; no. 4: 647–81; and 1904, no. 1: 34–70; and *Bolezn' N. V. Gogolia.*

109. Dr. Kachenovskii, *Bolezn' Gogolia: Kriticheskoe issledovanie* (St. Petersburg: Svet, 1906), 115.

110. This objection was later formulated by a Gogol scholar: "Some of Chizh's hypotheses may be valid, but he clearly weakens his case by what could be charitably termed ideological parochialism. At some point, Gogol's 'reactionary' views are adduced as incontrovertible proof of his psychosis—a reasoning which assumes a more organic relationship between liberalism and sanity than can be conclusively demonstrated." Erlich, *Gogol,* 212.

111. Nikolai Berdiaev, quoted in Edith W. Clowes, *The Revolution of Moral Con-*

sciousness: Nietzsche in Russian Literature, 1890–1914 (DeKalb, Ill.: Northern Illinois Univ. Press, 1988), epigraph, 1.

112. Lev Shestov, *Dostoevsky, Tolstoy, and Nietzsche* [1903] (Athens, Ohio: Ohio Univ. Press, 1969), 322.

113. D. S. Merezhkovskii, "Gogol" [1909], in *Izbrannye stat'i: Simvolizm, Gogol', Lermontov* (Munich: Wilhelm Fink, 1972), 241 (see also K. V. Mochul'skii, *Dukhovnyi put' Gogolia* [Paris: YMCA Press, 1934]); M. O. Shaikevich, "Psikhopatologicheskii metod v russkoi literaturnoi kritike," *Voprosy filosofii*, 1904, no. 3: 321.

114. G. Ia. Troshin, "Genii i zdorov'e N. V. Gogolia," *Voprosy filosofii*, 1905, no. 1: 37–82; no. 2: 186; no. 3: 333–83.

115. M. B. Mirskii, "Troshin, Grigorii Iakovlevich," in *Russkoe zarubezh'e: Zolotaia kniga emigratsii: Pervaia tret' XX veka: Entsiklopedicheskii biograficheskii slovar'* (Moscow: Rosspen, 1997), 629–31.

116. Troshin, "Genii i zdorov'e," 54. Troshin's reference to laughter echoed Gogol's own response to those who criticized his comedy *The Inspector General* for its lack of a positive hero: "I regret that no one noticed the honorable person who was in my play. Yes, there was one honorable, noble person acting in it through its entire length. This honorable, noble person was laughter." Quoted in Rufus W. Mathewson Jr., *The Positive Hero in Russian Literature*, 2d ed. (Stanford: Stanford Univ. Press, 1975), 18.

117. Troshin, "Genii i zdorov'e," 54.

118. On Nietzsche's reception in Russia, see two collections of essays edited by Bernice Glatzer Rosenthal: *Nietzsche in Russia* (Princeton: Princeton Univ. Press, 1986) and *Nietzsche and Soviet Culture: Ally and Adversary* (Cambridge: Cambridge Univ. Press, 1994).

119. I. A. Sikorskii, *O knige V. Veresaeva* Zapiski vracha (*Chto daet eta kniga literature, nauke i zhizni?*) (Kiev: Kushnerev, 1902), 10.

120. Shaikevich, *Psikhologiia i literatura,* 16–17, 14–15; Troshin quoted in ibid., 22.

121. Shaikevich, "Psikhopatologicheskii metod," 315.

122. Galai, *Liberation Movement,* 236.

123. E. I. Al'tshuller, quoted in Brown, "Professionalization," 383.

124. Brown, "Professionalization," 387–88.

125. In the St. Nicholas Hospital, where Troshin worked, nurses and wardens worked sixteen hours a day. In addition to their duties in the patients' wards, they were also personal servants to *fel'dshers* (physician's assistants) and did the hospital laundry. See "Khronika," *Sovremennaia psikhiatriia,* 1913, no. 10: 836–37.

126. Troshin and the hospital warden, G. Shults, were found "intellectually guilty' (*intellektual'nye vinovniki*); see "Khronika," *Sovremennaia psikhiatriia,* 1907, no. 10: 383; see also Brown, " Professionalization," 350.

127. Chizh, *Turgenev,* 34, 104.

128. V. F. Chizh, "Znachenie politicheskoi zhizni v etiologii dushevnykh boleznei," *Obozrenie psikhiatrii,* 1908, no. 1: 10; no. 3: 149–62.

129. Chizh, *Kriminal'naia,* 50.

130. The first report was by F. E. Rybakov, "Mental Disturbances in Connection with Recent Events," presented at the meeting of the Moscow Society of Psychiatrists on October 28, 1905. His colleagues questioned his interpretation of the presented case, arguing that it showed revolutionary events had simply stimulated the development of tangible symptoms in somebody who already had a disease. See "Iz Obshchestva nevropatologov i psikhiatrov v Moskve," *Obozrenie psikhiatrii,* 1906, no. 5: 388–89.

131. On "revolutionary psychosis," see Julie V. Brown, "Revolution and Psychosis: The Mixing of Science and Politics in Russian Psychiatric Medicine, 1905–13," *Russian Review* 46 (1987): 283–302. Earlier, army psychiatrists had reported a high percentage of mentally ill soldiers and officers and discussed whether the war had produced a special kind of mental illness, "war psychosis." As in the case of "prison psychosis," the discrimination of this diagnosis was above all a political issue.

132. Chizh, "Znachenie politicheskoi," 5–6.

133. The editor of the Moscow journal *Contemporary Psychiatry* (*Sovremennaia psikhiatriia*), P. B. Gannushkin, attacked Chizh's article as a product of his reactionary attitude. See Brown, "Revolution and Psychosis," 295.

134. M. A. Gershenzon, quoted in Lionel Kochan, *Russia in Revolution, 1890–1918* (London: Weidenfeld & Nicolson, 1966), 148.

135. V. G. Korolenko, "Tragediia velikogo iumorista (Neskol'ko myslei o Gogole)," in Kotov and Poliakov, *N. V. Gogol' v russkoi kritike,* 541–42.

136. Ibid., 594, 546.

137. Ermakov, *Ocherki,* 76. On Gogol's psychobiography, see Daniel Rancour-Laferrier, *Out from under Gogol's Overcoat: A Psychoanalytic Study* (Ann Arbor, Mich.: Ardis, 1982).

138. Gogol wrote to a friend, "God knows best whether the illness causes this condition in me or whether the illness develops just because I forced myself to put my mind into the state necessary for creative work; in any case I thought of my cure only in this sense, not that the suffering would become less, but that the life-giving moments of creating and being able to have the creation become word would return again to my soul." Quoted in Vsevolod Setchkarev, *Gogol: His Life and Works,* trans. Robert Kramer (London: Peter Owen, 1965), 75.

139. Friedrich Nietzsche, *Ecce Homo* [1908; written in 1888], trans. Anthony M. Ludovici (New York: Russell & Russell, 1964), 58. Chizh, who had also read and appreciated Nietzsche, completely overlooked his devastating criticism and his rebellion against accepted values. Every time Chizh quoted from Nietzsche, it was in support of his own moral stance. See, e.g., Chizh, *Uchebnik psikhiatrii,* 316; Chizh, "Znachenie politicheskoi," 157.

140. Philip Rieff, *Freud: The Mind of the Moralist* (Garden City, N.Y.: Anchor Books, 1961), 2.

141. Is it possible to say, with Robert A. Maguire, that the tendency to "relocate

the source of Gogol's art from the external to the internal world" marked the end of pathographies? (*Gogol from the Twentieth Century,* 19.) Indeed, the tradition of making illness responsible for the vicissitudes of Gogol's life almost disappeared. Late-twentieth-century scholars interpreted the events of Gogol's life as determined by factors within the world of literature, reattributing, for instance, his failure to write the second part of *Dead Souls* to the weaknesses of the dominant discourse of his time. Maguire's recent book on Gogol argues that the "so-called 'spiritual crisis' of his later years . . . was really a literary crisis." Gogol's death is interpreted as an escape into silence, which the writer conceived as a punishment for misusing words. See Robert A. Maguire, *Exploring Gogol* (Stanford: Stanford Univ. Press, 1994), xiii, 338–41.

Attempts to explain the "enigma of Gogol" by references to organic influences continued well into the twentieth century. In *The Sexual Labyrinth of Nikolai Gogol* (Chicago: Univ. of Chicago Press, 1976), Simon Kagarlinsky suggests that the answer lay in Gogol's homosexuality. Richard Peace attributes at least some features of Gogol's writing (which he calls "medieval") to his "neurotic personality": his art "offers 'psychology without psychology' to an author who dare not look deep within himself; it projects a bizarre outer world that is, in effect, an inner one." See Richard Peace, *The Enigma of Gogol: An Examination of the Writings of N. V. Gogol and Their Place in the Russian Literary Tradition* (Cambridge: Cambridge Univ. Press, 1981), 291. Attempts to examine Gogol from the medical point of view continue. See, e.g., V. E. Lerner, E. Vitsum, and G. M. Kotikov, "Bolezn' Gogolia i ego puteshestvie k sviatym mestam," *Nezavisimyi psikhiatricheskii zhurnal,* 1996, no. 1: 63–71.

Two. Dostoevsky

Epigraphs: Dostoevsky, Stavrogin's words to Tikhon in "At Tikhon's: Stavrogin's Confession," a chapter intended for *The Devils* (but not included in the original edition because of the editor's objection), quoted in Mikhail Bakhtin, *Problems of Dostoevsky's Poetics,* ed. and trans. Caryl Emerson (Minneapolis: Univ. of Minnesota Press, 1984), 60; Stefan Zweig, *Three Masters: Balzac, Dickens, Dostoeffsky,* trans. Eden Paul and Cedar Paul (New York: Viking, 1930), 204; and V. M. Bekhterev, from "Dostoevsky i khudozhestvennaia patologiia," speech at the State Institute of Medical Knowledge on February 24, 1924, quoted in S. Belov and N. Agitova, "V. M. Bekhterev o Dostoevskom," *Russkaia literatura,* 1962, no. 4: 139.

1. Joseph Frank, *Through the Russian Prism: Essays on Literature and Culture* (Princeton: Princeton Univ. Press, 1990), 153.

2. V. G. Belinsky, quoted in Vladimir Seduro, *Dostoevsky in Russian Literary Criticism, 1846–1956* (New York: Octagon Books, 1957), 9, 6. I draw here and later upon Seduro's account of Dostoevsky literary criticism.

3. Maikov quoted in ibid., 12.

4. Ibid.

5. Isaiah Berlin, *Russian Thinkers,* ed. Henry Hardy and Aileen Kelly (London: Penguin Books, 1994), 116.

6. For an exhaustive study of Dostoevsky's epilepsy, see James L. Rice, *Dostoevsky and the Healing Art: An Essay in Literary and Medical History* (Ann Arbor, Mich.: Ardis, 1985), esp. 200–79.

7. The characterization of Dostoevsky as a "polemicist par excellence" is based on Václav Černy, *Dostoevsky and His Devils* (Ann Arbor, Mich.: Ardis, 1975).

8. On the popularity of *The Diary of a Writer,* see Frank, *Through the Russian Prism,* 153–69. On the radicals' response to *The Devils,* see ibid., 138.

9. Mikhailovsky quoted in Seduro, *Dostoevsky,* 35–38.

10. On the persistence of this pattern in Soviet criticism of Dostoevsky, see Vladimir Seduro, *Dostoevsky's Image in Russia Today* (Belmont, Mass.: Nordland, 1975).

11. Prince Peter Kropotkin, *Ideals and Realities in Russian Literature* (New York: Alfred Knopf, 1915), 168–69.

12. On Chernyshevsky's novel, see Michael R. Katz and William G. Wagner, "Introduction," in *What Is to Be Done?* [1863], by Nikolai Chernyshevsky, trans. Michael R. Katz (Ithaca, N.Y.: Cornell Univ. Press, 1989), 1–36; see also Frank, *Through the Russian Prism,* 187–200.

13. Rufus W. Mathewson Jr., *The Positive Hero in Russian Literature,* 2d ed. (Stanford: Stanford Univ. Press, 1975), 18–19.

14. Vladimir Solov'ev, *"Tri rechi v pamiat' Dostoevskogo"* [1881–83], translated in *Literature and National Identity: Nineteenth-Century Russian Critical Essays,* edited by Paul Debreczeny and Jesse Zeldin (Lincoln: Univ. of Nebraska Press, 1970), 169–79; Eugène-Melchior de Vogüé, *Le roman russe,* 3d ed. (Paris: Plon-Nourrit, 1892). After publication of de Vogüé's influential book, reference to the psychological bias of Russian literature became a cliché of literary criticism. See, e.g., Ossip Lourié, *La psychologie des romanciers russes du XIXe siècle* (Paris: Félix Alcan, 1905).

15. Nikolai Mikhailovsky, *Dostoevsky: A Cruel Talent* [1882], trans. Spencer Cadmus (Ann Arbor, Mich.: Ardis, 1978), 12.

16. V. F. Chizh, *Dostoevsky kak psikhopatolog* (Moscow: M. Katkov, 1885). For a discussion of this book see Rice, *Dostoevsky,* 200–210.

17. Chizh, *Dostoevsky,* 4–5.

18. M. A. Antonovich, a journalist and Mikhailovsky's follower, quoted in Mathewson, *Positive Hero,* 20.

19. Chizh, *Dostoevsky,* 93.

20. *Obschestvo nevropatologov i psikhiatrov: Otchety za 1897–1900 gg.* (Moscow: Prostakov, 1901), 212.

21. Chizh, *Dostoevsky,* 113.

22. As James Rice has persuasively demonstrated, Dostoevsky was acquainted with major psychiatric works of the midcentury, some of which he borrowed from his physician at the time, S. D. Yanovsky, and often discussed with him. See Rice, *Dostoevsky,* 109–97.

23. Chizh, *Dostoevsky,* 120.

24. *Severnyi vestnik,* 1885, no. 7: 197–98, quoted in Rice, *Dostoevsky,* 210.

25. D. N. Ovsianiko-Kulikovskii, "Istoriia russkoi intelligentsii" [1911], in *Sobranie sochinenii* (The Hague: Mouton, 1969), 8, pt 2: 224, 238–39; Kropotkin, *Ideals and Realities,* 168–69.

26. Cesare Lombroso, *The Man of Genius* (London: Walter Scott, 1891), 359; Brandes quoted in James L. Rice, *Freud's Russia: National Identity in the Evolution of Psychoanalysis* (New Brunswick, N.J.: Transaction, 1993), 126; Rice, *Dostoevsky,* 105.

27. Dostoevsky quoted in Mathewson, *Positive Hero,* 352.

28. Ibid., 18–19, 90.

29. Merezhkovskii quoted in Seduro, *Dostoevsky,* 40–43.

30. Lev Shestov, "Dostoevsky and Nietzsche: The Philosophy of Tragedy" [1903], trans. Spencer Roberts, in Shestov's *Dostoevsky, Tolstoy, and Nietzsche* (Athens, Ohio: Ohio Univ. Press, 1969), 198–99.

31. Ibid., 316 (emphasis in original), 322.

32. Chizh, *Dostoevsky,* 88.

33. N. N. Bazhenov, *Gabriel Tarde: Lichnost', idei i tvorchestvo* (Moscow: Kushnerev, 1905), 4. This was the text of his speech given on September 31, 1905, at the meeting of the Moscow Society of Psychiatrists and Neuropathologists in memory of Gabriel Tarde (1843–1904).

34. Bazhenov's story as recalled by Tarde in "Foules et sectes au point de vue criminel," *Revue des deux mondes,* November 15, 1893, 349–87; also quoted in Athena Vrettos, *Somatic Fiction: Imagining Illness in Victorian Culture* (Stanford: Stanford Univ. Press, 1995), 81.

35. Tarde served as a magistrate in his native town of Sarlat until 1894, when he was promoted to head of the department of legal statistics at the Ministry of Justice. His academic career developed slowly: in 1890 he published his magnum opus in sociology, *Les lois de l'imitation,* and ten years later he was appointed to the prestigious chair of modern philosophy at the Collège de France. See Wolf Lepenies, *Between Literature and Science: The Rise of Sociology* (Cambridge: Cambridge Univ. Press, 1985), 47–92. For a discussion of Tarde's "Fragment de l'histoire future" (1876), see Lepenies, *Between Literature and Science,* 57–59.

36. On Lavrov, see Philip Pomper, *Peter Lavrov and the Russian Revolutionary Movement* (Chicago: Univ. of Chicago Press, 1972). Bazhenov's younger colleague and friend N. E. Osipov (discussed in Chapter 3), perhaps not knowing about Bazhenov's participation in The People's Will, saw his move to a provincial asylum as a heroic deed, a sacrifice of benefits that the European-educated psychiatrist could have received if he had remained in Moscow. N. E. Osipov, "Korsakov i Serbskii (Pervye professora psikhiatrii Moskovskogo universiteta)," in *Moskovskii universitet, 1755–1930: Iubileinyi sbornik,* ed. V. B. El'iashevich, A. A. Kizevetter, and M. M. Novikov (Paris: Sovremennye zapiski, 1930), 405–26.

37. A. G. Gerish and G. K. Ushakov, "Zhizn' i deiatel'nost' N. N. Bazhenova," *Zhurnal nevropatologii,* 1972, no. 8: 1238.

38. A. K. Streliukhin, "Zhizn' i deiatel'nost' N. N. Bazhenova, sviazannye s

Riazan'iu," in *Voprosy psikhonevrologii,* ed. A. K. Streliukhin and S. F. Semenov (Moscow: Minzdrav RSFSR, 1965), 15–23.

39. N. N. Bazhenov, *O prizrenii i lechenii dushevnobol'nykh v zemstvakh, i v chastnosti o novoi Riazanskoi psikhiatricheskoi lechebnitse* (St. Petersburg: M. M. Stasiulevich, 1887), 11.

40. A. G. Gerish, "Prioritet N. N. Bazhenova vo vvedenii v psikhiatricheskikh bol'nitsakh Rossii sistemy 'otkrytykh dverei,'" in *Materialy nauchno-prakticheskoi konferentsii vrachei psikhonevrologicheskikh uchrezhdenii g. Moskvy* (Moscow: Minzdrav RSFSR, 1970), 220.

41. N. N. Bazhenov to V. I. Iakovenko, July 28, 1889, quoted in R. M. Umanskaia and D. D. Fedotov, "Vzgliady N. N. Bazhenova na sistemu 'otkrytykh dverei' v psikhiatricheskikh bol'nitsakh," in *Voprosy psikhonevrologii,* 27.

42. Bazhenov quoted in Gerish, "Prioritet," 221.

43. Bazhenov's dissertation dealt with a common topic of the period, the role of autointoxication in nervous diseases. See N. N. Bazhenov, *O znachenii autointoksikatsii v patogeneze nervnykh simptomokompleksov* (Khar'kov: Gubernskaia uprava, 1894). He obtained his degree from Khar'kov University because both Petersburg and Moscow were closed to him.

44. "O priniatii v chislo privat-dotsentov Moskovskogo universiteta doktora meditsiny N. N. Bazhenova" (1902), in TsGIAM, f. 418, op. 63, d. 538.

45. Though puritans held the Literary-Artistic Circle in suspicion, the money from the night gambling often went to charity—to the Chekhov Fund for the Young Writers or to Moscow asylums. See L. V. Nikulin, *Gody nashei zhizni* (Moscow: Moskovskii rabochii, 1966), 311; V. R. Leikina-Svirskaia, *Russkaia intelligentsiia v 1900–1917 godakh* (Moscow: Mysl', 1981), 129; "Khronika," *Sovremennaia psikhiatriia,* 1907, no. 6: 191.

46. Andrei Bely, *Mezhdu dvukh revolutsii* (Moscow: Khudozhestvennaia literatura, 1990), 215–16.

47. Bazhenov even translated Baudelaire's "Correspondences" into Russian in order to demonstrate to a Russian audience the "oddity" of his metaphors, such as the one in which he compared "a smell with a green meadow or a sound of an oboe." In a book of poetry by Maurice Maeterlinck that contained thirty-three poems, Bazhenov counted twenty-five allusions to illness. See N. N. Bazhenov, *Simvolisty i dekadenty: Psikhiatricheskii etiud.* (Moscow: Mamontov, 1899), 8, 17.

48. Verlaine's "Effet de nuit," from his *Romances without Words* ("Il pleut dans mon coeur / Comme il pleut dans la ville"), fascinated Bazhenov, whereas "Serres chaudes" by Maeterlinck appeared a result of "perverse sensibility." Bazhenov, *Simvolisty,* 11, 28.

49. On Bazhenov's Pushkin Prize, see Gerish and Ushakov, "Zhizn'," 1238; on his inclusion in *Preparatory Sources,* see S. A. Vengerov, *Istochniki slovaria russkikh pisatelei* (St. Petersburg: Imperatorskaia Akademiia nauk, 1900), 1: 142. Bazhenov published his nonmedical work under the pen name Sleptsov-Teriaevskii (his wife's name was

Ol'ga Nikolaevna Sleptsova). See, e.g., O. N. Sleptsov-Teriaevskii, *Sinestezicheskii sposob izucheniia akkordov* (Petrograd: Sirius, 1915), an essay in which Bazhenov proposed the use of colored perception of sounds—synesthesia—as a mnemonic device for learning musical chords. The Bazhenovs eventually separated and Ol'ga Nikolaevna lived with their son, Nikolai (born in 1889), in Germany. See Muzei Preobrazhenskoi bol'nitsy, f. 103, l. 180.

50. Nikulin, *Gody,* 311.

51. V. F. Giliarovskii, "Lichnost' i deiatel'nost' N. N. Bazhenova (1856–1923) (Nekrolog)," *Zhurnal psikhologii,* 1923, no. 3: 11.

52. Gerish and Ushakov, "Zhizn'," 1238.

53. M. A. Krasnushkina, "Preobrazhenskaia bol'nitsa v period rukovodstva N. N. Bazhenovym," in *Sbornik nauchnykh trudov, posviashchennykh 150-letiiu Moskovskoi psikhonevrologicheskoi bol'nitsy N 3* (Moscow: Moskovskaia psikhonevrologicheskaia bol'nitsa N 3, 1963), 442. On Bazhenov's appointment, see "N. N. Bazhenov, glavnyi vrach Preobrazhenskoi bol'nitsy, March 1904–May 1917," in TsGIAM, f. 179, op. 37, d. 95.

54. R. M. Umanskaia and D. D. Fedotov, "Vzgliady N. N. Bazhenova na sistemu 'otkrytykh dverei,'" in Streliukhin and Semenov, *Voprosy psikhonevrologii,* 24.

55. Shmuel Galai, *The Liberation Movement in Russia, 1900–1905* (Cambridge: Cambridge Univ. Press, 1973), 267.

56. Mitskevich became involved in a Marxist group when he was a graduate student in medicine in Moscow. In 1894 he was arrested and exiled in Siberia. In 1899 he volunteered to work as a physician in the Kolyma region, beyond the Polar Circle, where he also collected material on so-called Polar hysteria among the native people. When he returned from exile at the end of 1903, he gave a talk on Polar hysteria at the Moscow Society of Psychiatrists. Mitskevich described in his memoirs how, after the talk, Bazhenov offered him a position in his private clinic. See S. I. Mitskevich, *Zapiski vracha-obshchestvennika (1888–1918),* 2d ed. (Moscow: Meditsina, 1969), 148. After the October Revolution, Mitskevich became one of the first historians of the Communist Party and a founder of the Museum of the Revolution in Moscow. On Lenin's attending a meeting, see Gerish and Ushakov, "Zhizn'," 1239.

57. Galai, *Liberation Movement,* 271.

58. N. N. Bazhenov, *Psikhologiia i politika* (Moscow: I. D. Sytin, 1906).

59. N. N. Bazhenov, *Psikhologiia kaznimykh* (Moscow: I. D. Sytin, 1906).

60. Joseph Frank, *Dostoevsky: The Seeds of Revolt, 1821–1849* (Princeton: Princeton Univ. Press, 1976), 109.

61. A. G. Gerish, "Uchastie professora N. N. Bazhenova v revolutsionnom dvizhenii 1905–07 godov," in *Materialy nauchno-prakticheskoi konferentsii,* 54–58. This particular conflict was caused by Bazhenov's trip in 1907 to Helsingfors (later, Helsinki), Finland, to the illegal congress of the Constitutional Democratic Party. See Muzei Preobrazhenskoi bol'nitsy, f. 103, l. 180.

62. M. V. Korkina, "N. N. Bazhenov (K 100-letiiu so dnia rozhdeniia)," *Zhurnal nevropatologii,* 1957, no. 8: 1033.

63. Other known Russian members of French lodges included the writer Ivan Turgenev and the grand duke Nikolai Mikhailovich, the tsar's uncle. But Turgenev died in 1883, and the grand duke was not ordained until the 1890s.

64. Among others, Lenin lectured at the school in 1903. See Ushakov and Gerish, "Zhizn'," 1237.

65. Probably owing to his Masonic connections, Bazhenov was awarded the Légion d'honneur; the order was signed in Paris on his birthday—August 8, 1905. See Muzei Preobrazhenskoi bol'nitsy, f. 103, ll. 1, 95. On the Moscow lodge, see Nina Berberova, *Liudi i lozhi: russkie masony XX stoletiia* (New York: Russica, 1986), 17. Berberova, daughter of a Russian Mason of that generation, reports that "the brothers" considered Bazhenov "too talkative" and thus not reliable. At the elections to the Russian Masonic Supreme Council in 1908, Bazhenov's candidature was blackballed (pp. 187–88). Unaware that Bazhenov returned to Russia in 1923, Berberova writes that he died in Belgium (p. 110). For more on the history of the Moscow lodge, see also A. Ia. Avrekh, *Masony i revoliutsiia* (Moscow: Politizdat, 1990), 50.

66. On the development of the so-called nervous clinics and sanatoria, see Edward Shorter's *From Paralysis to Fatigue: A History of Psychosomatic Illness in the Modern Era* (New York: Free Press, 1992), 213–20; and "Psychotherapy in Private Clinics in Central Europe, 1880–1913," in *Proceedings of the First European Congress on the History of Psychiatry and Mental Health Care, s-Hertogenbosch, The Netherlands, 24–26 October 1990,* ed. Leonie de Goei and Joost Vijselaar (Rotterdam: Erasmus, 1993), 39–50.

67. M. S. Micale, *Approaching Hysteria: Disease and Its Interpretations* (Princeton: Princeton Univ. Press, 1995), 276–77.

68. L. M. Rozenshtein, "Moskovskaia psikhiatricheskaia shkola i N. N. Bazhenov," *Klinicheskaia meditsina,* 1924, no. 2: 134.

69. N. Bajenoff and N. Osipoff, *La suggestion et ses limites* (Paris: Bloud et Cie, 1911). On Bazhenov's opinion about psychoanalysis, see Krasnushkina, "Preobrazhenskaia bol'nitsa," 442,

70. P. V. Rybakov, "Nekrolog N. N. Bazhenova," *Moskovskii meditsinskii zhurnal,* 1923, no. 2: 226.

71. "Ob"iavlenie o sanatorii N. N. Bazhenova i A. Marie v Choisy-le-Roy," in TsGIAM, f. 363, op. 1, d. 70, l. 185.

72. A. G. Gerish, "Perepiska N. N. Bazhenova ob organizatsii psikhiatricheskoi pomoshchi v pervuiu mirovuiu voinu," in *Voprosy kliniki, patogeneza i terapii psikhicheskikh zabolevanii,* ed. V. M. Banshchikov and I. A. Shishkin (Moscow: Moskovskaia gorodskaia psikhiatricheskaia bol'nitsa N 3, 1972), 31.

73. N. Bajenoff, *La révolution russe: Essai de psychologie sociale* (Paris: Bloud et Gay, 1919), 73. Bazhenov's donation of his personal library to the library of the Higher Women's Courses in December 1916 indicated his intention to stay away from Russia for a while. See TsGIAM, f. 363, op. 1, d. 70, l. 198.

74. Rozenshtein, "Moskovskaia psikhiatricheskaia shkola," 132.

75. John M. MacGregor, *The Discovery of the Art of the Insane* (Princeton: Princeton Univ. Press, 1989), chap. 11; Bazhenov (transliterated as "Bagenoff") is mentioned in ibid., p. 342, n. 29, with a (wrong) comment that he was a student of Marie.

76. Ibid., 178.

77. Réja [Meunier] quoted in ibid., 175.

78. Not all Bazhenov's geniuses were male. He referred to Maria Bashkirtseva, a very gifted Russian painter and author who died in her twenties. See his *Simvolisty,* 33. Meunier worked at the Villejuif Hospital when Auguste Marie was superintendent there, and he could have met Bazhenov through Marie. The publication of Bazhenov and Osipov's book, *La suggestion et ses limites,* in a series that Meunier published, also brought Meunier and Bazhenov into contact.

79. Bazhenov, *Simvolisty*; N. N. Bazhenov, "Bol'nye pisateli i patologicheskoe tvorchestvo," in *Psikhiatricheskie besedy na literaturnye i obshchestvennye temy* (Moscow: Mamontov, 1903), 10–40.

80. N. Bajenoff, *Gui de Maupassant et Dostoïewsky: Etude de psychopathologie comparée* (Lyon: A. Stork & Masson, 1904), 39.

81. Bazhenov, *Psikhiatricheskie,* 39. He often analyzed fragments of Dostoevsky's novels in his lectures at the Higher Women's Courses. One of his assistants there, T. E. Segalov (1881–1928), had written his medical dissertation on Dostoevsky's epilepsy. See Timofei Segaloff, *Die Krankheit Dostojewskys: Eine ärztlich-psychologische Studie mit einem Bildnis Dostojewskys.* (Munich: Ernst Reinhardt, 1907).

82. Bajenoff, *Maupassant et Dostoïewsky,* 4, 24.

83. Bazhenov, "Bol'nye pisateli," 27, 25.

84. Maupassant quoted in Bajenoff, *La révolution russe,* 31: "Depuis que s'agite notre courte pensée, l'homme est le même, ses sentiments, ses croyances, ses sensations sont les mêmes, il n'a point avancé, il n'a point reculé, il n'a point remué . . . Car la pensée de l'homme est immobile. Les limites précises, proches, infranchissables, une fois atteintes, elle tourne comme un cheval dans un cirque, comme une mouche dans une bouteille fermée, voletant jusqu'aux parois où elle se heurte toujours." Dostoevsky quoted in Mathewson, *Positive Hero,* 352.

85. Nordau quoted in Bazhenov, "Bol'nye pisateli," 36. In his lavish criticism of contemporary art, Nordau also made an exception of Dostoevsky, and he even contrasted Dostoevsky, as a moral writer, to those "egomaniacs" who delighted in describing morbid and immoral topics. "We have not a momentary doubt of the morality of the artist's emotions when we behold Callot's pictures of the horrors of war, or the bleeding, purulent saints of Zurbaran, or the murder scene in Dostoevsky's Raskol'nikov," Nordau wrote, and added, "These emotions are beautiful." Max Nordau, *Degeneration* (New York: D. Appleton, 1895); originally published as *Entartung* (1892); Nordau quoted here from the 1993 reprint (Lincoln: Univ. of Nebraska Press, 1993), 331.

86. Alex de Jonge, quoted in Frank, *Through the Russian Prism,* 183.

87. Frank, *Through the Russian Prism,* 183.

88. Dostoevsky to N. A. Lyubimov, assistant editor, July 8, 1866; quoted in Joseph Frank, *Dostoevsky: The Miraculous Years, 1865–1871* (Princeton: Princeton Univ. Press, 1995), 94–95.

89. Philip Rieff, *Freud: The Mind of the Moralist* (Garden City, N.Y.: Anchor Books, 1961), 50.

90. D. S. Merezhkovskii, quoted in Seduro, *Dostoevsky,* 45.

91. Rieff, *Freud,* 57. One of Dostoevsky's stories is titled "An Honest Thief."

92. P. J. Möbius, *Ausgewälte Werke,* vol. 1, *J. J. Rousseau* (Leipzig: Barth, 1909), xi.

93. Jan Goldstein, "Psychiatry," in *Companion Encyclopaedia of the History of Medicine,* ed. W. F. Bynum and Roy Porter (London: Routledge, 1993), 2: 1364.

94. Freud's comment on conventional psychiatry is quoted in S. L. Gilman, "Sexology, Psychoanalysis, and Degeneration: From a Theory of Race to a Race Theory," in *Degeneration: The Dark Side of Progress,* ed. J. E. Chamberlin and S. L. Gilman (New York: Columbia Univ. Press, 1985), 83. Freud found Dostoevsky's last novel, *The Brothers Karamazov,* especially valuable for psychoanalysis and therefore rediagnosed the writer's disorder. See Joseph Frank, "Freud's Case-History of Dostoevsky," in Frank's *Dostoevsky: Seeds of Revolt,* 379–92; Freud's letter to Zweig, October 19, 1920, is quoted on p. 381.

95. Chizh, *Dostoevsky,* 94; D. A. Amenitskii, "Psikhopatologiia Raskol'nikova, kak oderzhimogo naviazchivym sostoianiem," *Sovremennaia psikhiatriia,* 1915, no. 9: 388; N. E. Osipov, "*Dvoinik:* Peterburgskaia poema Dostoevskogo (Zapiski psikhiatra)," in *O Dostoevskom,* ed. A. L. Bem (Prague: Petropolis, 1929), 1: 39–64.

96. Nikolai Lossky, *Dostoevsky i ego khristianskoe miroponimanie* (New York: Izdatel'stvo imeni Chekhova, 1953), 329–30.

97. Bazhenov, "Bol'nye pisateli," 40.

98. Thomas Mann, "Dostojewski—mit Massen" [1945], in *Gesammelte Werke* (Hamburg: S. Fischer, 1974), 9: 666.

99. The Russian psychoanalysts who wrote about Dostoevsky, before Freud did so in 1928, are T. K. Rozental' and A. Kashina-Evreinova. See Rozental', "Stradanie i tvorchestvo Dostoevskogo (psikhoanaliticheskoe issledovanie)," *Voprosy izucheniia i vospitaniia lichnosti,* 1919, no. 1: 88–107; and Kashina-Evreinova, *Podpol'e geniia (seksual'nye istochniki tvorchestva Dostoevskogo)* (Petrograd: Tret'ia strazha, 1923). For a discussion of Russian Freudians and Dostoevsky, see Rice, *Dostoevsky,* esp. 210–24. The Moscow psychiatrist M. Iu. Lakhtin concluded that the "evolutionary meaning of suffering and religion" lay in the "limitless possibility for perfection" that they created. He wrote, "reconciling itself with earthly suffering . . . humankind creates conditions necessary to continue with life and to improve it." M. Iu. Lakhtin, "Stradaniia kak istochnik chelovecheskikh verovanii," *Voprosy nevrologii i psikhiatrii,* 1913, no. 11: 492.

100. M. P. Kutanin, "Bred i tvorchestvo," *Klinicheskii arkhiv,* 1929, no. 1: 3–35.

101. H. F. Ellenberger, "The Concept of *Maladie Créatrice*" [1964], in *Beyond the*

Unconscious: Essays of Henri F. Ellenberger in the History of Psychiatry, ed. M. S. Micale (Princeton: Princeton Univ. Press, 1993), 328, 329.

102. There is an extensive literature on this topic; see, e.g., Lionel Trilling, *The Liberal Imagination* (New York: Viking, 1945); George Pickering, *Creative Malady: Illness in the Lives and Minds of Charles Darwin, Florence Nightingale, Mary Baker Eddy, Sigmund Freud, Marcel Proust, Elisabeth Barret Browning* (New York: Oxford Univ. Press, 1974); Philip Sandblom, *Creativity and Disease: How Illness Affects Literature, Art, and Music,* 2d ed. (Philadelphia: G. F. Stickley, 1983). H. F. Ellenberger also mentions that illness might have played a creative role in the lives of Nietzsche, Freud, and Jung. He occasionally discusses the parallels between Nietzschean and Freudian thought; see Ellenberger, *The Discovery of the Unconscious: The History and Evolution of Dynamic Psychiatry* (London: Allen Lane, 1970), 271–79.

103. Herbert Dieckmann, cited in Penelope Murray, "Introduction," in *Genius: The History of an Idea,* ed. Penelope Murray (New York: Basil Blackwell, 1989), 2.

104. Max Nordau, "The Psychophysiology of Genius and Talent," in *Paradoxes,* trans. from the German (Chicago: L. Schick, 1886), 175. George L. Mosse defines nineteenth-century liberalism as concerned with progress through order, will, and rationality. See Mosse, "Max Nordau and His *Degeneration,*" introduction to *Degeneration,* by Max Nordau, trans. from 2d ed. of the German work (Lincoln: Univ. of Nebraska Press, 1993), xviii.

105. Nordau, *Entartung.* As George Bernard Shaw wrote sarcastically, Nordau "is so utterly mad on the subject of degeneration that he finds the symptoms of it in the loftiest geniuses as plainly as in the lowest jailbirds, the exception being himself, Lombroso, Krafft-Ebing, Dr. Maudsley, Goethe, Shakespeare, and Beethoven." G. B. Shaw, *The Sanity of Art: An Exposure of the Current Nonsense about Artists Being Degenerate* (London: Constable, 1911), 89.

106. Lombroso, *Man of Genius,* 209, 240.

107. Valentin Magnan and P.-M. Legrain, *Les Dégénérés (état mental et syndrôme épisodiques)* (Paris: Rueff, 1895); Henry Havelock Ellis, *The Criminal,* 3d ed. (London: Walter Scott, 1901), 160.

108. Nordau, "Psychophysiology of Genius," 134, 198.

109. Max Nordau, *Psikhofiziologiia geniia i talanta* (St. Petersburg: Vestnik znanii, 1908). This was published in English in 1886 (Nordau, "Psychophysiology of Genius") and in French in 1896: Max Nordau, *Paradoxes psychologiques* (Paris: Félix Alcan, 1896).

110. G. K. Chesterton called Nietzsche a "very timid thinker" because the German philosopher did "not even know in the least what sort of man he wants evolution to produce"; quoted in Patrick Bridgwater, *Nietzsche in Anglosaxony: A Study of Nietzsche's Impact on English and American Literature* (Leicester, U.K.: Leicester Univ. Press, 1972), 19.

111. Frank, *Dostoevsky: Miraculous Years,* 481.

112. Bazhenov, *Simvolisty,* 33.

113. Bajenoff, *Maupassant et Dostoïewsky,* 36: "Quand, en étudiant le psychomé-

canisme du génie, on emploie la terminologie psychiatrique, on commet la faute logique de la *petitio principii;* on implique tout de suite l'idée de maladie, de réversion ancestrale, de dégénérescence . . . Si nous acceptons pour la psychologie de l'homme aussi bien que pour n'importe quelle catégorie de faits biologiques la suprématie de la loi d'évolution progressive, pourquoi ne parlerions-nous pas plutôt de 'progénérescence' que de 'dégénérescence' et d' 'apostérisme' plutôt que d'atavisme?"

Three. Tolstoy and the Beginning of Psychotherapy in Russia

Epigraph: "Case Records of the Inhabitants of Yasnaya Polyana" were supposedly composed by Lev Tolstoy himself. See S. N. Tolstoy, *Ocherki bylogo,* 3d ed. (Tula: Priokskoe knizhnoe izdatel'stvo, 1965), 175.

1. D. S. Merezhkovskii, *L. Tolstoy i Dostoevsky,* 3d ed. (St. Petersburg: M. V. Pirozhkov, 1902–3); Stefan Zweig, *Drei Dichter ihres Lebens: Casanova, Stendhal, Tolstoi* (Leipzig: Insel-verlag, 1928).

2. P. I. Biriukov, *Biografiia L'va Nikolaevicha Tolstogo* (Moscow: Gosizdat, 1922), 3: 296.

3. K. P. Pobedonostsev to Alexander III, November 1, 1891, quoted in N. N. Apostolov, *Zhivoi Tolstoy: Zhizn' L'va Nikolaevicha Tolstogo v vospominaniiakh i perepiske* (St. Petersburg: Lenizdat, 1995), 375–76. The Holy Sinod was the highest official organ of the Russian Orthodox Church; its head, the Ober-Procurator, was appointed by the tsar.

4. Turgenev quoted in S. Rozanova, "Introduction," in *Perepiska Tolstogo s russkimi pisateliami,* ed. S. Rozanova (Moscow: Khudozhestvennaia literatura, 1962), vii.

5. L. N. Tolstoy, "What Then Must We Do?" [1885], trans. Aylmer Maude, in *Tolstoi Centenary Edition* (London: Humphrey Milford, 1934), 277.

6. S. A. Tolstaia (1879), quoted in S. N. Tolstoy, *Ocherki bylogo,* 72; S. N. Tolstoy's statement in ibid., 80.

7. N. Ch., "Psikhopatologicheskie proiavleniia novoi very grafa L'va Tolstogo," *Iuzhnyi krai,* no. 3378, 3381, 3383 (1890).

8. Isaiah Berlin, *Russian Thinkers,* ed. Henry Hardy and Aileen Kelly (London: Penguin Books, 1994), 45; N. K. Mikhailovsky, *Literaturnye vospominaniia i sovremennaia smuta* (St. Petersburg: Vol'f, 1900), 1: 253, 201, 221.

9. Berlin, *Russian Thinkers,* 126.

10. V. I. Lenin, "Lev Tolstoy kak zerkalo russkoi revoliutsii" (1908), quoted in *Lenin i Tolstoy,* ed. S. M. Breitburg (Moscow: Izdatel'stvo Kommunisticheskoi Akademii, 1928), 50. *Tolstovets* was a name for a follower of Tolstoy, someone who sought to fulfill his teaching in practice, usually tried to live a peasant's life, and was a pacifist and a vegetarian. Lenin saw Tolstoy's contradictions as a reflection of the peasants' contradictory situation after the 1860s' reforms, when they were liberated from serfdom but not made individual owners of land.

11. Cesare Lombroso writing for *Peterburgskaia gazeta* 236 (1908), as quoted in

Apostolov, *Zhivoi Tolstoy,* 429; Apostolov, *Zhivoi Tolstoy,* 431. In *Man of Genius* (London: Walter Scott, 1891), Lombroso mentioned Tolstoy in the chapter "Neurosis and Insanity in Genius," not in the chapter "Degeneration and Genius": "philosophic skepticism had led him into a condition approximating to madness; let us add, to *folie du doute*" (p. 50).

12. Apostolov, *Zhivoi Tolstoy,* 414–15.

13. Daniel Pick, "Lombroso and the Politics of Criminal Science in Post-Unification Italy," *History Workshop Journal,* no. 21 (spring 1986): 61.

14. Max Nordau, *Entartung* [1892], 2 vols., 3d ed. (Berlin: C. Dunker, 1896); translated as *Degeneration* (New York: D. Appleton, 1895). Nordau devoted the fourth chapter, "Tolstoism," of the second volume of his book to the phenomenon of "confused thinking" and "unrealistic love for the neighbors."

15. Max Nordau, *Dégénérescence,* 5th ed., trans. Auguste Dietrich (Paris: Félix Alcan, 1899), 1: 296 (French translation of *Entartung* [1892]).

16. L. N. Tolstoy, "The Memoirs of a Madman" [1912; written 1884–86], in *Tolstoi Centenary Edition* (London: Humphrey Milford, 1934), 15: 210; further quotations, 212–14; 224–25.

17. N. E. Osipov, "Zapiski sumashedshego, nezakonchennoe proizvedenie L. N. Tolstogo: k voprosy ob emotsii boiazni," *Psikhoterapiia,* 1913, no. 3: 5; further quotations, 6, 8, 11, 20.

18. N. E. Osipov, "Analiz romana grafa L. N. Tolstogo, *Semeinoe schast'e*" (1929), in TsGALI, f. 2299, op. 1, ed. khr. 19, l. 17.

19. N. E. Osipov, "Genii i nevroz L'va Tolstogo" (October 16, 1928), in ibid., ed. khr. 13, l. 26.

20. N. E. Osipov, "Dushevnaia bolezn' L'va Tolstogo" (1929), in ibid., ed. khr. 18, l. 28.

21. The reaction of Russian audiences to *Degeneration* was ambivalent. Within two years of the original publication, two Russian translations appeared and received mixed reviews. See Max Nordau's *Vyrozhdenie,* trans. R. I. Sementkovskii (St. Petersburg: Pavlenkov, 1894); and *Vyrozhdenie,* trans. V. Genkevich (Kiev: Ioganson, 1894). Despite many angry articles with titles that spoke for themselves—e.g., "Genius under Psychiatric Trial" (A–t, "Genii na sude psikhiatra," *Novoe vremia,* 6380 [December 1, 1894])—there were also sympathetic reviews praising Nordau's literary style and "critical thinking." Some of the reviewers regarded *Degeneration* as a major offense not only to Tolstoy but also to other artists; see, e.g., V. Chechott, "Max Nordau o Vagnere," *Kievlianin,* no. 337 (1895).

22. V. A. Rudnev [editor of *Contemporary Notes (Sovremennye zapiski)*], to [Osipov's friend] M. P. Polosin, October 21, 1927, in TsGALI, f. 2299, op. 1, ed. khr. 88; M. O. Wulff to N. E. Osipov, February 8, 1931, in ibid., ed. khr. 44, l. 2.

23. L. N. Tolstoy, *War and Peace* [1865–69] (London: Penguin Books, 1964), 2: 776–77.

24. Berlin, *Russian Thinkers,* 240.

25. *Tolstoy's Diaries,* ed. and trans. R. F. Christian (London: HarperCollins, 1994), 6 [April 17, 1847].

26. In the process of writing a book-length essay, "The Notion of Life," in which he presented his view in a systematically logical form, Tolstoy had thoughts that, as he wrote to a friend, "can be expressed by means of art only." See Biriukov, *Biografiia,* 67.

27. Ovsianiko-Kulikovskii quoted in Alexander Vucinich, *Science in Russian Culture, 1861–1917* (Stanford: Stanford Univ. Press, 1970), 39.

28. Apostolov, *Zhivoi Tolstoy,* 466. Tolstoy reported to his biographer an episode in which Chernyshevsky had come to talk to him about his writings: "very embarrassed, he began to say that Lev Nikolaevich has talent and literary skills, but he does not know what to write about . . . It is necessary to write in a critical way [*oblichitel'no*]." Quoted in Rozanova, *Perepiska Tolstogo,* 460.

29. This observation was made by Mikhailovsky himself, see his *Literaturnye vospominaniia,* 220–21.

30. Dostoevsky put these words in the mouth of Dmitrii, one of the Karamazov brothers; quoted in Mikhail Bakhtin, *Problems of Dostoevsky's Poetics,* ed. and trans. Caryl Emerson (Minneapolis: Univ. of Minnesota Press, 1984), 61. "Bernard" here refers to the physiologist Claude Bernard, a proponent of experiment and a materialist outlook.

31. *Tolstoy's Diaries,* 322 [March 21, 1898].

32. Tolstoy's deathbed warning quoted in Daniel P. Todes, *Darwin without Malthus: The Struggle for Existence in Russian Evolutionary Thought* (New York: Oxford Univ. Press, 1989), 44. For an account of Tolstoy's views on Darwin, see ibid., 43–44.

33. *Tolstoy's Diaries* 369 [April 14, 1903] and 214 [April 22, 1889].

34. Tolstoy, "What Then Must We Do?" 277.

35. The article, by M. Ia. Kapustin, was written in response to Tolstoy's essay "The First Step," in which he started the polemic on vegetarianism and alcohol and tobacco. See *Tolstoy's Diaries,* 280 [May 3, 1894].

36. Ibid., 4 [March 17, 1847].

37. Tolstoy to P. D. Golokhvastov (1876), quoted in Harold K. Schefski, "Tolstoj's Case against Doctors," *Slavic and East European Journal,* 22, no. 4 (1978): 569.

38. It was said that Tolstoy's son, Lev (Lyova), suffered from neurasthenia. See *Tolstoy's Diaries,* 525 [1893].

39. L. N. Tolstoy to T. L. Sukhotina-Tolstaia (April 15, 1902), quoted in Schefski, "Tolstoj's Case," 569.

40. L. N. Tolstoy, *The Death of Ivan Ilych* [1886], trans. Aylmer Maude (New York: New American Library, 1960), 121.

41. *Tolstoy's Diaries,* 364 [September 20, 1902]. Tolstoy's relationship with medicine is the subject of numerous works, most of which deal with the descriptions of illnesses in his fiction. In 1994 alone, the following articles appeared: A. M. Basom, "Anna Karenina and Opiate Addiction," *Pharmacy in History* 36 (1994), 132–40;

M. Benezech, "*La sonate à Kreutzer* ou la jalousie homicide selon Tolstoi," *Annales médico-psychologiques,* no. 5 (1994); M. J. Hurst and D. L. Hurst, "Tolstoy's Description of Tourette Syndrome in *Anna Karenina,*" *Journal of Child Neurology* 4 (1994): 366–67; David Pike, "Vronsky's Teeth," *Lancet* 344 (1994): 1784; A. F. Sanford et al., "Reading Literary Theory, Reading *Ivan Ilych:* Old Wine in New Wineskins," *Caduceus* 3 (1994): 161–78. Articles of another type contain an account of Tolstoy's contacts with physicians and his views on medicine: M. L. Gomon, "L. N. Tolstoi i khar'kovskoe meditsinskoe obschestvo," *Klinicheskaia meditsina* 71 (1993): 174–79; N. N. Kostruba, "Psikhiatriia v tvorchestve i zhizni L. N. Tolstogo," *Zhurnal nevropatologii,* 1992, no. 2: 110–15; N. E. Osipov, "Psikhoterapiia v literaturnykh proizvedeniiakh L. N. Tolstogo (otryvok iz raboty 'Tolstoy i meditsina')," *Psikhoterapiia,* 1911, no. 1: 1–21; P. E. Zablu-dovskii and Z. M. Konius, "Lev Nikolaevich Tolstoi i voprosy meditsinskogo dela," *Klinicheskaia meditsina* 63 (1985): 140–43.

42. Tolstoy quoted in Ernest J. Simmons, *Leo Tolstoy* (London: John Lehmann, 1949), 719.

43. Tolstoy probably would have agreed with Makovitskii's unpretentious final diagnosis: "the moral suffering he had been enduring and the exhaustion caused by his difficult journey had weakened his heart and nervous system to such extent that the illness immediately took a serious form that led to a fatal ending." D. P. Makovit-skii, "Lev Nikolaevich's Departure from Yasnaya Polyana," in *Reminiscences of Lev Tolstoy by His Contemporaries* (Moscow: Foreign Language Publishing House, 1969), 260.

44. Berlin, *Russian Thinkers,* 45. On Tolstoy's conception of history, see Henry Gifford, "Tolstoy and Historical Truth," in *Russian Thought and Society, 1800–1917: Essays in Honour of Eugene Lampert,* ed. Roger Bartlett (London: the contributors, 1984), 114–28.

45. Kutuzov quoted in Gifford, "Tolstoy," 128; Prince Andrei's words from Tolstoy, *War and Peace,* 1: 886.

46. N. E. Osipov, "Tolstoy i meditsina" (November 1, 1928), in TsGALI, f. 2299, op. 1, ed. khr. 14, l. 44.

47. The founders of community medicine, E. A. Osipov, I. I. Molesson, and F. F. Erisman, worked for the Moscow Region *zemstvo,* where they founded a health care department and contributed to the improvement of the sanitary situation in this most populated area of Russia. Together with N. I. Pirogov, a liberal-minded physician who fell out of favor with the tsarist government, they were highly respected by their colleagues and became models for many in the medical profession. See Nancy Mandelker Frieden, *Russian Physicians in an Era of Reform and Revolution, 1856–1905* (Princeton: Princeton Univ. Press, 1981).

48. The writer and doctor A. P. Chekhov was one of those who made *zemstvo* medicine so morally attractive. He was a *zemstvo* physician after he graduated from the medical department of Moscow University. When he was already a famous writer, he returned to the *zemstvo* and treated peasants from twenty-five villages and small towns of Serpukhov District without salary. In 1892 he worked during the cholera

epidemic under the same conditions. A year earlier, he wrote in his diary, "A desire to serve public welfare should be a need of the soul, a condition of one's personal happiness; if it does not originate here, but comes from theoretical or other reasons, it is not the same." Quoted in N. M. Pirumova, *Zemskaia intelligentsiia i ee rol' v obshchestvennoi bor'be do nachala XX v.* (Moscow: Nauka, 1986), 224.

49. Author of the memoir is quoted in ibid., 22.

50. Frieden, *Russian Physicians, 17.*

51. Nevertheless, the ideological, professional, and personal were interwoven in the real lives of *zemstvo* physicians, and F. F. Erisman (1842–1915) is a good example. Erisman, a Swiss physician, met and married N. P. Suslova (1843–1918), a Russian medical student, when she studied in Zurich. Suslova graduated in 1867 and became the first female doctor in Russia. The main motive for the choice of her career, however, was an ideological one: she sought to join the revolutionary activity and turned to the medical profession in search of emancipation from her family and gender. According to Erisman's Russian biographer, Suslova opened to Erisman "wide prospects of medical work for public benefit, and persuaded him to move to Russia." He went to Petersburg and made contacts with public health physicians, received permission to conduct a series of medical-statistical investigations, and then returned to Central Europe to study with the hygienist Max von Pettenkofer in Munich. In 1875 Erisman settled in Russia, and E. A. Osipov soon invited him to work in the Moscow Provincial Sanitary Bureau; together with Osipov and Molesson, Erisman acquired fame as "the father of Russian community medicine." See V. A. Bazanov, *F. F. Erisman (1842–1915)* (Leningrad: Meditsina, 1966); "Pamiati professora F. F. Erismana," *Voprosy psikhologii,* 1963, no. 2: 189; Frieden, *Russian Physicians,* 99–100.

52. The author of the book was V. O. Portugalov, a member of the Populist movement in the 1860s and a *zemstvo* physician in the 1870s. Quoted in Pirumova, *Zemskaia intelligentsiia,* 91–92.

53. M. S. Karpova, quoted in ibid., 92.

54. Frieden, *Russian Physicians,* 228.

55. On the strike, see Samuel D. Kassow, *Students, Professors, and the State in Tsarist Russia* (Berkeley: Univ. of California Press, 1989), 91–119.

56. While abroad, Osipov married, but the marriage lasted less than a year. He divorced in 1903 in Moscow and married again in 1905. See A. L. Bem, F. M. Dosuzhkov, and N. O. Lossky, eds., *Zhizn' i smert': Sbornik rabot v pamiat' N. E. Osipova* (Prague: Petropolis, 1935), 12.

57. V. P. Karpov, *Osnovnye cherty organicheskogo ponimaniia prirody* (Moscow: Put', 1913).

58. The fragment of this uncompleted work "Organicheskaia naturfilosofiia v sovremennoi russkoi nauke" was published under the title "Life and Death." See N. E. Osipov, "Zhizn' i smert'," in Bem, Dosuzhkov, and Lossky, *Zhizn' i smert',* 67–78.

59. Osipov probably remembered his childhood when later he wrote, "the mentally sane should govern, and not the mentally ill, as is sometimes the case on the his-

torical stage or in the closed life of ordinary people in distant provinces." Quoted in F. N. Dosuzhkov, "Nikolai Evgrafovich Osipov kak psikhiatr," in Bem, Dosuzhkov, and Lossky, *Zhizn' i smert'*, 31. Osipov's mother is not mentioned anywhere else in the personal documents that were available for this research; it is known only that she died in Moscow in 1920, while her son was trying to leave Russia via the Black Sea.

60. L. M. Rozenshtein, "V. P. Serbskii—klassik Moskovskoi psikhiatricheskoi shkoly," *Psikhogigienicheskie issledovaniia* (Moscow: Gos. Nauchnyi Institut nevro-psikhicheskoi profilaktiki, 1928), 1, pt. 1: 7–16.

61. See *Nevrologicheskii vestnik* 14 (1907): 143–44; A. G. Gerish, *P. B. Gannushkin* (Moscow: Meditsina, 1975), 26–28.

62. Julie Vail Brown, "The Professionalization of Russian Psychiatry" (Ph.D. diss., Univ. of Pennsylvania, 1981), 347.

63. All the physicians left, with one exception: Fedor Rybakov stayed and was appointed director by Kasso; Moscow psychiatrists did not allow him to speak at their meetings. See N. E. Osipov, "Korsakov i Serbskii (Pervye professora psikhiatrii Moskovskogo universiteta)," in *Moskovskii universitet, 1755–1930: Iubileinyi sbornik*, ed. V. B. El'iashevich, A. A. Kizevetter, and M. M. Novikov (Paris: Sovremennye zapiski, 1930), 424.

64. Though respect and admiration for Korsakov were in many cases genuine, his image was also used to ascribe legendary status to the Moscow school of psychiatry. See Julie V. Brown, "Heroes and Non-Heroes: Recurring Themes in the Historiography of Russian-Soviet Psychiatry," in *Discovering the History of Psychiatry*, ed. M. S. Micale and Roy Porter (New York: Oxford Univ. Press, 1994), 297–307.

65. Osipov, "Korsakov i Serbskii," 410.

66. Dosuzhkov, "Nikolai Evgrafovich Osipov," 27.

67. Heinrich Rickert, *Kulturwissenschaft und Naturwissenschaft*, 5th ed. (Tübingen: Mohr, 1921), 63.

68. Windelband taught in Zurich, where Osipov worked on his medical dissertation; while there, Osipov had discussions about neo-Kantian philosophy with Friedrich Erisman, at that time a professor in Zurich.

69. N. E. Osipov, "O logike i metodologii psikhiatrii," *Zhurnal nevropatologii*, 1912, no. 2–3: 465. Little Fridays were started as biweekly conferences for the physicians of the clinic; in 1908 they were opened to physicians from other institutions as well as to nonphysicians and were attended also by biologists, psychologists, and sociologists. After 1911 Little Fridays were held at the Moscow Society of Psychiatrists, eventually becoming an independent association. Osipov's talk opened the first session in the new location; other contributors included: M. M. Asatiani ("The Mechanism of Symptom Development in One Case of Hysteria"), L. M. Rozenshtein ("The Demonstration of Mr. A.'s Phenomenal Counting Ability"), D. G. Konovalov ("Emergence of the Enthusiastic Sects"), V. P. Karpov ("Inheritance in the Light of New Biological Data"), and others. See N. E. Osipov, "Moskovskii psikhiatricheskii kruzhok 'Malye piatnitsy,'" *Zhurnal nevropatologii*, 1912, no. 2–3: 456–87.

70. Osipov, "O logike," 460.

71. N. E. Osipov, "Dvulikost' i edinstvo meditsiny," in *Russkii narodnyi universitet v Prage: Nauchnye trudy* (Prague: Russkii narodnyi universitet, 1929), 2: 175–92.

72. Osipov, "Psikhoterapiia v literaturhykh proizvedeniiakh," 5.

73. Osipov, "Dvulikost'," 192.

74. N. E. Osipov, "Nevrasteniia," in Bem, Dosuzhkov, and Lossky, *Zhizn' i smert'*, 106.

75. Kostruba, "Psikhiatriia," 112.

76. For a list of psychiatrists read by Tolstoy, see the commentaries to L. N. Tolstoy, *Polnoe sobranie sochinenii* (Moscow: Khudozhestvennaia literatura, 1936), 38: 584–85.

77. T. L. Sukhotina-Tolstaia, *Vospominaniia* (Moscow: Khudozhestvennaia literatura, 1976), 434, 435.

78. The article, "On the Psychiatric Question" (1899), was by an author identified only as A.M. It reported that psychiatrists incarcerated innocent, healthy people in asylums for personal gain and described in detail one such case when harsh measures were used to teach the patient obedience. See Brown, "Professionalization," 255.

79. L. N. Tolstoy, "O bezumii" [1910], in *Polnoe sobranie sochinenii*, 38: 411.

80. S. A. Tolstaia, *Dnevniki* (Moscow: Khudozhestvennaia literatura, 1978), 2: 211.

81. Tolstoy escaped into the sanitary colony "for neurotics" organized by Dr. Ogranovich in the countryside near Zvenigorod, Moscow region, in 1888. See S. A. Tolstaia, *Dnevniki, Part 2: 1891–1897* (Moscow: Sabashnikovy, 1929), 108, 236.

82. For a discussion of these changes, see, e.g., Julie V. Brown, "Psychiatrists and the State in Tsarist Russia," in *Social Control and the State,* ed. Stanley Cohen and Andrew Scull (New York: M. Robertson, 1983), 267–87.

83. Quoted in John F. Hutchinson, *Politics and Public Health in Revolutionary Russia, 1890–1918* (Baltimore: Johns Hopkins Univ. Press, 1990), 54–61.

84. V. F. Chizh, "Pis'mo redaktoru," *Nevrologicheskii vestnik*, 1895, no. 3: 174; also quoted in Julie V. Brown, "Professionalization and Radicalization: Russian Psychiatrists Respond to 1905," in *Russia's Missing Middle Class: The Professions in Russian History,* ed. Harley D. Balzer (Armonk, N.Y.: M. E. Sharpe, 1996), 145.

85. K. R. Evgrafov, quoted in T. I. Iudin, *Ocherki istorii otechestvennoi psikhiatrii* (Moscow: Medgiz, 1951), 322. Similar criticism was addressed to laboratory research in bacteriology, which, in the opinion of the old *zemstvo* physicians, distracted young physicians from practical work. See Hutchinson, *Politics,* 56.

86. E. N. Dovbnia and L. M. Rozenshtein, *Pervyi s"ezd russkikh nevropatologov i psikhiatrov* (Moscow: Shtab Moskovskogo voennogo okruga, 1911), app.

87. William H. Parry-Jones, *The Trade in Lunacy, A Study of Private Madhouses in England in the Eighteenth and Nineteenth Centuries* (London: Routledge, 1972), 33.

88. Edward Shorter, "Private Clinics in Central Europe, 1850–1933," *Social History of Medicine,* 1990, no. 3: 159–95.

89. The sanitary colony of M. P. Ogranovich was established in the Crimea, 1883–87. See "Proshenie vracha Mikhaila Petrovicha Ogranovicha o razreshenii emu otkryt' v imenii grafa S. D. Sheremeteva 'Aliaukhovo' Zvenigorodskogo uezda sanitarnuiu koloniiu dlia malokrovnykh i nervnykh bol'nykh" (October 15, 1893–January 27, 1897), in TsGIAM, f. 1, op. 2, d. 2704. M. Ia. Droznes's sanatorium was founded in Odessa in about 1890; see M. Ia. Droznes, *Osnovy ukhoda za nervno- i dushevnobol'nymi, vyrabotannye v vide opyta dlia sluzhebnogo personala chastnoi lechebnitsy dlia nervno- i dushevnobol'nykh doktora M. Ia. Droznesa v Odesse* (Odessa: Isakovich & Beilenson, 1897).

90. V. K. Rot, "Obshchestvennoe popechenie o nervno-bol'nykh: Ustroistvo spetsial'nykh sanatorii," in *Trudy Vtorogo s"ezda otechestvennykh psikhiatrov* (Kiev: Kul'zhenko, 1907), 479.

91. N. N. Bazhenov, *Proekt zakonodatel'stva o dushevno-bol'nykh i ob"iasnitel'naia zapiska k nemu* (Moscow: Gorodskaia tipografiia, 1911).

92. S. S Korsakov, "Ob ustroistve chastnykh lechebnits," *Zhurnal nevropatologii,* 1901, no. 5–6: 937–65.

93. Anne Digby, *Madness, Morality, and Medicine: A Study of the York Retreat, 1796–1914* (Cambridge: Cambridge Univ. Press, 1985), 34. Locke quoted in ibid., 59. The Russians had shared the worldwide admiration of the York Retreat since the beginning of the nineteenth century. Samuel Tuke reported in his memoirs that when Grand Duke Nicholas, future Emperor of Russia, visited the retreat in 1814, he was so impressed that he exclaimed frequently, "C'est parfait! C'est admirable!"; ibid., 256.

94. It seems that Korsakov learned to appreciate the "unifying woman's role" while working in a private clinic owned by Maria Becker. After Korsakov's death, Becker continued to help with the clinic, and young physicians called her the "*babushka* [granny] of Russian psychiatry." See Osipov, "Korsakov i Serbskii," 410.

95. Parry-Jones, *Trade in Lunacy,* 33.

96. In the case of one patient, it was stated, "When medicine, mechanical restraint, hydrotherapy and medical distraction had all failed to quiet her over a period of ten months after her admission it was decided to try animal magnetism as last resort." Quoted in Digby, *Madness,* 138.

97. "Svidetel'stvo o poilticheskoi blagonadezhnosti N. E. Osipova" (December 1907), in TsGIAM, f. 1, op. 2, d. 3097, l. 10.

98. The increasing interest in private clinics in the early 1900s was probably the reason why the journal published Korsakov's paper presented at the meeting of Moscow Society of Psychiatrists and Neuropathologists fifteen years earlier. Russian psychiatrists used the metaphor "lay monasteries," which was also used by Möbius and Freud. See, e.g., S. S. Stupin, "K voprosu o narodnykh sanatoriiakh dlia nervno-bol'nykh," *Zhurnal nevropatologii,* 1904, no. 3: 367.

99. Osipov, "Psikhoterapiia v literaturnykh proizvedeniiakh."

100. Lev Tolstoy, *Anna Karenina* [1875–76], trans. Aylmer Maude (New York: Norton, 1970), 108; also quoted in Schefski, "Tolstoj's Case," 570.

101. Tolstoy, *War and Peace*, 779.

102. Ibid, 777–78.

103. Schefski, "Tolstoj's Case," 572.

104. N. E. Osipov, "Mysli i somneniia po povodu odnogo sluchaia 'degenerativnoi psykhopatii,'" *Psikhoterapiia*, 1911, no. 5: 189–215.

105. Dubois quoted in Edward Shorter, *From Paralysis to Fatigue: A History of Psychosomatic Illness in the Modern Era* (New York: Free Press, 1993), 247. The statement by the sanatorium director (N. A. Vyrubov) is from an advertisement for the Kriukovo sanatorium, in *Sovremennaia psikhiatria*, 1909, no. 1: inside front cover.

106. B. S. Greidenberg, "Psikhologicheskie osnovy nervno-psikhicheskoi terapii," in *Trudy Pervogo s"ezda Russkogo soiuza psikhiatrov i nevropatologov, Moskva, 4-11.9.1911,* ed. N. A. Vyrubov et al. (Moscow: Shtab Moskovskogo voennogo okruga, 1914), 138.

107. Tolstoy quoted in N. E. Osipov, "O naviazchivoi ulybke," *Zhurnal nevropatologii*, 1912, no. 4: 578.

108. Osipov, "Nevrasteniia," 106. Osipov was not the only person to emphasize the similarity between Tolstoy and Dubois. The psychologist N. Iurman also compared rational therapy with Tolstoy's moral teaching, although critically: "the psychotherapists, like Dubois and Iarotskii, see a panacea in moral and altruistic education, repeating in a scientific form the moralizing sermons of such critics of science and medicine, as Tolstoy." N. Iurman, "[Review of] *Vopros o nravstvennom pomeshatel'stve v svete panidealisticheskoi psikhologii sovesti,* [by] K. Ia. Grinberg," *Psikhiatricheskaia gazeta*, 1916, no. 7: 126–27.

109. H. F. Ellenberger, *The Discovery of the Unconscious: The History and Evolution of Dynamic Psychiatry* (London: Allen Lane, 1970), 804.

110. Recent studies of psychoanalysis in Russia have assumed that the development of psychotherapy was dominated by psychoanalysis. A. M. Etkind, for instance, argues that Russian physicians eagerly embraced Freud's theories and that, in the early twentieth century, psychoanalysis penetrated Russian culture and everyday life; see Alexander Etkind, *Eros nevozmozhnogo: Istoriia psikhoanaliza v Rossii* (St. Petersburg: Meduza, 1993). My aim in this chapter is to show that the reception of psychoanalysis was much more cautious and not at all at the expense of other psychotherapies.

111. Vogt quoted in Greidenberg, "Psikhologicheskie," 137.

112. N. E. Osipov, "O nevroze boiazni (*Ängstneurose*)," *Zhurnal nevropatologii*, 1901, no. 5–6: 797.

113. O. B. Fel'tsman, "Vpechatleniia o poezdke k Dubois (Pis'mo iz-za granitsy)," *Psikhoterapiia*, 1910, no. 1: 49; O. B. Fel'tsman, "O psikhoanalyze i psikhoterapii," *Sovremennaia psikhiatriia*, 1909, no. 1: 257–69.

114. N. Bajenoff and N. Osipoff, *La suggestion et ses limites* (Paris: Bloud et Cie, 1911); N. E. Osipov, "O bol'noi dushe," *Zhurnal nevropatologii*, 1913, no. 5–6: 661.

115. N. A. Vyrubov, "Psikhoterapevticheskie vzgliady S. S. Korsakova," *Psikhoterapiia*, 1910, no. 3: 1–10; N. A. Vyrubov, *Psikhoterapevticheskie zadachi sanatoriia dlia nevrotikov* (Moscow: Kushnerev, 1910), 4.

116. In a personal communication of February 21, 1995, V. I. Ovcharenko informed me that though the sanatorium was abolished after the October Revolution, the building still displays objects with engraved psychoanalytic and Christian inscriptions from the years of the sanatorium. See also Etkind, *Eros nevozmozhnogo*, 158.

117. "A mal psychique traitment psychique"; Dubois quoted in Shorter, *From Paralysis*, 257.

118. Freud's famous Russian patient, the Wolf-Man, initially intended to consult Dubois. He and his doctor, Leonid Droznes, were on their way to Bern, but Droznes suggested they make a stop to see Freud in Vienna. See Magnus Ljunggren, "Psychoanalytic Breakthrough in Russia on the Eve of the First World War," in *Russian Literature and Psychoanalysis,* ed. Daniel Rancour-Laferriere (Amsterdam: John Benjamins, 1989), 189.

119. Jung by that time had already heard about Osipov. See S. Freud to C. G. Jung, January 2, 1910, in *Freud/Jung Letters,* 282–83; Dosuzhkov, "Nikolai Evgrafovich Osipov," 33.

120. N. E. Osipov, "Beseda s Dubois," *Zhurnal nevropatologii*, 1910, no. 5–6: 1773.

121. J.-J. Déjerine and E. Gauckler, *Funktsional'nye proiavleniia psikhonevrozov i ikh lechenie psikhoterapieiu* [*Les manifestations fonctionnelles des psychonévroses: leur traitement par la psychothérapie*], trans. V. P. Serbskii (Moscow: Kosmos, 1912).

122. N. E. Osipov, "Psikhologicheskie i psikhopatologicheskie vzgliady Freud'a," *Zhurnal nevropatologii*, 1908, no. 3–4: 564–84; "Psikhologiia kompleksov," *Zhurnal nevropatologii*, 1908, no. 6: 1021–74. In 1911 Moshe Wulff informed his European readers that in Russia Osipov reported on "practically all of Freud's writings"; see Wulff's "Die russische psychoanalytische Literatur bis zum Jahre 1911," *Zentralblatt für Psychoanalyse: Medizinische Monatsschrift für Seelenkunde*, 1911, no. 7–8: 364–71.

123. Freud's comments on Osipov (1910) quoted in Hans Lobner and Vladimir Levitin, "A Short Account of Freudism: Notes on the History of Psychoanalysis in the USSR," *Sigmund Freud House Bulletin*, 1978, no. 1: 7–8.

124. On the introduction of psychoanalysis in Russia, see Jacques Marti, "La psychanalyse en Russie et en Union Soviétique de 1909 à 1930," *Critique,* no. 346 (1976): 216–17; Etkind, *Eros nevozmozhnogo,* chaps. 1–4; V. I. Ovcharenko, *Psikhoanaliticheskii glossarii* (Minsk: Vysheishaia shkola, 1995); Martin Miller, *Freud and the Bolsheviks: Psychoanalysis in Imperial Russia and the Soviet Union* (New Haven: Yale Univ. Press, 1998).

125. N. A. Vyrubov, "Psikho-analiticheskii metod Freud'a i ego lechebnoe znachenie," *Zhurnal nevropatologii*, 1909, no. 1–2: 28.

126. Osipov, "Psikhologiia kompleksov," 1046; N. E. Osipov, "Eshche o psikho-analyze," *Psykhoterapiia*, 1910, no. 4–5: 169.

127. Marti, "La psychanalyse," 201.

128. N. E. Osipov, "O 'panseksualizme' Freuda," *Zhurnal nevropatologii*, 1911, no. 5–6: 749–56.

129. N. E. Osipov, "Basni Krylova: K psikhologii literaturnogo tvorchestva" (December 10, 1924), in TsGALI, f. 2299, op. 1, ed. khr. 3, l. 69.

130. Osipov's comments on the two psychotherapies are in "Eshche o psikho-analize," 169 (division of labor); "Beseda s Dubois," 1781 (complementarity); and "Eshche o psikhoanalize," 172 (both therapies directed to same end). This latter understanding was probably closer to the original language of Freud's writings, which, as Bruno Bettelheim pointed out, were sometimes misunderstood when translated into English. See Bruno Bettelheim, *Freud and Man's Soul* (New York: Alfred A. Knopf, 1983), 3–5. The German word *Seele* was translated as *mind* or *mental* and therefore "scientized," whereas the Russian, *dusha,* is a more exact translation.

131. Osipov, "O bol'noi dushe," 673.

132. Osipov, "Analiz romana grafa Tolstogo, *Semeinoe schast'e,*" l. 26.

133. N. E. Osipov, "Analiz povesti L. N. Tolstogo *Detstvo*" (1929), in TsGALI, f. 2299, op. 1, ed. khr. 21, ll. 3, 1.

134. N. E. Osipov, "Voina i mir" (1928–1929), in ibid., ed. khr. 15, l. 9.

135. Osipov, "Analiz povesti Tolstogo *Detstvo,*" l. 6.

136. Serbskii quoted in Marti, "La psychanalyse," 201.

137. Freud to Jung, January 2, 1910, 283. Ironically, once psychoanalysis was accepted, it began to structure psychiatrists' imagination and, in particular, it led Osipov to analyze Tolstoy as neurotic in Freud's terms.

138. Osipov's analysis appeared in German as N. Ossipoff, *Tolstois* Kindheitserin-nerungen: *Ein Beitrag zur Freud Libidotheorie* (Leipzig: Imago-Bucher, II, 1923). His comment on the Provisional Government is quoted in M. P. Polosin, "Doktor med-itsiny Nikolai Evgrafovich Osipov (1877–1934)," in Bem, Dosuzhkov, and Lossky, *Zhizn' i smert'*, 12.

139. G. Fedorov, *Puteshestvie bez santimentov (Krym, Gallipoli, Stambul)* (1926), quoted in E. I. Pivovar et al., *Rossiiskaia emigratsiia v Turtsii, Iugo-vostochnoi i Tsentral'noi Evrope 20-kh godov (grazhdanskie bezhentsy, armiia, uchebnye zavedeniia)* (Moscow: Historical and Archival Institute of RGGU, 1994), 91–93.

140. In Soviet Russia in 1920, over 60 percent of civil servants had only a primary school level of education. See E. P. Serapionova, *Rossiiskaia emigratsiia v Chekhoslovatskoi respublike (20-30-e gody)* (Moscow: Russian Academy of Sciences, 1995), 6.

141. Before 1917 there were two public (or "People's") universities in Moscow, similar to the British and American university extension programs. One of them, the Shaniavskii University, was run by the City Council "to disseminate advanced scientific education and instill a love of science and knowledge among the people."

Quoted in Joseph Bradley, "Voluntary Associations, Civic Culture, and *Obshestven-nost'* in Moscow," in *Between Tsar and People: Educated Society and the Quest for Public Identity in Late Imperial Russia,* ed. Edith W. Clowes, Samuel D. Kassow, and James L. West (Princeton: Princeton Univ. Press, 1991), 144.

142. See N. O. Lossky, *History of Russian Philosophy* (London: Allen & Unwin, 1952); M. M. Novikov, *Ot Moskvy do N'iu-Iorka: Moia zhizn' v nauke i politike* (New York: Izdatel'stvo imeni Chekhova, 1952).

143. The museum collections grew gradually, with donations from Russian émi-grés from all over the world; they were taken to Russia after the Red Army entered Czechoslovakia at the end of the Second World War.

144. S. P. Postnikov, *Russkie v Prage, 1918–1928* (Prague: Postnikov, 1928). This activity in part continued the movement for regional autonomy, stimulated by the increased interest in the national culture during the second half of the nineteenth century. See Bradley, "Voluntary Associations."

145. Eugenia Fischer, "Czechoslovakia," in *Psychoanalysis International: A Guide to Psychoanalysis throughout the World,* ed. Peter Kutter (Stuttgart: Frommann, 1992), 1: 36.

146. Stepan Vereshchaka, "Russkii psikhiatricheskii kruzhok v Prage," in Bem, Dosuzhkov, and Lossky, *Zhizn' i smert',* 55–57.

147. V. V. Nabokov, *The Defence* [1929], trans. Michael Scammell (Oxford: Oxford Univ. Press, 1986). Marina Tsvetaeva is quoted in Serapionova, *Rossiiskaia emigratsiia,* 78; editorial quoted on p. 166.

148. Serapionova, *Rossiiskaia emigratsiia,* 83.

149. "M. P. Polosin," in Moscow Cultural Foundation. Archive of Russian Emi-gration.

150. The titles of Troshin's works, as they appear in the Troshin papers in the Archive of Russian Emigration, are (my translations) "Pushkin and the Psychology of Creativity," "Mental Illness in Pushkin's Work," "Pushkin and Philosophy," "Push-kin and His Attempt to Emigrate," and "Pushkin Studies in Russia and outside Rus-sia." Osipov's activities are described in "Publichnye vystupleniia N. E. Osipova v Prage," in Bem, Dosuzhkov, and Lossky, *Zhizn' i smert',* 60–64.

151. E. A. Liatskii to N. E. Osipov, November 6, 1927, in TsGALI, f. 2299, op. 1, ed. khr. 47, l. 1.

152. N. E. Osipov, "Dostoevsky i psikhiatry" (December 1923), in ibid., ed. khr. 1, l. 7.

153. Fischer, "Czechoslovakia," 36, 39–41.

154. N. E. Osipov, "Vsevolod Mikhailovich Garshin" (1928), in TsGALI, f. 2299, op. 1, ed. khr. 17, l. 51.

155. Liatskii to Osipov, November 6, 1927.

156. A. L. Bem, "Razvertyvanie sna (*Vechnyi muzh* Dostoevskogo)," in *Uchenye zapiski, osnovannye Russkoi uchebnoi collegiei v Prage* (Prague, 1924), 1: 45–59; N. E. Osi-

pov, "Novyi podkhod k Dostoevskomu: Raboty A. L. Bema" (November 13, 1929), in TsGALI, f. 2299, op. 1, ed. khr. 26, l. 14.

157. A. L Bem to N. E. Osipov, May 10, 1931, in TsGALI, f. 2299, op. 1, ibid., ed. khr. 42, l. 40.

158. Carlo Ginzburg, "Morelli, Freud and Sherlock Holmes: Clues and Scientific Method," *History Workshop Journal,* no. 9 (1980): 5–36.

159. Responses in the West also varied. The neurologist Kurt Goldstein, for instance, turned to courage for a response to the "shocks of existence." See Anne Harrington, *Reenchanted Science: Holism in German Culture from Wilhelm II to Hitler* (Princeton: Princeton Univ. Press, 1996), 156.

160. On Spektorskii, see "Spektorskii Evgenii Vasilievich," in *Filosofy Rossii XIX–XX Stoletii: Biografii, idei, trudy,* ed. P. V. Alekseev et al. (Moscow: Kniga i Biznes, 1993), 173. On Lapshin, see N. O. Lossky, *Istoriia russkoi filosofii* (Moscow: Izdatel'skaia gruppa "Progress," 1994), 180–84.

161. Before the Revolution, N. O. Lossky (1870–1965) taught philosophy at St. Petersburg University. He was expelled with other Russian intellectuals in 1922 and moved to Prague, where he worked at the Russian People's University. In 1942 he moved to Belgrade, and later to the United States. He called his conception "metaphysical personalism." Lossky's comment on Freud is from his *History of Russian Philosophy,* 330. V. V. Zen'kovskii (1881–1962) moved to Belgrade after the Revolution, and then to Prague, where he was a director of the Pedagogical Institute. He wrote on philosophical psychology, history of philosophy, and literature (my translations of the titles): *The Problem of Psychical Causality* (1914), "The Hierarchical Structure of the Soul" (1929), and *N. V. Gogol* (1961). B. P. Vysheslavtsev (1877–1954), professor of the philosophy of law at Moscow University, was expelled from Russia in 1922. In Paris he worked in the Russian section of the YMCA Press, then lived in Switzerland. He published abroad his main books: *The Heart of Man in the Indian and Christian Mysticism* (Paris: YMCA Press, 1929) and *The Ethics of Transfigured Eros* (Paris: YMCA Press, 1932). Lossky's comment on Vysheslavtsev is from Lossky, *History of Russian Philosophy,* 387.

162. Freud's letters to Osipov are published by Miller as an appendix to his *Freud and the Bolsheviks,* 169–74.

163. Fischer, "Czechoslovakia," 37.

164. Dosuzhkov, "Nikolai Evgrafovich Osipov," 44.

165. See Lapshin's (my translations of the titles) *The Laws of Thought and the Forms of Knowledge* (1906), *Artistic Creativeness* (1922), and *The Philosophy of Inventiveness and Invention in Philosophy* (1922). He was expelled from Soviet Russia in 1922 and settled in Prague, where he published essays on Russian literature and art, including "Tolstoy's Metaphysics" (1929), "Dostoevsky's Metaphysics" (1931), and *Russian Music* (1948).

166. N. O. Lossky, "N. E. Osipov kak filosof," in Bem, Dosuzhkov, and Lossky, *Zhizn' i smert',* 50.

167. N. O. Lossky, *History of Russian Philosophy,* 331.

168. N. E. Osipov, "Strashnoe u Gogolia i Dostoevskogo," in Bem, Dosuzhkov, and Lossky, *Zhizn' i smert',* 135; N. E. Osipov, "Revoliutsiia i son" [1927], in *Russkii narodnyi universitet v Prage: Nauchnye trudy* (Prague: Russkii narodnyi universitet, 1931), 4: 175–203. Similarly, Nikolai Berdiaev, a religious philosopher, interpreted history as a drama of love and irrational freedom in which a victory for irrational freedom results in chaos, in Non-Being.

169. Tolstoy quoted in Biriukov, *Biografiia,* 68; N. E. Osipov, "Život a smrt," in *Russkii narodnyi universitet v Prage: Nauchnye trudy* (Prague: Russkii narodnyi universitet, 1928), 1: 138–46. A Russian translation of this Czech version of Osipov's paper appeared as "Zhizn' i smert'," in Bem, Dosuzhkov, and Lossky, *Zhizn' i smert',* 67–78.

Four. Decadents, Revolutionaries, and the Nation's Mental Health

Epigraphs: D. S. Merezhkovskii, "Lermontov: Poet sverkhchelovechestva," in *Izbrannye stat'i: Simvolizm, Gogol', Lermontov* (Munich: Wilhelm Fink, 1972), 332; and I. A. Sikorskii, "Biologicheskie voprosy v psikhologii i psikhiatrii," *Voprosy nervnopsikhicheskoi meditsiny,* 1904, no. 1: 113.

1. Emile Durkheim, *Suicide: A Study in Sociology* [1897] (London: Routledge & Kegan Paul, 1952), 77.

2. Henry Havelock Ellis, *The Genius of Europe* (Westport, Conn.: Greenwood, 1951), 204. Not everybody agreed with this opinion. The main theoretician of decadence, Paul Bourget, was as pessimistic about the Slavs as about the French and Germans. He believed that, unlike the "solitary and bizarre neuroses" of French decadents or Schopenhauer's tragic mood, social pessimism in Russia took the form of nihilism. See Jean Pierrot, *The Decadent Imagination, 1880–1900,* trans. Derek Coltman (Chicago: Univ. of Chicago Press, 1981), 16.

3. I. A. Sikorskii, "Uspekhi russkogo khudozhestvennogo tvorchestva: Rech' v torzhestvennom zasedanii II-go s"ezda otechestvennykh psikhiatrov v Kieve," *Voprosy nervno-psikhicheskoi meditsiny,* 1905, no. 3: 497–504; no. 4: 617–18.

4. Peter Henry, "Introduction," in *From the Reminiscences of Private Ivanov and Other Stories,* by Vsevolod Garshin, trans. Peter Henry, Liv Tudge, Donald Rayfield, and Philip Taylor (London: Angel Books, 1988), 11.

5. This argument is supported by Roger Keys, among others; see his *The Reluctant Modernist: Andrei Belyi and the Development of Russian Fiction: 1902–1914* (Oxford: Clarendon, 1996), esp. 25–35.

6. John E. Bowlt, "Through the Glass Darkly: Images of Decadence in Early-Twentieth-Century Russian Art," *Journal of Contemporary History* 17 (1982): 96–97.

7. Quoted in Jeffrey Brooks, "Popular Philistinism and the Course of Russian Modernism," in *Literature and History: Theoretical Problems and Russian Case-Studies,* ed. Gary Soul Morson (Stanford: Stanford Univ. Press, 1986), 101.

8. The term *decadent* was supposedly first used in the Russian press in 1889 by an

art critic. See Bowlt, "Through the Glass," 93. On Briusov and the symbolist movement in Russia, see Joan Delaney Grossman, *Valery Briusov and the Riddle of Russian Decadence* (Berkeley: Univ. of California Press, 1985); Martin P. Rice, *Valery Briusov and the Rise of Russian Symbolism* (Ann Arbor, Mich.: Ardis, 1975).

9. V. M. Doroshevich, *Dekadent* (1912), quoted in Louise McReynolds, "V. M. Doroshevich: The Newspaper Journalist and the Development of Public Opinion in Civil Society," in *Between Tsar and People: Educated Society and the Quest for Public Identity in Late Imperial Russia,* ed. Edith W. Clowes, Samuel D. Kassow, and James L. West (Princeton: Princeton Univ. Press, 1991), 239.

10. I. A. Sikorskii, "Russkaia psikhopaticheskaia literatura, kak material dlia ustanovleniia novoi klinicheskoi formy—*Idiophrenia paranoides,*" *Voprosy nervno-psikhicheskoi meditsiny,* 1902, no. 1: 47; F. E. Rybakov, *Sovremennye pisateli i bol'nye nervy: Psikhiatricheskii etiud* (Moscow: V. Richter, 1908), 14, 15.

11. Rybakov, *Sovremennye pisateli,* 3; G. I. Rossolimo, *Iskusstvo, bol'nye nervy i vospitanie* (Moscow: G. I. Prostakov, 1901), 38; Rybakov, *Sovremennye pisateli,* 6.

12. See Murray G. H. Pittock, *Spectrum of Decadence: The Literature of the 1890s* (London: Routledge, 1993), 26.

13. Rossolimo, *Iskusstvo,* 37.

14. M. O. Shaikevich, "Psikhopatologicheskii metod v russkoi literaturnoi kritike," *Voprosy filosofii,* 1904, no. 3: 328–30; "psychological automatism" was the term used by L. Sheinis; ibid., 327.

15. M. Shaikevich, "Psikhopatologicheskie cherty geroev Maksima Gor'kogo," *Vestnik psikhologii,* 1904, no. 1: 55; no. 2: 40–50; no. 3: 124–41.

16. Sikorskii, "Uspekhi russkogo," 618.

17. Ibid., 499–500; M. P. Nikinin, "Chekhov kak izobrazitel' bol'noi dushi," *Vestnik psikhologii,* 1905, no. 1: 7, 13; Rossolimo quoted in I. D. Ermakov, "Desiatyi Pirogovskii s"ezd v Moskve, 25.IV–2.V.1907," *Zhurnal nevropatologii,* 1907, no. 2–3: 554.

18. Sikorskii, "Uspekhi russkogo," 504.

19. Newspaper headline quoted in Orlando Figes, *A People's Tragedy: The Russian Revolution, 1891–1924* (London: Jonathan Cape, 1996), 181. On the 1905 revolution, see, e.g., Abraham Ascher, *The Revolution of 1905: Russia in Disarray* (Stanford: Stanford Univ. Press, 1988); Roberta Thompson Manning, *The Crisis of the Old Order in Russia: Gentry and Government* (Princeton: Princeton Univ. Press, 1982).

20. V. V. Vorob'ev, "Degeneraty i ikh obshchestvennoe znachenie," in *Otchety Moskovskogo obshchestva nevropatologov i psikhiatrov za 1901–1902 gg.* (Moscow: Kushnerev, 1902), 10.

21. To provide assistance to wounded strikers and other victims of the street fighting, some members of the radical All-Russian Union of Medical Personnel organized an unofficial Red Cross committee. See John F. Hutchinson, *Politics and Public Health in Revolutionary Russia, 1890–1918* (Baltimore: Johns Hopkins Univ. Press, 1990), 211.

22. See Julie V. Brown, "Social Influences on Psychiatric Theory and Practice in Late Imperial Russia," in *Health and Society in Revolutionary Russia,* ed. Susan Gross Solomon and John F. Hutchinson (Bloomington: Indiana Univ. Press, 1990), 42.

23. J. F. Hutchinson shows that the medical profession was divided between two models for a health care system, locally and centrally oriented; see his *Politics,* xix–xx. Veresaev quoted in Nancy Mandelker Frieden, *Russian Physicians in an Era of Reform and Revolution, 1856–1905* (Princeton: Princeton Univ. Press, 1981), 199.

24. On the history and bibliography of this discussion, see V. L. L'vov-Roga-chevskii, "V. Veresaev," in *Die Russische Literatur des 20. Jahrhunderts,* ed. S. A. Vengerov (Munich: Wilhelm Fink, 1972), 145–72.

25. I. A. Sikorskii, *O knige V. Veresaeva* Zapiski Vracha *(Chto daet eta kniga literature, nauke i zhizni?)* (Kiev: Kushnerev, 1902).

26. On the history of attitudes towards the proneness of different races to diseases, see John M. Efron, *Defenders of the Race: Jewish Doctors and Race Science in Fin-de-Siècle Europe* (New Haven: Yale Univ. Press, 1994); Douglas A. Lorimer, *Colour, Class, and the Victorians: English Attitudes to the Negro in the Mid-Nineteenth Century* (Leicester: Leicester Univ. Press, 1978); Edward Shorter, *From the Mind into the Body: The Cultural Origins of Psychosomatic Symptoms* (New York: Free Press, 1994).

27. Robert A. Nye, *Crime, Madness, and Politics in Modern France: The Medical Concept of National Decline* (Princeton: Princeton Univ. Press, 1984), 140, 142.

28. Ibid., 317–18.

29. Ellis, *Genius of Europe,* 90

30. Alfred Fouillée, *Esquisse psychologique des peuples européens,* 4th ed. (Paris: Félix Alcan, 1903), 412: "Plus passive qu'active, plus résistante qu'entreprenante, plus entraînée que volontaire, plus résignée que révoltée, plus respectueuse de la force qu'impérieuse et forte."

31. N. I. Mukhin, "Neirasteniia i degeneratsiia," *Arkhiv psikhiatrii,* 1888, no. 1: 49, 67; V. M. Bekhterev, "Voprosy vyrozhdeniia i bor'ba s nim," *Obozrenie psikhiatrii,* 1908, no. 9: 518–21. See also a report of Bekhterev's talk in "Khronika," *Obozrenie psikhiatrii,* 1908, no. 8: 510–11.

32. M. Iu. Lakhtin, "Patologicheskii al'truizm v literature i zhizni," *Voprosy nevrologii i psikhiatrii,* 1912, no. 7: 294; Tutyshkin's opinion in Julie V. Brown, "Revolution and Psychosis: The Mixing of Science and Politics in Russian Psychiatric Medicine, 1905–1913," *Russian Review* 46 (1987): 298; B. S. Greidenberg, "Psikhologicheskie osnovy nervno-psikhicheskoi terapii," in *Trudy Pervogo s"ezda Russkogo soiuza psikhiatrov i nevropatologov, Moskva, 4–11.9.1911,* ed. N. A. Vyrubov et al. (Moscow: Shtab Moskovskogo voennogo okruga, 1914), 118–41.

33. D. A. Amenitskii, "Analiz geroia *Mysli* Leonida Andreeva (K voprosu o paranoidnoi psikhopatii)," *Sovremennaia psikhiatriia,* 1915, no. 5: 248–49; Dr. V. M. B–r, "*Gamlet* Shekspira s mediko-psikhologicheskoi tochki zreniia," *Arkhiv psikhiatrii,* 1897, no. 2: 99.

34. W. F. Bynum and Michael Neve, "Hamlet on the Couch," in *The Anatomy of*

Madness: Essays in the History of Psychiatry, ed. W. F. Bynum, Roy Porter, and Michael Shepherd (London: Tavistock, 1985), 1: 297; Henry Maudsley, *The Physiology and Pathology of the Mind* (London: Macmillan, 1867), 153–54. Maudsley's book was translated into Russian by I. Isain as *Fiziologiia i patologiia dushi* (St. Petersburg: Bakst, 1871).

35. A. N. Kremlev, "K voprosu o 'bezumii' Gamleta," *Voprosy psikhologii*, 1905, no. 4: 298; Ellis, *Genius of Europe,* 133; B–r, "*Gamlet* Shekspira," 103, 107.

36. Sikorskii, "Uspekhi russkogo khudozhestvennogo tvorchestva," 613 (emphasis in original).

37. N. A. Dobroliubov, "What Is Oblomovitism?" [1859], in *Belinsky, Chernyshevsky, and Dobroliubov: Selected Criticism,* ed. and intro. Ralph E. Matlaw (Bloomington: Indiana Univ. Press, 1976), 148.

38. One such hero was the title character of Pushkin's *Eugene Onegin,* a novel in verse that one critic called the "encyclopedia of Russian life" of the first third of the nineteenth century. Alexander Pushkin, *Eugene Onegin* [1833], trans. Charles Johnston, intro. John Bayley (Harmondsworth, U.K.: Penguin Books, 1979), 52:

> The illness with which he'd been smitten
> should have been analyzed when caught,
> something like *spleen,* that scourge of Britain,
> or Russian *chondria,* for short;
> it mastered him in slow gradation;
> thank God, he had no inclination
> to blow his brains out, but in stead
> to life grew colder than the dead.
> So, like Child Harold, glum, unpleasing,
> he stalked the drawing-rooms, remote
> from Boston's cloth or gossip's quote;
> no glance so sweet, no sigh of teasing,
> no, nothing caused his heart to stir,
> and nothing pierced his senses' blur.

39. P. P. Kapterev, "Detstvo Il'i Il'icha Oblomova: Psikhologo-pedagogicheskii etiud o prichinakh proiskhozhdeniia i razvitiia leni," *Zhenskoe obrazovanie,* 1891, no. 3: 248–66. Alternative models for education varied from enforced studies of the mother tongue and Russian literature at school to the hardening of will in Boy Scout groups. The former model was advocated by the liberally minded nationalist; the latter was introduced by the hard-liners of both conservative and radical beliefs. The Boy Scout movement was imported by the tsar himself, who sent his army officers to Britain for instruction. All the same, boy-scouting found support with the Social Democrats: a psychiatrist Tutyshkin, who later joined the Bolshevik party, praised the hard-will style of education as the only means to fight the "Oblomovitism" of Russian youth. See P. P. Tutyshkin, "Sovremennye voprosy pedagogicheskoi psikhologii

i psikhiatrii," in Vyrubov et al., *Trudy Pervogo s"ezda,* 768. For an example of Boy Scout literature by a medical doctor, see A. K. Anokhin, *Sputnik iunogo razvedchika: Organizatsiia i zaniatiia s iunymi razvedchikami* (Kiev: I. I. Samonenko, 1916).

40. For the English translation of the essay, first published in 1860, see I. S. Turgenev, *Hamlet and Don Quixote: An Essay,* trans. Robert Nichols (London: Henderson, 1930). For a discussion of Turgenev's essay and its effect on Russian intellectual and literary life, see L. M. Lotman, *Realizm russkoi literatury 60-kh godov XIX veka (Istoki i esteticheskoe svoeobrazie)* (Leningrad: Nauka, 1974), esp. chaps. 1 and 3.

41. On the reception of *Don Quixote* in Russia, see Iurii Aikhenval'd, *Don Kikhot na russkoi pochve* (New York: Chalidze, 1982).

42. Peter Henry, *A Hamlet of His Time: Vsevolod Garshin: The Man, His Works, and His Milieu* (Oxford: Willem A. Meeuws, 1983), 167; see chap. 7 for the history, interpretations, and reception of *The Red Flower.* For an English translation of Garshin's story, see Garshin, *From the Reminiscences of Private Ivanov.*

43. Uspenskii, quoted in Henry, *Hamlet,* 166; Mikhailovsky quoted in ibid., 166–67. After choosing the heading for this section, I learned that Joseph Frank had already used a similar phrase in the title of his essay, "The Search for a Positive Hero," in *Through the Russian Prism: Essays on Literature and Culture* (Princeton: Princeton Univ. Press, 1990), 75–82.

44. Ellis, *Genius of Europe,* 179.

45. I. A. Sikorskii, "Krasnyi tsvetok: Rasskaz Vsevoloda Garshina," *Vestnik klinicheskoi i sudebnoi psikhiatrii i nevropatologii,* 1884, no. 1: 348.

46. Garshin's comments on Sikorskii are from "Pis'ma," in *Polnoe sobranie sochinenii v trekh tomakh* (Moscow: Academia, 1934), 3: 304, 339. Sikorskii's book was *Education in Infancy* (*Vospitanie v vozraste pervogo detstva* [1884]), 3d ed. (St. Petersburg: A. E. Riabchenko, 1904).

47. Fausek quoted in P. M. Zinov'ev, *Dushevnye bolezni v kartinakh i obrazakh* (Moscow: Sabashnikovy, 1927), 131, 128–29. Zinov'ev was quoting from Fausek's "Reminiscences" ("Vospominaniia," in *Polnoe sobranie sochinenii,* by V. M. Garshin [St. Petersburg: A. F. Marks, 1910], 28–63) while giving his own accents to the story. For a biographer's account of these events, see Henry, *Hamlet,* chap. 5.

48. N. N. Bazhenov, "Dushevnaia drama Garshina," in *Psikhiatricheskie besedy na literaturnye i obshchestvennye temy* (Moscow: Mamontov, 1903), 122.

49. M. Iu. Lakhtin, *Patologicheskii al'truizm v literature i zhizni* (Moscow: Snegirev, 1912), 6, 16. Other psychiatrists who wrote (or thought about writing) on Garshin were Moshe Wulff and N. E. Osipov. Both of them had the chance to observe a member of Garshin's family who was repeatedly admitted to the Moscow University Clinic and whose disorder was diagnosed as manic-depression. See "N. E. Garshina's Case Record," in the Archive of the Psychiatric Clinic imeni S. S. Korsakova, of Moscow Medical Academy.

50. M. Iu. Lakhtin, "Patologicheskii al'truizm v literature i zhizni," *Voprosy nevrologii i psikhiatrii,* 1912, no. 7: 294.

51. On Elena as a female version of the positive hero, see Rufus W. Mathewson Jr., *The Positive Hero in Russian Literature,* 2d ed. (Stanford: Stanford Univ. Press, 1975).

52. M. I. Konorov, "Don-Kikhot kak tsel'naia patologicheskaia lichnost'," *Voprosy psikhologii,* 1906, no. 4: 305–18; no. 6: 494–506.

53. On Gorky, see Richard Hare, *Maxim Gorky: Romantic Realist and Conservative Revolutionary* (London: Oxford Univ. Press, 1962).

54. Shaikevich, "Psikhopatologicheskie," 131–32.

55. N. Vavulin, *Bezumie, ego smysl i tsennost': Psikhologicheskie ocherki* (St. Petersburg: Vaisberg & Gershunin, 1913), 126.

56. Iu. V. Kannabikh, "Zametki o 'normal' nom' i 'nenormal' nom' (skhema)," *Psikhoterapiia,* 1913, no. 2: 7–8; A. A. Tokarskii, "Strakh smerti," *Voprosy filosofii,* 1897, no. 40: 977 (this article was discussed in Tolstoy's family; see S. A. Tolstaia, *Dnevniki* [Moscow: Khudozhestvennaia literatura, 1978], 1: 363); A. I. Iarotskii, *Idealism kak fiziologicheskii faktor* (Iur'ev: K. Matissen, 1908), 284, 183.

57. Joan Burbick, *Healing the Republic: The Language of Health and the Culture of Nationalism in Nineteenth-Century America* (Cambridge: Cambridge Univ. Press, 1994), 240.

58. Anson Rabinbach argues that physicians reserved the category of "traumatic neurasthenia" for working-class patients, and it was not identical with the neurasthenia of middle-class patients. Anson Rabinbach, *The Human Motor: Energy, Fatigue, and the Origins of Modernity* (Berkeley: Univ. of California Press, 1992), 158.

59. Beard and Mitchell quoted in Burbick, *Healing the Republic,* 225.

60. William Marrs, quoted in Tom Lutz, *American Nervousness, 1903: An Anecdotal History* (Ithaca, N.Y.: Cornell Univ. Press, 1991), 7.

61. N. N. Bazhenov, "Vneuniversitetskaia deiatel'nost' i znachenie S. S. Korsakova, kak vracha i uchitelia," in *Psikhiatricheskie besedy,* 2.

62. Bazhenov quoted in M. Iu. Lakhtin, *Chastnaia lechebnitsa dlia dushevno-bol'nykh voinov: Otchet s 19.5.1905 po 1.1. 1906* (Moscow: Russkii trud, 1906).

63. S. S. Stupin, "K voprosu o narodnykh sanatoriiakh dlia nervno-bol'nykh," *Zhurnal nevropatologii,* 1904, no. 3: 363.

64. "Sektsiia nervnykh i dushevnykh boleznei IX-go s'ezda Obshchestva russkikh vrachei v pamiat' N. I. Pirogova," *Zhurnal nevropatologii,* 1904, no. 1–2: 269.

65. V. K. Rot, "Obshchestvennoe popechenie o nervno-bol'nykh. Ustroistvo spetsial'nykh sanatorii" [talk given in 1905], in *Trudy vtorogo s"ezda otechestvennykh psikhiatrov* (Kiev: Kul'zhenko, 1907), 481; M. Ia. Droznes, "Vazhneishie zadachi sovremennoi prakticheskoi psikhiatrii," in *Trudy vtorogo s"ezda otechestvennykh psikhiatrov,* 213; Mitskevich quoted in I. D. Ermakov, "Desiatyi Pirogovskii s"ezd v Moskve, 25.IV–2.V.1907," *Zhurnal nevropatologii,* 1907, no. 2–3: 551.

66. Yet some years earlier Tutyshkin was involved in establishing, within the Khar'kov Public Hospital, a sanatorium for people with nervous and mental illnesses who could not afford private clinics. See P. P. Tutyshkin, "Ob ustroistve obshchestvennykh (zemskikh, gorodskikh) lechebnits-pansionatov dlia nervno i dushevno-

bol'nykh, to est' uchrezhdenii dvoiako-smeshannogo tipa," *Zhurnal nevropatologii,* 1902, no. 1–2: 206–10.

67. Rot quoted in Ermakov, "Desiatyi Pirogovskii s"ezd," 551.

68. See Manning, *Crisis of the Old Order,* 106–37.

69. A. O. Edel'shtein, *Psikhiatricheskie s"ezdy i obshchestva za polveka (K istorii med-itsinskoi obshchestvennosti, 1887–1936)* (Moscow: Medgiz, 1948), 22.

70. A selected bibliography for I. A. Sikorskii includes *Psikhopaticheskii etiud* (Kiev: Universitet Sv. Vladimira, 1892); "O velikikh uspekhakh i vozrastaiushchem znachenii psikhiatrii i nevrologii sredi nauk i v zhizni," *Voprosy nervno-psikhicheskoi meditsiny,* 1899, no. 1: 1–14; "Znachenie gigieny vospitaniia v vozraste pervogo detstva," *Vestnik klinicheskoi,* 1899, no. 2: 59–128; "Biologicheskie voprosy v psikhologii i psikhiatrii," *Voprosy nervno-psikhicheskoi meditsiny,* 1904, no. 1: 79–114; *Vseobshchaia psikhologiia s fiziognomikoi* (Kiev: Kul'zhenko, 1904); and *Sbornik nauchno-literaturnykh statei po voprosam obshchestvennoi psikhologii, vospitatel'noi i nervno-psikhicheskoi gigieny,* 5 vols. (Kiev: F. A. Ioganson, 1900–1904): (my translations of the titles) vol. 1, *Psychological Features of Great Men: Herbert Spencer, Adam Mickievicz, Pushkin, Saltykov, S. P. Botkin, Father Ioann Kronshtadskii;* vol. 2, *The Soul and the Brain of Great Men: Gambetta, Tur-genev, and Helmholtz;* vol. 3, *Success of Russian Art and its Significance for Social Life;* and vol. 5, *Russian Women-Doctors.*

71. Sikorskii, "Uspekhi russkogo," 497.

72. Edel'shtein, *Psikhiatricheskie s"ezdy,* 19.

73. On Taine's views of the French Revolution, see Jaap van Ginneken, *Crowds, Psychology, and Politics, 1871–1889* (Cambridge: Cambridge Univ. Press, 1992), 42.

74. Sikorskii, "Uspekhi russkogo," 619. Trusting in his nationalist convictions, Sikorskii contrasted formal classical education with one rooted in the "native soil." His view stemmed from the early Slavophile idea that "outside the national soil there is no firm ground; outside the national, there is nothing real, vital; and every good idea, every institution not rooted in the national historical soil or grown organically from it, turns sterile and becomes old rag" (Ivan Aksakov, quoted in Richard Pipes, *Russia under the Old Regime* [New York: Charles Scribner's Sons, 1974], 276). Several years later, in the period of political reaction, Sikorskii's nationalism led him to become a prosecution witness at the trial of a Jew accused in a ritual murder. See I. A. Sikorskii, *Ekspertiza po delu ob ubiistve Andriushi Iushchinskogo* (St. Petersburg: A. S. Suvorin, 1913). The majority of the intelligentsia, including psychiatrists, scorned this trial; the jury finally acquitted the accused, Beilis.

75. Sikorskii, "Uspekhi russkogo," 622.

76. Manning, *Crisis of the Old Order,* 329.

77. See Laura Engelstein, *The Keys to Happiness: Sex and the Search for Modernity in Fin-de-Siècle Russia* (Ithaca, N.Y.: Cornell Univ. Press, 1992), 259–60; N. N. Ba-zhenov, *Psikhologiia i politika* (Moscow: I. D. Sytin, 1906), 13–18.

78. See Frieden, *Russian Physicians,* 319.

79. Iakovenko quoted in Brown, "Revolution and Psychosis," 292–93; M. Zhu-

kovskii, "O vliianii obshchestvennykh sobytii na razvitie dushevnykh zabolevanii," *Vestnik psikhologii*, 1907, no. 3: 161–63.

80. V. P. Serbskii, "Russkii soiuz psikhiatrov i nevropatologov im. S. S. Korsakova," in Vyrubov et al., *Trudy Pervogo s"ezda,* 83. Serbskii quoted K. D. Bal'mont's poem "I Wish" ("Khochu"; 1902); see Konstantin Bal'mont, *Stikhotvoreniia* (Moscow: Khudozhestvennaia literatura, 1990), 122.

81. On the strike, see Samuel D. Kassow, *Students, Professors, and the State in Tsarist Russia* (Berkeley: Univ. of California Press, 1989), 352–402.

82. Serbskii, "Russkii soiuz psikhiatrov," 83.

83. F. E. Rybakov to V. P. Serbskii, October 1911, in Muzei Moskovskoi Meditsinskoi Akademii, f. 525/34, op. 1, ed. khr. 44. The order about Rybakov's appointment was signed April 10, 1911. The young physician who acted in the story was L. M. Rozenshtein, who left soon after Serbskii and returned to the clinic only after Rybakov's retirement in 1919. On this conflict, see also A. O. Edel'shtein, "Psikhiatricheskaia klinika imeni Korsakova za 50 let," in *Piat'desiat let Psikhiatricheskoi klinike imeni Korsakova* (Moscow: Pervyi Moskovskii meditsinskii institut, 1940), 9–23.

84. Rybakov to Serbskii, October 1911. In 1917, after Nicholas II's abdication, the Provisional Government issued an order to reestablish pre-Kasso professors in their positions. Rybakov received his retirement, but Serbskii died shortly after the order was issued. The Soviet Ministry of Public Health, Narkomzdrav, granted Rybakov a pension, but he continued to be active under the new regime and, together with A. N. Bernstein and A. P. Nechaev, organized the Psycho-Neurological Museum in Moscow, a research and training institution modeled after Bekhterev's famous Psycho-Neurological Institute. Rybakov died in Moscow in 1920. See "Formuliarnyi spisok F. E. Rybakova," in Muzei Moskovskoi Meditsinskoi Akademii, f. 523/132, op. 2. ed. khr. 12.

85. M. O. Gurevich, "Moskovskaia psikhiatricheskaia klinika v istorii otechestvennoi psikhiatrii," in *Piat'desiat let,* 3–8.

86. F. E. Rybakov, "Alkogolizm i dushevnoe rasstroistvo," in *Otchety Moskovskogo obshchestva nevropatologov i psikhiatrov za 1897–1901 gg.* (Moscow: G. I. Prostakov, 1901), 210; F. E. Rybakov, *Ob organizatsii ambulatorii dlia alkogolikov* (St. Petersburg: Ia. Trei, 1904).

87. S. A. Liass, quoted in "Vtoroi s"ezd nevropatologov i psikhiatrov" (editorial), *Obozrenie psikhiatrii*, 1906, no. 2: 152.

88. F. E. Rybakov, *Atlas dlia eksperimental'no-psikhologicheskogo issledovaniia lichnosti s podrobnym opisaniem i ob"iasneniem tablits: Sostavlen primenitel'no k tseli pedagogicheskogo i vrachebno-diagnosticheskogo issledovaniia* (Moscow: I. D. Sytin, 1910).

89. "Khronika," *Sovremennaia psikhiatriia*, 1910, no. 8: 242

90. On early psychiatric and neurological tests, see Milos Bondy, "Psychiatric Antecedents of Psychological Testing (before Binet)," *Journal of the History of the Behavioral Sciences*, 46, no. 2 (1974): 180–94. For a history of mental testing with a pathological perspective, see John M. Reisman, *A History of Clinical Psychology*, 2d ed. (New

York: Hemisphere, 1991). On A. N. Bernstein's objective approach, see his *Eksperimental'no-psikhologicheskaia metodika raspoznavaniia dushevnykh boleznei* (Moscow: S. P. Iakovlev, 1908); and *Eksperimental'no-psikhologicheskie skhemy dlia izucheniia narushenii u dushevno-bol'nykh* (Moscow: S. P. Iakovlev, 1910). For a discussion of the development of Kraepelin's clinical as opposed to symptomatological approach and the role of psychological data, see G. E. Berrios and Renata Hauser, "The Early Development of Kraepelin's Ideas on Classification: A Conceptual History," *Psychological Medicine* 18 (1988): 813–21.

On G. I. Rossolimo's tests, see his "Profili psikhologicheski nedostatochnykh detei (opyt eksperimental'no-psikhologicheskogo issledovaniia stepenei odarennosti)," *Sovremennaia psikhiatriia*, 1910, no. 9–10: 377–412. Unlike Rybakov, Rossolimo was one of those who resigned his position (as professor of neurology) at Moscow University) in support of his colleagues in 1911. In 1914 he organized and headed a private Institute for Child Neurology and Psychology, the first in Russia. The Soviet government adopted Rossolimo's tests for mass psychological testing in schools. See G. I. Rossolimo, "Metodika massovogo issledovaniia po 'psikhologicheskomu profiliu' i pervonachal'nye dannye," *Zhurnal nevropatologii*, 1925, no. 1: 45–58.

91. "Korrespondentsiia iz sektsii nervnykh i dushevnykh boleznei X-go Pirogovskogo s"ezda, 26.04.1907," *Sovremennaia psikhiatriia*, 1907, no. 3: 138. See also the debate on school tests between the leading experimental psychologists G. I. Chelpanov and A. P. Nechaev: G. I. Chelpanov, "Zadachi sovremennoi psikhologii," *Voprosy filosofii*, 1909, no. 4: 285–308; and Nechaev's response in "Otvet Chelpanovu," *Voprosy filosofii*, 1909, no. 5: 805–10.

92. F. E. Rybakov, "Granitsy sumasshestviia," in *Otchety*, 5–6; Rybakov, *Sovremennye pisateli*, 21.

93. The Freud–Jung letters mentioning Asatiani are evoked by James Rice as an illustration of Freud's stereotypes of Russia; see James Rice, *Freud's Russia: National Identity in the Evolution of Psychoanalysis* (New Brunswick, N.J.: Transaction, 1993), 67. On Asatiani, see A. D. Zurabashvili and I. T. Mentetashvili, "Vydaiushchiisia psikhiatr M. M. Asatiani," *Zhurnal nevropatologii*, 1952, no. 4: 72–73.

94. C. G. Jung to S. Freud, 1909, in *The Freud/Jung Letters: The Correspondence between Sigmund Freud and C. G. Jung*, ed. William McGuire (London: Hogarth, 1974), 225–27.

95. M. M. Asatiani, "Sovremennoe sostoianie voprosa teorii i praktiki psikhoanaliza po vzgliadam Junga," *Psikhoterapiia*, 1910, no. 3: 124.

Five. The Institute of Genius

Epigraphs: Leon Trotsky, *Literature and Revolution* [1923], trans. Rose Strunsky (Ann Arbor: Univ. of Michigan Press, 1975), 256; and P. I. Karpov, *Tvorchestvo dushevnobol'nykh i ego vliianie na razvitie nauki, iskusstva i tekhniki* (Moscow: GIZ, 1926), 17.

1. Richard Stites, *Revolutionary Dreams: Utopian Vision and Experimental Life in the Russian Revolution* (New York: Oxford Univ. Press, 1989), 251.

2. The Moscow Institute of Brain was formed in 1928 from the reorganization of a laboratory founded in 1924 to study Lenin's brain; see Monika Spivak, "Maiakovskii v Institute mozga," *Logos*, 2000, no. 3: 139–48. The Central Institute of Labor was founded in 1920; see Kendall Bailes, "Alexei Gastev and the Soviet Controversy over Taylorism," *Soviet Studies* 29 (1977): 373–94; I. E. Sirotkina, "Tsentral'nyi institut truda—voploshchenie utopii?" *Voprosy istorii estestvoznaniia i tekhniki*, 1991, no. 2: 67–72; Stites, *Revolutionary Dreams*, 145–64. The Psychoanalytic Institute was set up in 1923; see V. I. Ovcharenko, *Psikhoanaliticheskii glossarii* (Minsk: Vysheishaia shkola, 1994).

3. Nicholas II abdicated in favor of his son on March 2/March 15 (Old Russian calendar/Gregorian calendar). See, e.g., memoirs of Nicolas de Basili, *The Abdication of Emperor Nicholas II of Russia* (Princeton, N.J.: Kingston, 1984).

4. W. Bruce Lincoln, *Passage through Armageddon: The Russians in War and Revolution, 1914–1918* (New York: Simon & Schuster, 1986), 403.

5. "Konferentsiia vrachei psikhiatrov i nevropatologov, sozvannaia Pravleniem Soiuza psikhiatrov v Moskve 10–12 aprelia 1917 goda," *Sovremennaia psikhiatriia*, 1917, no. 2: 195–96.

6. P. E. Snesarev, quoted in ibid.

7. Advocating centralization seemed to be a "natural" way to deal with emergencies. As John F. Hutchinson shows, it led to, among other things, the foundation of the first Soviet Ministry of Public Health, Narkomzdrav, in the summer of 1918. Facing the danger of a cholera epidemic, the Soviet government did what physicians of the old regime would have done: it established a strong centralized agency to direct medical and sanitary affairs and to coordinate antiepidemic measures. See John F. Hutchinson, *Politics and Public Health in Revolutionary Russia, 1890–1918* (Baltimore: Johns Hopkins Univ. Press, 1990), 202.

8. In Chekhov's play *The Cherry Orchard* (1904), the new owners cut down the orchard cultivated by generations of their aristocratic predecessors, to build commercially.

9. "Konferentsiia vrachei," 182–83, 192.

10. Ibid., 185.

11. The February Revolution took place from February 27 to March 2 by the Old Russian calendar, which is March 12–15 by the Gregorian calendar; likewise, the October Revolution took place on October 25 by the Old Russian calendar, or November 7 by the Gregorian calendar.

12. Similarly, as Paul Weindling comments, during the 1919 political upheaval in Germany, "medical campaigners for social hygiene had a clear aim: a national Ministry of Health headed by a doctor"; unlike their Russian counterparts, they were unsuccessful. Paul Weindling, *Health, Race, and German Politics between National Unification and Nazism, 1870–1945* (Cambridge: Cambridge Univ. Press, 1989), 344.

13. On the history of Soviet public health and its affinities with pre-revolutionary community medicine, see Nancy Mandelker Frieden, *Russian Physicians in an Era of Reform and Revolution, 1856–1905* (Princeton: Princeton Univ. Press, 1981); Susan Gross Solomon and John F. Hutchinson, eds., *Health and Society in Revolutionary Russia* (Bloomington: Indiana Univ. Press, 1990); Hutchinson, *Politics*. On psychiatrists in particular, see Julie Vail Brown, "The Professionalization of Russian Psychiatry: 1857–1922" (Ph.D. diss., Univ. of Pennsylvania, 1981).

14. The Council of Medical Collegia was founded in January and Narkomzdrav in July 1918. For further discussion of the early history of Soviet public health care, see Neil B. Weissman, "Origins of Soviet Health Administration: Narkomzdrav, 1918–1928," in Solomon and Hutchinson, *Health and Society,* 97–120.

15. "Ot Russkogo soiuza psikhiatrov i nevropatologov v Sovet vrachebnykh kollegii" (May 1918), in GARF, f. 482, op. 1, d. 81, ll. 1, 3–4.

16. The Psychiatric Commission undertook an extremely difficult task. Inspections of local hospitals involved dangerous trips in the countryside, ruined by the Civil War. Even in Moscow traveling was a problem, and the commission had to solicit the government to give the psychiatrists traveling by trams to survey the hospitals permission to enter trams at the front door to escape the queues (passengers were required to enter through the rear door only). See "Nevro-psikhiatricheskaia podsektsiia lechebnoi sektsii Narkomzdrava" (June 14, 1918–December 24, 1919), in GARF, f. 482, op. 1, d. 22, l. 15.

17. L. A. Prozorov, "Nastoiashchee polozhenie dela psikhiatricheskoi pomoshchi v SSSR," *Zhurnal nevropatologii,* 1925, no. 1: 93–104.

18. "Nevro-psikhiatricheskaia podsektsiia," l. 28.

19. "Nevropsikhiatricheskaia podsektsiia: Pitanie dushevnobol'nykh" (1921), in GARF, f. 482, op. 1, d. 540, ll. 36–45.

20. L. A. Prozorov, "Polozhenie dela psikhiatricheskoi pomoshchi v SSSR," *Zhurnal nevropatologii,* 1926, no. 2: 97–106.

21. "Protokol zasedaniia Organizatsionnoi podkomissii Narkomzdrava" (November 30, 1918), in GARF, f. 482, op. 1, d. 495, l. 2.

22. Rozenshtein was "co-opted" (appointed without elections) to the commission on November 30, 1918; see ibid. On Rozenshtein, see Iu. V. Kannabikh, L. A. Prozorov, and I. G. Ravkin, "L. M. Rozenshtein, ego nauchnaia i obshchestvennaia deiatel'nost," *Sovetskaia psikhonevrologiia,* 1934, no. 3: 7–14; D. E. Melekhov and A. V. Grosman, "L. M. Rozenshtein i period stanovleniia sovetskoi sotsial'noi psikhiatrii," in *Klinicheskie aspekty sotsial'noi readaptatsii psikhicheski bol'nykh,* ed. R. F. Semenov (Moscow: Institut psikhiatrii, 1976), 235–43; D. N. Pisarev, "L. M. Rozenshtein," *Sovetskaia psikhonevrologiia,* 1934, no. 3: 5–6; A. G. Gerish, "Rozenshtein, Lev Markovich," in *Bol'shaia meditsinskaia entsiklopediia* (Moscow: Sovetskaia entsiklopediia, 1984), 22: 1079–80.

23. A. O. Edel'stein, "L. M. Rozenshtein i Moskovskaia psikhiatricheskaia shkola,"

in *Problemy nevrastenii i nevrozov,* ed. L. M. Rozenshtein, S. I. Zander, and S. I. Gol'd-berg (Moscow: GIZ meditsinskoi literatury, 1935), 19.

24. L. M. Rozenshtein, "V. P. Serbskii—klassik Moskovskoi psikhiatricheskoi shkoly," in *Psikhogigienicheskie issledovaniia* (Moscow: Gos. Nauchnyi Institut nevro-psikhicheskoi profilaktiki, 1928), 1, pt. 1: 7–16; "Moskovskaia psikhiatricheskaia shkola i N. N. Bazhenov," *Klinicheskaia meditsina,* 1924, no. 4: 131–35; "P. B. Gannushkin kak psikhiatr epokhi," in *Trudy Psikhiatricheskoi kliniki Pervogo MMI. Pamiati Gannushkina* (Moscow: Gosizdat, 1934), 4: 13–19.

25. Rozenshtein, "V. P. Serbskii," 11.

26. Rozenshtein contributed to these discussions with publications in the re-cently founded journal *Psikhoterapiia.* See his "[Review of] *Neurasthenies et psycho-névroses,* [by] Hippolyte Bernheim" and a report from the Eleventh Congress of the Pirogov Society on the discussion of hysteria, in *Psikhoterapiia,* 1910, no. 3: 134–35; no. 6: 265–68.

27. Gerish, "Rozenshtein," 1079–80.

28. L. M. Rozenshtein, "O sovremennykh psikhiatricheskikh techeniiakh v So-vetskoi Rossii," in *Moskovskii Gosudarstvennyi nevro-psikhiatricheskii dispanser: Psikho-gigienicheskie i nevrologicheskie issledovaniia,* ed. L. M. Rozenshtein (Moscow: Narkomz-drav RSFSR, 1928), 119.

29. See Kannabikh et al., "L. M. Rozenshtein," 14.

30. S. S. Stupin, "K voprosu ob obshchestvennom lechenii i prizrenii alkogo-likov," *Sovremennaia psikhiatriia,* 1907, no. 11: 400; L. M. Rozenshtein, "K voprosu o lechenii alkogolikov (o protivoalkogol'nykh dispanserakh)," *Zhurnal nevropatologii,* 1915–16, no. 4–5–6: 519–27, quoted in N. V. Ivanov, "Vozniknovenie i razvitie otech-estvennoi psikhiatrii" (M.D. diss., Moscow, 1954), 579.

31. On general dispensaries, see John E. Pater, *The Making of the National Health Service* (London: King Edward's Hospital Fund for London, 1981), esp. 2–3; Ronald D. Cassel, *Medical Charities, Medical Politics: The Irish Dispensary System and the Poor Law, 1836–1872* (Woolbridge, U.K.: Boydell, 1997), esp. 130–31. On tuberculosis dis-pensaries, see F. B. Smith, *The Retreat of Tuberculosis, 1850–1950* (London: Croom Helm, 1988), 66–67; for French and German developments, see Pierre Guillaume, *Du désespoir au salut: les tubercouleux aux 19ᵉ et 20ᵉ siècles* (Paris, 1986), 187–215; Paul Wein-dling, "The Modernization of Charity in Nineteenth-Century France and Ger-many," in *Medicine and Charity before the Welfare State,* ed. Jonathan Barry and Colin Jones (London: Routledge, 1991), 190–206. For a discussion of German tuberculosis dispensaries as models, see Weindling, *Health,* 179–81.

32. Smith, *Retreat,* 67. The aim of tuberculosis dispensaries is from D. J. Wil-liamson (1911), quoted in ibid.

33. N. A. Vyrubov, "Po psikhiatricheskim bol'nitsam Shotlandii," *Sovremennaia psikhiatriia,* 1913, no. 9: 694.

34. Adolf Meyer, "The Aims of a Psychiatric Clinic" [1913], in *The Commonsense Psychiatry of Adolf Meyer: Fifty-two Selected Papers,* ed. Alfred Lief (New York: McGraw-

Hill, 1948), 367. On the U.S. mental hygiene movement and Meyer's role in it, see Johannes C. Pols, "Managing the Mind: The Culture of American Mental Hygiene, 1920–1950" (Ph.D. diss., Univ. of Pennsylvania, 1997).

35. "In 1913, as a member of the International Congress of Physicians in London, I was present at a discussion between Adolf Meyer of Baltimore and the Scotch psychiatrists as to the best method of developing psychiatry. History has shown the correctness of the view of Adolf Meyer and American psychiatry." L. Rozenshtein, "Public-Health Service and Mental Hygiene in the U.S.S.R.," *Mental Hygiene* 4 (1931): 739–43.

36. See a discussion of war neurosis in *Sovremennaia psikhiatriia*, 1915, no. 1: 48. For the history of shell shock, see Martin Stone, "Shellshock and the Psychologists," in *The Anatomy of Madness: Essays in the History of Psychiatry,* ed. W. F. Bynum, Roy Porter, and Michael Shepherd (London: Tavistock, 1985), 2: 242–71; Anthony Babington, *Shell Shock: A History of the Changing Attitudes to War Neurosis* (London: Leo Cooper, 1997).

37. P. M. Avtokratov, "Prizrenie, lechenie i evakuatsiia dushevnobol'nykh vo vremia russko-iaponskoi voiny v 1904–905 godakh," *Obozrenie psikhiatrii,* 1906, no. 10: 665–68. See also "P. M. Avtokratov: Nekrolog," *Sovremennaia psikhiatriia,* 1915, no. 3: 153–54.

38. "Khronika," *Sovremennaia psikhiatriia,* 1915, no. 1: 48.

39. M. O. Shaikevich, "Eshche o psikhozakh v voiskakh," *Sovremennaia psikhiatriia,* 1913, no. 10: 790, 795.

40. P. M. Zinov'ev, "Privat-dotsent T. E. Segalov," *Klinicheskaia meditsina* 22 (1928): 226; T. E. Segalov's "K voprosu o sushchnosti kontuzii sovremennymi artilleriiskimi snariadami (*Morbus decompressionis*)," *Sovremennaia psikhiatriia,* 1915, no. 3: 103–17; and "K voprosu ob organicheskikh i funktsional'nykh zabolevaniiakh pri kontuzii artilleriiskimi snariadami. Stat'ia vtoraia," *Sovremennaia psikhiatriia,* 1915, no. 6: 263–70.

41. Shaikevich, "Eshche o psikhozakh," 795. For an example of those accepting Segalov's explanation, see G. Ia. Troshin, *Travmaticheskii nevroz po materialam tekushchei voiny* (Moscow: Shtab Moskovskogo voennogo okruga, 1916).

42. Rozenshtein quoted in Kannabikh et al., "L. M. Rozenshtein," 11. On the censorship, see D. N. Pisarev, "L. M. Rozenshtein."

43. Rozenshtein, "O sovremennykh psikhiatricheskikh techeniiakh," 119–20.

44. Though patriotic, Rozenshtein appreciated foreign developments in psychiatry and called the mental hygiene movement in the West a "factor of world significance." Quoted in Kannabikh et al., "L. M. Rozenshtein," 8.

45. L. M. Rozenshtein, "K psikhopatologii krainego golodaniia (nekrofagiia i antropofagiia)," a reference to this talk in [A. Kozhevnikov], "O deiatel'nosti Obshchestva nevropatologov i psikhiatrov v Moskve," *Zhurnal nevropatologii,* 1925, no. 1: 123–31.

46. Susan Gross Solomon, "Social Hygiene and Soviet Public Health, 1921–1930," in Solomon and Hutchinson, *Health and Society,* 189.

47. Ibid., 180. On social medicine in Germany, see Weindling, *Health,* esp. chaps. 3 and 6; on sanitary utopias, 76–80.

48. The 1919 statement is reported in *Postanovleniia KPSS i sovetskogo pravitel'stva ob okhrane zdorov'ia naroda* (1958), quoted in Weissman, "Origins of Soviet Health Administration," 106.

49. N. A. Semashko, "O zadachakh obshchestvennoi nevrologii i psikhiatrii," *Sotsial'naia gigiena,* 1924, no. 3–4: 93.

50. A colleague of Rozenshtein later interpreted his outpatient service as an "embryonic dispensary." L. L. Rokhlin, "Programma kursa psikhogigieny," *Sovetskaia psikhonevrologiia,* 1934, no. 3: 94.

51. V. I. Lenin, quoted in Stites, *Revolutionary Dreams,* 49; P. M. Zinov'ev, *K voprosu ob organizatsii nevro-psikhiatricheskikh dispanserov (razvitie myslei vtoroi chasti doklada na Vtorom Vserossiiskom soveshchanii po voprosam psikhiatrii i nevrologii, [November 12–17, 1923])* (Moscow, 1924), 1–4.

52. P. M. Zinov'ev, *K voprosu.*

53. "Proekt rezoliutsii Vtorogo Vserossiiskogo soveshchaniia psikhiatrov i nevropatologov" (1922), in GARF, f. 482, op. 1, d. 194, ll. 38–39.

54. L. M. Rozenshtein, *Psikhicheskie faktory v etiologii dushevnykh boleznei* (Moscow: Gosizdat, 1923).

55. "Otchet o rabote Moskovskogo gorodskogo nevropsikhiatricheskogo dispansera za 1926," in GARF, f. 482, op. 1, d. 619, l. 38.

56. As Neil B. Weissman remarks, "While almost the entire network of medical facilities was transferred to local financing (even in Moscow, Semashko argued, 'you can count our institutions on one hand!'), the basic agencies of sanitation and the campaign against social disease remained on the state budget." Weissman, "Origins of Soviet Health Administration," 110.

57. "Otchet o rabote Moskovskogo gorodskogo," ll. 38–48.

58. This work was supervised by Segalov, the same physician who in 1917 called for psychiatrists to be flexible and adapt their strategies to the new authorities.

59. E. I. Lotova, "Pervyi eksperiment po dispanserizatsii (Iz istorii dispanserizatsii v Moskve v dvadtsatykh godakh)," *Sovetskaia meditsina,* 1985, no. 5: 119–22.

60. L. Rozenshtein, "The Development of Mental Hygiene in Russia (USSR)," *Mental Hygiene* 3 (1930): 646.

61. I. A. Berger and I. D. Dobronravov, "O gigienicheskoi dispanserizatsii," *Zhurnal nevropatologii,* 1925, no. 2: 56–57.

62. L. M. Rozenshtein, quoted in T. I. Iudin, *Ocherki istorii otechestvennoi psikhiatrii* (Moscow: Medgiz, 1951), 376.

63. Berger and Dobronravov, "O gigienicheskoi dispanserizatsii," 70.

64. A. B. Zalkind, "The Fundamentals and the Practice of Mental Hygiene in Adolescence and Youth in Soviet Russia," *Mental Hygiene* 3 (1930): 647.

65. "Chem budet zanimat'sia Moskovskii gorodskoi nevropsikhiatricheskii dis-

panser v 1927/28 gg.," in GARF, f. 482, op. 1, d. 619, ll. 53–58. On the history of psychotherapy in Russia and the Soviet Union, see Ivanov, "Vozniknovenie i razvitie."

66. L. Rokhlin, "College of Mental Hygiene in the Ukraine (USSR)," *Mental Hygiene* 3 (1930): 662–63.

67. "Otchet o rabote Instituta nevro-psikhiatricheskoi profilaktiki za 1928–1929 gg.," in GARF, f. 482, op. 10, d. 1748, ll. 42–49.

68. Rozenshtein taught at the First Moscow Medical University. In Khar'kov, the chair at the Psychoneurological College was occupied by L. L. Rokhlin, who was also director of a research institute of social psychoneurology and mental hygiene within the Khar'kov Psychoneurological Academy. See L. L. Rokhlin, "O prepodavanii psikhogigieny," *Sovetskaia psikhonevrologiia*, 1934, no. 3: 58–90.

69. "Protokol Moskovskogo Soveta Narodnykh Komissarov, June 2, 1926: Khodataistvo o vkliuchenii v smetu nevropsikhiatricheskikh dispanserov," in GARF, f. 259, op. 10a, d. 61, ed. khr. 6. Rozenshtein and colleagues' project was comparable with the one suggested under the Mental Retardation Facilities and Community Mental Health Centers Construction Act passed by the U.S. government some forty years later; its long-term goal—never to be realized—was to establish a national network of two thousand centers. See Ellen Herman, *The Romance of American Psychology: Political Culture in the Age of Experts* (Berkeley: Univ. of California Press, 1995), 253.

70. V. A. Grombakh, "Moskovskaia psikhiatricheskaia organizatsiia," *Zhurnal nevropatologii*, 1925, no. 1: 107.

71. N. A. Semashko, "O zadachakh obshchestvennoi nevrologii i psikhiatrii," *Sotsial'naia gigiena*, 1924, no. 3–4: 93.

72. Grombakh, "Moskovskaia psikhiatricheskaia organizatsiia," 111.

73. See Frankwood E. Williams, *Russia, Youth, and the Present-Day World: Further Studies in Mental Hygiene* (New York: Farrar & Rinehart, 1934); Pols, "Managing the Mind," 379–82.

74. On utopianism in post-revolutionary Russia, see Stites, *Revolutionary Dreams;* on the role of psychologists and psychiatrists in the "new man project," see Raymond A. Bauer, *The New Man in Soviet Psychology* (Cambridge: Harvard Univ. Press, 1952); Alexander M. Etkind, *Eros of the Impossible: The History of Psychoanalysis in Russia,* trans. Noah Rubins and Maria Rubins (Boulder, Colo.: Westview, 1997); David Joravsky, "The Construction of the Stalinist Psyche," in *Cultural Revolution in Russia, 1928–1931,* ed. Sheila Fitzpatrick (Bloomington: Indiana Univ. Press, 1978), 105–28. On psychotechnics in the Soviet Union, see Lewis H. Siegelbaum, "*Okhrana Truda:* Industrial Hygiene, Psychotechnics, and Industrialization in the USSR," in Solomon and Hutchinson, *Health and Society,* 224–45.

75. G. V. Segalin, "Institut genial'nogo tvorchestva," *Klinicheskii arkhiv*, 1928, no. 1: 53.

76. G. V. Segalin, "O zadachakh evropatologii kak otdel'noi otrasli psikhopatologii," *Klinicheskii arkhiv*, 1925, no. 1: 10.

77. This part of the project—providing a favorable environment—was added later, when the neuropsychiatric dispensaries had become an everyday reality. Segalin, "Institut genial'nogo."

78. Michael David-Fox, *Revolution of the Mind: Higher Learning among the Bolsheviks, 1918–1929* (Ithaca, N.Y.: Cornell Univ. Press, 1997), 56, citing *Piat' let raboty Tsentral'noi komissii po uluchsheniiu byta uchenykh pri Sovete narodnykh komissarov RSFSR (TsEKUBU), 1921–1926* (Moscow: Izdanie TsEKUBU, 1927), 3–16.

79. On education and enlightenment as Soviet ideals, see David-Fox, *Revolution of the Mind;* Sheila Fitzpatrick, *The Commissariat of Enlightenment: Soviet Organization of Education and the Arts under Lunacharsky, October 1917–1921* (Cambridge: Cambridge Univ. Press, 1971); Robert Tucker, "Lenin's Bolshevism as a Culture in the Making," in *Bolshevik Culture: Experiment and Order in the Russian Revolution,* ed. Abbott Gleason et al. (Bloomington: Indiana Univ. Press, 1985).

80. Segalin, "Institut genial'nogo tvorchestva," 55–56.

81. Ibid., 57–59.

82. Glavlit, the Main Administration for Literary and Publishing Affairs, was founded within the People's Commissariat of Education in 1922. See Herman Ermolaev, *Censorship in Soviet Literature, 1917–1991* (Lanham, Md.: Rowman & Littlefield, 1997), 3.

83. B. Ia. Vol'fson, "'Panteon mozga' Bekhtereva i 'Insitut genial'nogo tvorchestva' Segalina," *Klinicheskii arkhiv,* 1928, no. 1: 52. For a discussion of Rossolimo's later years, see Vas. Khoroshko, "Pamiati professora G. I. Rossolimo," *Klinicheskaia meditsina* 22 (1928): 223–25.

84. Weindling, *Health,* 231.

85. Ibid., 141–154, 234, 123. On Otto Weininger, see Chandak Sengoopta, "The Unknown Weininger: Science, Philosophy, and Cultural Politics in Fin-de-Siècle Vienna," *Central European History* 4 (1997): 453–93.

86. The painting and most of Segalin's literary archive were lost after the war, when he moved from the Urals. His last medical work on "precancer syndrome" is dated 1948. This and other biographical information about Segalin is from Iu. Sorkin, "Polivalentnyi chelovek," *Nauka Urala,* no. 12 (1992): 4–5.

87. In 1921 Rüdin began compiling a "total register of population" for these purposes, and five years later the Reich Ministry of the Interior gave the Genealogical Department, which he headed, official status and the right to consult state and criminal records. In 1930 German psychiatrists had data on 800,000 individuals and set about the task of producing for each person a "psycho-biogram," which would correlate his or her physical and mental qualities and allow a classification using Kretschmer's typology. See Weindling, *Health,* 384–85.

88. Vol'fson, "'Panteon mozga,'" 52. In 1926 Segalin's journal published an article by A. A. Kapustin reporting on his dissections of the brains of the famous physicians S. S. Korsakov, A. Ia. Kozhevnikov, and P. I. Bakmet'ev, which were kept in the collection of Rossolimo's Neurological Institute. See A. A. Kapustin, "O mozge

uchenykh v sviazi s problemoi vzaimootnosheniia mezhdu velichinoi mozga i oda-rennost'iu," *Klinicheskii arkhiv*, 1926, no. 2: 107–14.

89. Sorkin, "Polivalentnyi," 4.

90. See, e.g., Walther Riese, "Bolezn' Vinsenta Van Goga," *Klinicheskii arkhiv*, 1927, no. 2: 137–46.

91. *Klinicheskii arkhiv genial'nosti i odarennosti (evropatologii), posviashchennyi vopro-sam patologii genial'no-odarennoi lichnosti, a takzhe voprosam odarennogo tvorchestva, tak ili inache sviazannogo s psikhopatologicheskimi uklonami: Vykhodit otdel'nymi vypuskami ne menee 4 raz v god pod redaktsiei osnovatelia etogo izdaniia doktora meditsiny G. V. Segalina, zaveduiushchego psikhotekhnicheskoi laboratoriei i prepodavatelia Ural'skogo universiteta.* I borrow Mark Adams's translation of the title; see Mark B. Adams, "Eugenics in Russia, 1900–1940," in *The Wellborn Science: Eugenics in Germany, France, Brazil, and Russia,* ed. Mark B. Adams (New York: Oxford Univ. Press, 1990), 167.

92. Segalin, "Institut genial'nogo tvorchestva," 57.

93. T. I. Iudin, "[Review of] *Norm und Entartung der Menschen,* [by] Kurt Hilde-brandt," *Russkii evgenicheskii zhurnal*, 1924, no. 1: 72.

94. L. S. Vygotsky and P. M. Zinov'ev, "Genial'nost'," in *Bol'shaia meditsinskaia entsiklopediia* (Moscow: Sovetskaia entsiklopediia, 1929), 6: 612. On Morselli, see Patrizia Guarneri, "Between Soma and Psyche: Morselli and Psychiatry in Late-Nineteen-Century Italy," in *The Anatomy of Madness: Essays in the History of Psychia-try* ed. W. F. Bynum, Roy Porter, and Michael Shepherd (London: Routledge, 1988), 3: 102–24.

95. Karpov, *Tvorchestvo dushevnobol'nykh,* 7; Segalin, "Institut genial'nogo," 56.

96. Weindling, *Health,* 151, 335.

97. On tracing Euler's genealogy, see "Rodoslovnye Gertsena, Lermontova, Chaadaeva, Kropotkina, Tolstogo, Raevskogo, Razumovskikh, Repninykh i Volkon-skikh, Pushkina, Euler'a, Trubetskikh, Puni i dr. 1921," in ARAN, f. 450, op. 4, d. 26, ll. 115–16. On Dostoevsky and others, see "Evgenicheskie zametki: Russkoe ev-genicheskoe obshchestvo v 1923 godu," *Russkii evgenicheskii zhurnal*, 1924, no. 1: 60.

98. A. G. Galach'ian and T. I. Iudin, "Opyt nasledstvenno-biologicheskogo anal-iza odnoi maniakal'no-depressivnoi sem'i," *Russkii evgenicheskii zhurnal*, 1924, no. 3–4: 321–42. Though Mark Adams remarks that eugenics in Russia was launched "not as a part of psychiatry or hygiene, but as a socially responsible, socially relevant branch of the new experimental biology," he lists a number of psychiatrists who played an important role in it. See Adams, "Eugenics in Russia," 158–59, 166–67.

99. [Ernst Kretschmer], "Doklad Kretschmera v Miunkhenskom obshchestve po gigiene ras 11.11.1926 na temu 'genial'nost' i vyrozhdenie,'" *Klinicheskii arkhiv*, 1927, no. 2: 177; Ernst Kretschmer, *The Psychology of Men of Genius,* trans. R. B. Cattell (London: Kegan Paul, Trench, Truber, 1931), 16.

100. Vygotsky and Zinov'ev, "Genial'nost'," 614.

101. N. K. Kol'tsov, "O potomstve velikikh ludei," *Russkii evgenicheskii zhurnal*, 1928, no. 4: 164, 175–76.

102. Iu. A. Filipchenko, "Statisticheskie resul'taty ankety po nasledstvennosti sredi uchenykh Peterburga," *Izvestiia Buro po evgenike*, 1922, no. 1: 5–22; D. M. D'iakonov and L. L. Lus, "Raspredelenie i nasledovanie spetsial'nykh sposobnostei," *Izvestiia Buro po evgenike*, 1922, no. 1: 72–104; Iu. A. Filipchenko, "Nashi vydaiushchiesia uchenye," *Izvestiia Buro po evgenike*, 1922, no. 1: 37; Iu. A. Filipchenko, "Rezul'taty obsledovaniia leningradskikh predstavitelei iskusstva," *Izvestiia Buro po evgenike*, 1924, no. 2: 28.

103. G. V. Segalin, "Patogenez i biogenez velikikh liudei," *Klinicheskii arkhiv*, 1925, no. 1: 28–29.

104. The "Indiana idea" was the name given by the Russian psychiatrist Liublinskii to the U.S. program of sterilization. See Mark B. Adams, "Eugenics as Social Medicine in Revolutionary Russia," in Solomon and Hutchinson, *Health and Society*, 211–12.

105. The main spokesman for eugenic sterilization was M. V. Volotskoi, see his "O polovoi sterilizatsii nasledstvenno defektivnykh," *Russkii evgenicheskii zhurnal*, 1922–24, no. 2: 201–22.

106. "Diskussiia po povodu doklada M. V. Volotskogo v zasedanii Evgenicheskogo obshchestva 30.XII.1921," *Russkii evgenicheskii zhurnal*, 1922–24, no. 2: 222.

107. Segalin, "O zadachakh," 11; Segalin, "K patogenezu leningradskikh uchenykh i deiatelei iskusstv," *Klinicheskii arkhiv*, 1928, no. 3: 20.

108. N. V. Popov, "K voprosu o sviazi odarennosti s dushevnoi bolezn'iu (po povodu rabot doktora Segalina i drugikh)," *Russkii evgenicheskii zhurnal*, 1927, no. 3–4: 145–46, 150, 154. Haeckel's "biogenetic law" stated that ontogeny (the growth of the embryo) recapitulates philogeny (the evolutionary history of the species). See, e.g., P. J. Bowler, *The Fontana History of the Environmental Sciences* (London: Fontana, 1992), 337–39.

109. N. K. Kol'tsov, "Rodoslovnye nashikh vydvizhentsev," *Russkii evgenicheskii zhurnal*, 1926, no. 3–4: 142–43.

110. Kol'tsov's desire to present eugenics in this way was suggested to me by Kirill Rossiianov in a personal communication, April 7, 1998.

111. August Forel, "Europathologie und Eugenik," *Klinicheskii arkhiv*, 1928, no. 1: 51.

112. Quoted in Gleb Struve, *Russian Literature under Lenin and Stalin, 1917–1953* (Norman, Okla.: Univ. of Oklahoma Press, 1971), 14.

113. The pre-revolutionary critics referred to here are Chizh (see Chapter 1) and Sikorskii. Sikorskii enthusiastically wrote about Pushkin's "international or all-human psyche" following Dostoevsky's famous remark about Pushkin's exceptional sensitivity to the soul of other nations. Sikorskii attributed this quality to the fact that Pushkin had Ethiopian ancestors. I. A. Sikorskii, *Antropologicheskaia i psikhologicheskaia genealogiia Pushkina* (Kiev: Kul'zhenko, 1912).

114. P. M. Zinov'ev, "O zadachakh patograficheskoi raboty," in *Trudy Psikhiatricheskoi kliniki Pervogo MMI. Pamiati Gannushkina* (Moscow: Gosizdat, 1934), 4:

413, 411; L. M. Rozenshtein, "Psikhopatologiia myshleniia pri maniakal'no-depressivnom psikhoze i osobye paralogicheskie formy maniakal'nogo sostoianiia," *Zhurnal nevropatologii*, 1926, no. 7: 5–28; I. B. Galant, "Evroendokrinologiia velikikh russkikh pisatelei i poetov," *Klinicheskii arkhiv*, 1927, no. 1: 50; no. 3: 203–42. In the early 1920s, the gland-based typologies were popular in Europe as well as on the other side of the Atlantic. According to German E. Berrios, the U.S. psychiatrist L. Berman "believed that since 'a single gland can dominate the life history of an individual' it was possible to identify 'endocrine types' such as adrenal, pituitary, thyroid, thymo-centric, and gonado-centric." German E. Berrios, *The History of Mental Symptoms: Descriptive Psychopathology since the Nineteenth Century* (Cambridge: Cambridge Univ. Press, 1996), 434.

115. N. A. Iurman, "Bolezn' Dostoevskogo," *Klinicheskii arkhiv*, 1928, no. 1: 62.

116. Ibid.; T. K. Rozental', "Stradanie i tvorchestvo Dostoevskogo (psikhoanaliticheskoe issledovanie)," *Voprosy izucheniia i vospitaniia lichnosti*, 1919, no. 1: 88–107; G. V. Segalin, "Evropatologiia genial'nykh epileptikov: Formy i kharakter epilepsii u velikikh liudei," *Klinicheskii arkhiv*, 1926, no. 3: 143–87.

117. Ia. V. Mints, "Alexander Blok (patograficheskii ocherk)," *Klinicheskii arkhiv*, 1928, no. 3: 53.

118. V. S. Grinevich, "Iskusstvo sovremennoi epokhi v svete patologii," *Klinicheskii arkhiv*, 1928, no. 1: 49. Grinevich died of consumption in 1928, at the age of twenty-four. See "Nekrolog V. S. Grinevicha," *Klinicheskii arkhiv*, 1928, no. 3: 79.

119. Struve, *Russian Literature*, 26.

120. In this account of Semashko's articles of 1926, I draw on Constantin V. Ponomareff, *Sergey Esenin* (Boston: Twayne, 1978), 154–55.

121. When celebrated in the post-Soviet atmosphere of glasnost, Esenin's centenary in 1995 became an occasion for "sensational" biographical discoveries. Two recent works, one by a former criminal investigator and the other by an Esenin scholar, who interviewed psychiatrists, give diametrically opposed interpretations of the reasons why Esenin was in the clinic. See Eduard Khlystalov, *13 ugolovnykh del Sergeia Esenina: Po materialam sekretnykh arkhivov i spetskhranov* (Moscow: Rusland, 1994), esp. 62–64; and Anatolii Panfilov, *Esenin bez tainy: bolezni poeta i tragediia 28 dekabria 1925 g.: poiski i issledovaniia* (Moscow: Narodnaia kniga, 1994).

122. I. B. Galant, "O dushevnoi bolezni S. Esenina," *Klinicheskii arkhiv*, 1926, no. 2: 132; V. S. Grinevich, "K patografii Esenina," *Klinicheskii arkhiv*, 1927, no. 1: 94.

123. In his criticism of attempts to "pathologize" Jesus Christ, Albert Schweitzer (*The Psychiatric Study of Jesus: Exposition and Criticism* [1911], trans. and intro. Charles R. Joy [Boston: Beacon, 1948]), responded to three authors: George de Loosten (Dr. Georg Lomer), *Jesus Christ from the Standpoint of Psychiatry* (1905); William Hirsch, *Conclusions of a Psychiatrist* (1912); and Charles Binet-Sanglé, *The Insanity of Jesus,* four volumes of which were published between 1910 and 1915. The Russian psychiatrist P. B. Gannushkin also examined the ecstasy of religious believers as pathology; see his "La volupté, la cruauté et la religion," *Annales médico-psychologiques* 14 (1901): 353–75,

translated into Russian as "Sladostrastie, zhestokost' i religiia," in *Izbrannye trudy,* ed. O. B. Kerbikov (Moscow: Meditsina, 1964), 80–94. On the militant atheism in post-revolutionary Russia, see, e.g., Stites, *Revolutionary Dreams,* 105–9.

124. Ia. V. Mints, "Iisus Khristos—kak tip dushevnobol'nogo," *Klinicheskii arkhiv,* 1927, no. 3: 245.

125. I. B. Galant, "O suitsidomanii Maksima Gor'kogo: Lichnost' M. Gor'kogo v svete sovershennogo im v dekabre 1887 goda pokusheniia na samoubiistvo," *Klinicheskii arkhiv,* 1925, no. 3: 93–109; I. B. Galant, "O psikhopatologii snovidnoi zhizni (*Traumleben*) Maksima Gor'kogo: O dvukh snakh M. Gor'kogo i tolkovanii ikh L'vom Tolstym," *Klinicheskii arkhiv,* 1925, no. 3: 111–14. Galant dedicated a lengthy article on Gorky's portrayal of psychoses to the thirty-fifth anniversary of the writer's work; see I. B. Galant, "Psikhozy v tvorchestve Maksima Gor'kogo," *Klinicheskii arkhiv,* 1928, no. 2: 5–112.

126. G. V. Segalin, "Obshchaia simptomatologiia evro-aktivnykh (tvorcheskikh) pristupov," *Klinicheskii arkhiv,* 1926, no. 1: 3–78.

127. G. V. Segalin, "Evropatologiia lichnosti i tvorchestva L'va Tolstogo," *Klinicheskii arkhiv,* 1919, no. 3–4: 5–148; V. I. Rudnev, "*Zapiski sumasshedshego* L. Tolstogo," *Klinicheskii arkhiv,* 1929, no. 1: 69; G. V. Segalin, "*Zapiski sumasshedshego* L'va Tolstogo kak patograficheskii dokument," *Klinicheskii arkhiv,* 1929, no. 1: 73–78.

128. Voronskii (1923) quoted in Robert A. Maguire, *Red Virgin Soil: Soviet Literature in the 1920s* (Princeton: Princeton Univ. Press, 1968), 280–81. The older Marxist was L. I. Aksel'rod-Ortodoks, quoted in ibid., 299.

129. On the jubilee, see S. L. Frank, "Tolstoi i bol'shevism" [1928], in *Russkoe mirovozzrenie* (St. Petersburg: Nauka, 1996), 455–59.

130. N. I. Balaban, "O patologicheskom v lichnosti L'va Tolstogo: Kriticheskii ocherk," *Sovetskaia psikhonevrologiia,* 1933, no. 3: 108–11.

131. See, e.g., Ia. G. Oppengeim, *Rekonstruktsiia zdravookhraneniia i edinyi dispanser* (Moscow: Mosoblispolkom, 1930); N. A. Semashko, *Health Protection in the U.S.S.R.* (London: Victor Gollancz, 1934).

132. V. I. Smirnov, ed., *Sotsialisticheskaia rekonstruktsiia zdravookhraneniia* (Moscow: GIZ, 1930), 5. As was often the case, Soviet hygienists looked to their German colleagues for a model. Paul Weindling comments that the idea of health passports appeared in Germany prior to 1914. See Weindling, *Health,* 384–85. An idea for "psychophysiological passports," introduced by Emmanuel Enchmen just after the Bolshevik Revolution, may provide a Russian parallel to the health passports recommended by German hygienists. Yet his idea was severely criticized by top Bolshevik officials, and Enchmen never had a chance to develop his "theory of new biology." See David Joravsky, *Soviet Marxism and Natural Science, 1917–1932* (New York: Columbia Univ. Press, 1961), 93–97.

133. G. V. Segalin, "Izobretateli kak tvorcheskie nevrotiki (evronevrotiki)," *Klinicheskii arkhiv,* 1929, no. 2: 70–72.

134. See the discussion of the Soviet health care system in Jerome Davis, ed., *The*

New Russia: Between First and Second Five-Year Plan (New York: John Day, 1933); Arthur Newsholme and John Adam Kingsbury, *Red Medicine: Socialized Health in Soviet Russia* (Garden City, N.Y.: Doubleday, Doran, 1934); Henry E. Sigerist, *Socialized Medicine in the Soviet Union* (New York: Norton, 1937). As a publisher's note to Sigerist's book warned the reader, "though objective, . . . [the book] implies the feasibility of socialist medicine under proper conditions, such as obtained in the Soviet Union." See also Frankwood Williams on mental hygiene in the Soviet Union in *Soviet Russia Fights Neurosis* (London: Routledge, 1934).

135. *Zdravookhranenie v gody vosstanovleniia i sotsialisticheskoi rekonstruktsii narodnogo khoziaistva SSSR, 1925–1940: Sbornik dokumentov i materialov* (Moscow: Meditsina, 1973), 174–76. In January 1928, Rozenshtein's Neuropsychiatric Dispensary was upgraded into an institute. See "Protokol zasedaniia kollegii Narkomzdrava ot 13.01.1928," in GARF, f. 482, op. 1, d. 618, ll. 2–3.

136. Christopher M. Davis, "Economics of Soviet Public Health, 1928–1932: Development Strategy, Resource Constraints, and Health Plans," in Solomon and Hutchinson, *Health and Society*, 146–74.

137. Kannabikh et al., "L. M. Rozenshtein," 8.

138. Zinov'ev, *K voprosu ob organizatsii*, 5. Zinov'ev only paraphrased Adolf Meyer, who had mentioned that mental hygiene should focus on "that type of case," which "might be by no means . . . willing to consider himself, or would not be considered by others, as sufficiently disturbed mentally to require removal to a state hospital or asylum." See Meyer, "Aims of a Psychiatric Clinic," 360. Unlike Meyer, who until the end of his life had a high professional standing, Zinov'ev was forced to leave his university position. He reportedly disappeared from Moscow in the mid-1930s and appeared in the republic of Azerbaidjan, where he held a chair of psychiatry in a medical college. See "Petr Mikhailovich Zinov'ev: Nekrolog," *Zhurnal nevropatologii*, 1966, no. 2: 324–25.

139. Kannabikh et al., "L. M. Rozenshtein," 8.

140. A. B. Zalkind, "Mental-Hygiene Activities in Russia (USSR)," *Mental Hygiene* 3 (1930): 650; G. A. Tiganova, "K voprosu o polozhenii invalidov voiny v RSFSR," *Zhurnal nevropatologii*, 1927, no. 3: 330.

141. Yet, as late as 1933, the entry on "Psychohygiene" by L. M. Rozenshtein, L. Rokhlin, and A. Edel'shtein in the *Major Medical Encyclopedia* (*Bol'shaia meditsinskaia entsiklopediia* [Moscow: OGIZ, 1933], 27: 749–62) mentioned sympathetically the names of American, French, and German leaders of the mental hygiene movement.

142. Rozenshtein's successor, V. A. Vnukov, appointed in June 1935, was previously director of the Moscow University Psychiatric Clinic, but he also had a worthy record as a party *apparatchik*. See "Pasport Gosudarstvennogo nauchno-issledovatel'skogo instituta nevro-psikhiatricheskoi profilaktiki im. professora V. V. Kramera" (1928), in GARF, f. 482, op. 28, d. 208, ll. 2–5. Despite the defeat of mental hygiene,

it left an indelible mark on the organization of psychiatry. In post-Soviet Russia, neuropsychiatric dispensaries still remain the basis of the mental health system.

143. Weindling, *Health,* 451–52, 579. Karl Kautsky (1854–1938) was a German socialist and, early in his life, a Marxist.

144. Adams, "Eugenics as Social Medicine," 218, 219.

145. Soviet biology of this period has received much attention from historians; see Loren R. Graham, *Science, Philosophy, and Human Behavior in the Soviet Union* (New York: Columbia Univ. Press, 1987); Joravsky, *Soviet Marxism*; N. L. Krementsov, *Stalinist Science* (Princeton: Princeton Univ. Press, 1997); E. S. Levina, *Vavilov, Lysenko, Timofeev-Resovskii: Biologiia v SSSR: istoriia i istoriografiia* (Moskva: AIRO-XX, 1995); Alexander Vucinich, *Science in Russian Culture* (Stanford: Stanford Univ. Press, 1963).

146. There is an abundant literature on this period; see, e.g., Herman Ermolaev, *Soviet Literary Theories, 1917–1934: The Genesis of Socialist Realism* (Berkeley: Univ. of California Press, 1963); Max Hayward and Leopold Labedz, eds., *Literature and Revolution in Soviet Russia, 1917–62: A Symposium* (London: Oxford Univ. Press, 1963); Maguire, *Red Virgin Soil.*

147. A. A. Zhdanov, *Sovetskaia literatura—samaia ideinaia, samaia peredovaia literatura v mire* (1934), quoted in Struve, *Russian Literature,* 262.

148. On pre-revolutionary roots of socialist realism, see Rufus W. Mathewson Jr., *The Positive Hero in Russian Literature,* 2d ed. (Stanford: Stanford Univ. Press, 1975).

149. Evgenii Zamiatin (1921), quoted in Ermolaev, *Censorship,* 47.

150. Fadeev quoted in Ermolaev, *Soviet Literary Theories,* 148; Cesare Lombroso, *The Man of Genius* (London: Walter Scott, 1910), ix.

151. Zinov'ev, "O zadachakh patograficheskoi raboty," 415–16; P. B. Gannushkin, *Klinika psikhopatii: ikh statika, dinamika, sistematika* (Moscow: Sever, 1933), 55, also quoted in D. A. Amenitskii, "Epilepsiia v tvorcheskom osveshchenii F. M. Dostoevskogo," in *Trudy Psikhiatricheskoi kliniki Pervogo MMI. Pamiati Gannushkina* (Moscow: Gosizdat, 1934), 4: 430–31. On Gannushkin, see A. G. Gerish, *P. B. Gannushkin* (Moscow: Meditsina, 1975).

152. P. B. Gannushkin, "O psikhoterapii i psikhoanalize," in *Izbrannye trudy,* ed. O. B. Kerbikov (Moscow: Meditsina, 1964), 284.

153. P. B. Gannushkin, "Postanovka voporsa o granitsakh dushevnogo zdorov'ia" (1908), in *Izbrannye trudy,* 108. As an example of "sociography," Robert Maquire (*Red Virgin Soil,* 301) mentions G. Zalkind's *G. P. Kamenev (1772–1803) (Opyt imushchestvennoi kharakteristiki pervogo russkogo romantika)* (Kazan', 1926).

154. A fragment of Ermakov's manuscript on Dostoevsky was published as "Psikhoanaliz u Dostoevskogo," *Rossiiskii psikhoanaliticheskii vestnik,* 1994, no. 3–4: 145–54. On Ermakov, see M. I. Davydova and A. V. Litvinov, "Ivan Dmitrievich Ermakov," *Rossiiskii psikhoanaliticheskii vestnik,* 1991, no. 1: 115–27; M. M. Davydova, "Nezavershennyi zamysel: K istorii izdaniia trudov Z. Freida v SSSR," *Sovetskaia bibliografiia,* 1989, no. 3: 61–70.

155. On Marxism and psychoanalysis, see Elisabeth Roudinesco, *La bataille de cent*

ans: Histoire de psychanalyse en France, Vol. 2: 1925–1985 (Paris: Seuil, 1986), esp. 50–70; V. M. Leibin, ed., *Zigmund Freid, psikhoanaliz i russkaia mysl'* (Moscow: Respublika, 1994).

156. E. Iu. Solov'ev, "Biograficheskii analiz kak vid istoriko-filosofskogo issledovaniia," *Voprosy filosofii*, 1981, no. 9: 140–41.

157. V. N. Iuzhakov, "Patografiia kak zabytyi aspekt sotsiokul'turnykh issledovanii v psikhiatrii," *Nezavisimyi psikhiatricheskii zhurnal*, 1994, no. 3: 55–62. Iuzhakov's manifesto also contained a pathography, of the painter M. A. Vrubel'. His call for a revival of the genre was heard, and the next two pathographies appeared in the same journal in 1996; see V. E. Lerner, E. Vitsum, and G. M. Kotikov, "Bolezn' Gogolia i ego puteshestvie k sviatym mestam," *Nezavisimyi psikhiatricheskii zhurnal*, 1996, no. 1: 63–71; and A. V. Shuvalov, "Patograficheskii ocherk o Daniile Kharmse," *Nezavisimyi psikhiatricheskii zhurnal*, 1996, no. 2: 74–78.

BIBLIOGRAPHY

Archival Sources

Arkhiv Rossiiskoi akademii nauk (Archive of the Russian Academy of Sciences), f. 450, op. 4.

Gosudarstvennyi arkhiv Rossiiskoi Federatsii (State Archive of the Russian Federation), f. 259, op. 10a; f. 482, op. 1; f. 482, op. 10; f. 482, op. 28.

Moskovskii kul'turnyi fond. Arkhiv russkoi emigratsii, sostavlennyi A. M. Okunevym (Moscow Cultural Foundation. Archive of Russian Emigration, comp. A. M. Okunev. F. 175. Personalia).

Muzei Moskovskoi Meditsinskoi Akademii, f. 523/132, op. 2; f. 525/34.

Muzei Preobrazhenskoi bol'nitsy. F. 103. Arkhiv N. N. Bazhenova. 1904–16.

Tsentral'nyi gosudarstvennyi arkhiv literatury i iskusstva (Central State Archive of Literature and Arts), f. 2299, op. 1.

Tsentral'nyi gosudarstvennyi arkhiv istorii i arkhitektury Moskvy (Central State Archive of the History and Architecture of Moscow), f. 1, op. 2; f. 363, op. 1; f. 418, op. 63.

Published Primary Sources

Amenitskii, D. A. "Analiz geroia *Mysli* Leonida Andreeva (K voprosu o paranoidnoi psikhopatii)." *Sovremennaia psikhiatriia*, 1915, no. 5: 223–51.

———. "Epilepsiia v tvorcheskom osveshchenii F. M. Dostoevskogo." In *Trudy Psikhiatricheskoi kliniki Pervogo MMI. Pamiati Gannushkina*. Vol. 4: 417–31. Moscow: Gosizdat, 1934.

———. "Psikhopatologiia Raskol'nikova, kak oderzhimogo naviazchivym sostoianiem." *Sovremennaia psikhiatriia*, 1915, no. 9: 373–88.

Anokhin, A. K. *Sputnik iunogo razvedchika: Organizatsiia i zaniatiia s iunymi razvedchikami*. Kiev: I. I. Samonenko, 1916.

Apostolov, N. N. *Zhivoi Tolstoy: Zhizn' L'va Nikolaevicha Tolstogo v vospominaniiakh i perepiske*. St. Petersburg: Lenizdat, 1995.

Asatiani, M. M. "Sovremennoe sostoianie voprosa teorii i praktiki psikhoanaliza po vzgliadam Jung'a." *Psikhoterapiia*, 1910, no. 3: 117–24.

A–t. "Genii na sude psikhiatra." *Novoe vremia*, no. 6380 (December 1, 1894).

Avtokratov, P. M. "Prizrenie, lechenie i evakuatsiia dushevnobol'nykh vo vremia russko-iaponskoi voiny v 1904–905 godakh." *Obozrenie psikhiatrii, nevrologii i eksperimental'noi psikhologii*, 1906, no. 10: 665–68.

Bajenoff, N. *Gui de Maupassant et Dostoïewsky: Etude de psychologie comparée*. Lyon: A. Stork & Masson, 1904.

————. *La révolution russe: Essai de psychologie sociale.* Paris: Bloud et Gay, 1919.

Bajenoff, N., and N. Osipoff. *La suggestion et ses limites.* Paris: Bloud et Cie, 1911.

Bakhtin, Mikhail. *Problems of Dostoevsky's Poetics.* Edited and translated by Caryl Emerson. Introduction by Wayne C. Booth. Theory and History of Literature, vol. 8. Minneapolis: University of Minnesota Press, 1984.

Balaban, N. I. "O patologicheskom v lichnosti L'va Tolstogo. Kriticheskii ocherk." *Sovetskaia psikhonevrologiia*, 1933, no. 3: 108–11.

Bazhenov, N. N. *Bolezn' i smert' Gogolia.* Moscow: Kushnerev, 1902.

————. "Bolezn' i smert' Gogolia." *Russkaia mysl'*, 1902, no. 1: 133–49; no. 2: 52–71.

————. "Bol'nye pisateli i patologicheskoe tvorchestvo." In *Psikhiatricheskie besedy na literaturnye i obshchestvennye temy*, 10–40. Moscow: Mamontov, 1903.

————. "Dr. N. N. Bazhenov on Gogol." In *The Completion of Russian Literature*, edited by Andrew Field, 83–99. New York: Atheneum, 1971. Abridged translation of N. N. Bazhenov, *Bolezn' i smert' Gogolia* (1902).

————. "Dushevnaia drama Garshina." In *Psikhiatricheskie besedy na literaturnye i obshchestvennye temy*, 104–22. Moscow: Mamontov, 1903.

————. *Gabriel Tarde: Lichnost', idei i tvorchestvo.* Moscow: Kushnerev, 1905.

————. *O prizrenii i lechenii dushevnobol'nykh v zemstvakh, i v chastnosti o novoi Riazan-skoi psikhiatricheskoi lechebnitse.* St. Petersburg: M. M. Stasiulevich, 1887.

————. *O znachenii autointoksikatsii v patogeneze nervnykh simptomokompleksov.* Khar'kov: Gubernskaia uprava, 1894.

————. *Proekt zakonodatel'stva o dushevno-bol'nykh i ob"iasnitel'naia zapiska k nemu.* Moscow: Gorodskaia tipografiia, 1911.

————. *Psikhiatricheskie besedy na literaturnye i obshchestvennye temy.* Moscow: Mamontov, 1903.

————. *Psikhologiia kaznimykh.* Moscow: I. D. Sytin, 1906.

————. *Psikhologiia i politika.* Moscow: I. D. Sytin, 1906.

————. *Simvolisty i dekadenty: Psikhiatricheskii etiud.* Moscow: Mamontov, 1899.

————. "Vneuniversitetskaia deiatel'nost' i znachenie S. S. Korsakova, kak vracha i uchitelia." In *Psikhiatricheskie besedy na literaturnye i obshchestvennye temy.* Moscow: Mamontov, 1903.

————. "Vtoroi mezhdunarodnyi kongress po kriminal'noi antropologii." *Voprosy filosofii i psikhologii*, 1889, no. 2: 17–41.

Bekhterev, V. M. *Avtobiografiia (posmertnaia).* Moscow: Ogonek, 1928.

————. "Dostoevsky i khudozhestvennaia psikhopatologiia." Reprinted in S. Belov and N. Agitova, "V. M. Bekhterev o Dostoevskom," *Russkaia literatura*, 1962, no. 4: 134–41.

————. "Voprosy vyrozhdeniia i bor'ba s nim." *Obozrenie psikhiatrii, nevrologii i eksperimental'noi psikhologii*, 1908, no. 9: 518–21.

Belinsky, G. V. "Letter to N. V. Gogol." In *Belinsky, Chernyshevsky, and Dobroliubov: Selected Criticism*, edited and with an introduction by Ralph E. Matlaw, 83–92. Bloomington: Indiana University Press, 1976. Letter dated 1847.

Bely, Andrei. *Mezhdu dvukh revolutsii.* Moscow: Khudozhestvennaia literatura, 1990.

Bem, A. L. "Razvertyvanie sna (*Vechnyi muzh* Dostoevskogo)." In *Uchenye zapiski, osnovannye Russkoi uchebnoi kollegiei v Prage.* Vol. 1: 45–59. Prague, 1924.

Berberova, Nina. *Liudi i lozhi: russkie masony XX stoletiia.* New York: Russica, 1986.

Berger, I. A., and I. D. Dobronravov. "O gigienicheskoi dispanserizatsii." *Zhurnal nevropatologii i psikhiatrii imeni S. S. Korsakova,* 1935, no. 2: 49–72.

Bernstein, A. N. *Eksperimental'no-psikhologicheskaia metodika raspoznavaniia dushevnykh boleznei.* Moscow: S. P. Iakovlev, 1908.

———. *Eksperimental'no-psikhologicheskie skhemy dlia izucheniia umstvennykh narushenii u dushevnobol'nykh.* Moscow: S. P. Iakovlev, 1910.

B–r, Dr. V. M. "*Gamlet* Shekspira s mediko-psikhologicheskoi tochki zrenia." *Arkhiv psikhiatrii, neirologii i sudebnoi psikhologii,* 1897, no. 2: 39–107.

Cattell, James McKeen. *An Education in Psychology: James McKeen Cattell's Journal and Letters from Germany and England, 1880–1888,* selected and edited by Michael M. Sokal. Cambridge: MIT Press, 1981.

Chechott, V. "Max Nordau o Vagnere." *Kievlianin,* no. 337 (1895).

Chelpanov, Georgii. "Izmerenie prosteishikh umstvennykh aktov." *Voprosy filosofii i psikhologii,* 1896, no. 9–10: 19–57.

———. *Obzor noveishei literatury po psikhologii (1890–1896).* Kiev: Universitet Sv. Vladimira, 1897.

———. "Zadachi sovremennoi psikhologii." *Voprosy filosofii i psikhologii,* 1909, no. 4: 285–308.

Chernyshevsky, N. G. "[Review of] Zapiski o zhizni Nikolaia Vasil'evicha Gogolia, St. Petersburg, 1856." In *N. V. Gogol' v russkoi kritike,* edited by A. K. Kotov and M. Ia. Poliakov, 391–406. Moscow: Khudozhestvennaia literatura, 1953. First published 1856.

Chizh, V. F. "Appertseptivnye protsessy u dushevno-bol'nykh." *Arkhiv psikhiatrii, neirologii i sudebnoi psikhologii,* 1886, no. 1–2: 1–32.

———. *Bolezn' N. V. Gogolia.* Moscow: Kushnerev, 1904.

———. "Bolezn' N. V. Gogolia." *Voprosy filosofii i psikhologii,* 1903, no. 2: 262–313; no. 3: 418–68; no. 4: 647–81; 1904, no. 1: 34–70.

———. *Dostoevsky kak psikhopatolog.* Moscow: M. Katkov, 1885.

———. "Eksperimental'noe issledovanie vnimaniia vo vremia sna." *Obozrenie psikhiatrii, nevrologii i eksperimental'noi psikhologii,* 1896, no. 9: 671–75.

———. "Eksperimental'nye issledovaniia po metodu komplikatsii, ob appertseptsii prostykh i slozhnykh predstavlenii (iz laboratorii professora Wundta)." *Vestnik klinicheskoi i sudebnoi psikhiatrii i nevropatologii,* 1885, no. 1: 58–87.

———. "Intellektual'nye chuvstvovaniia u dushevno-bol'nykh." *Nevrologicheskii vestnik,* 1896, no. 1: 27–52; no. 2: 69–88; no. 3: 1–18.

———. "Izmerenie vremeni elementarnykh psikhicheskikh protsessov u dushevno-bol'nykh (iz kliniki professora Flechsig'a." *Vestnik klinicheskoi i sudebnoi psikhiatrii i nevropatologii,* 1885, no. 2: 41–66.

————. "K ucheniu ob organicheskoi prestupnosti." *Arkhiv psikhiatrii, neirologii i sudebnoi psikhologii*, 1893, no. 1: 137–76.

————. *Kriminal'naia antropologiia*. Odessa: G. Beilenson & I. Iurovskii, 1895.

————. *Metodologiia diagnoza*. St. Petersburg: Prakticheskaia meditsina, 1913.

————. "Metody nauchnoi psikhologii." *Arkhiv psikhiatrii, neirologii i sudebnoi psikhologii*, 1894, no. 1: 46–59.

————. "Nravstvennost' dushevno-bol'nykh." *Voprosy filosofii i psikhologii*, 1891, no. 3: 122–48.

————. "O bolezni Gogolia: Lektsia, chitannaia 20 marta 1903 g. v Iur'evskom obshchestve estestvoispytatelei." *Saratovskii listok* 70 (1903).

————. "Obozrenie sochinenii po kriminal'noi antropologii." *Arkhiv psikhiatrii, neirologii i sudebnoi psikhologii*, 1893, no. 3: 105–18.

————. "Otvet Kaplanu (Po povodu stat'i g. Kaplana: 'Pliushkin i Starosvetskie pomeshchiki')." *Voprosy filosofii i psikhologii*, 1903, no. 4: 755–59.

————. "Pis'mo redaktoru." *Nevrologicheskii vestnik*, 1895, no. 3: 174.

————. "Pliushkin, kak tip starcheskogo slaboumiia." *Vrachebnaia gazeta*, 1902, no. 10: 217–20.

————. "Pochemu vozzreniia prostranstva i vremeni postoianny i nepremenny?" *Voprosy filosofii i psikhologii*, 1896, no. 3: 229–64.

————. "Psikhologiia fanatizma." *Voprosy filosofii i psikhologii*, 1905, no. 1: 1–36; no. 2: 149–86.

————. *Pushkin kak ideal dushevnogo zdorov'ia*. Iur'ev: Tipografiia universiteta, 1899.

————. "Shirota vospriiatiia u dushevno-bol'nykh." *Arkhiv psikhiatrii, neirologii i sudebnoi psikhologii*, 1890, no. 1–2: 23–38.

————. *Turgenev kak psikhopatolog*. Moscow: Kushnerev, 1899.

————. *Uchebnik psikhiatrii*. St. Petersburg: Sotrudnik, 1911.

————. "Vremia assotsiatsii u zdorovykh i dushevno-bol'nykh." *Nevrologicheskii vestnik*, 1894, no. 2: 95–116.

————. "Znachenie bolezni Pliushkina (po povodu stat'i d-ra Ia. Kaplana: 'Pliushkin. Psikhologicheskii razbor ego')." *Voprosy filosofii i psikhologii*, 1902, no. 4: 872–88.

————. "Znachenie politicheskoi zhizni v etiologii dushevnykh boleznei." *Obozrenie psikhiatrii, nevrologii i eksperimental'noi psikhologii*, 1908, no. 1: 1–12; no. 3: 149–62.

————, ed. *O razvitii eticheskikh vozzrenii*. *Iz lektsii Wundt'a*. Moscow: Universitetskaia tipografiia (M. Katkov), 1886.

Darwin, Charles. *The Descent of Man, and Selection in Relation to Sex*. With an introduction by John Tyler Bonner and Robert M. May. Princeton: Princeton University Press, 1981. First published 1871.

Davis, Jerome, ed. *The New Russia: Between First and Second Five-Year Plan*. New York: John Day, 1933.

Déjerine J.-J., and E. Gauckler. *Funktsional'nye proiavleniia psikhonevrozov i ikh lechenie psikhoterapieiu* [*Les manifestations fonctionnelles des psychonévroses: leur traitement par la psychothérapie*]. Translated by V. P. Serbskii. Moscow: Kosmos, 1912.

D'iakonov, D. M., and L. L. Lus. "Raspredelenie i nasledovanie spetsial'nykh sposobnostei." *Izvestiia Buro po evgenike*, 1922, no. 1: 72–104.

"Diskussiia po povodu doklada M. V. Volotskogo v zasedanii Evgenicheskogo obshchestva 30.XII.1921." *Russkii evgenicheskii zhurnal*, 1922–24, no. 2: 220–22.

Dobroliubov, N. A. "What Is Oblomovitism?" In *Belinsky, Chernyshevsky, and Dobroliubov: Selected Criticism*, edited and with an introduction by Ralph E. Matlaw, 133–75. Bloomington: Indiana University Press, 1976. First published 1859.

Dosuzhkov, F. N. "Nikolai Evgrafovich Osipov kak psikhiatr." In *Zhizn' i smert'*, edited by A. L. Bem, F. M. Dosuzhkov, and N. O. Lossky, 25–45. Prague: Petropolis, 1935.

Dovbnia, E. N., and L. M. Rozenshtein. *Pervyi s"ezd russkikh nevropatologov i psikhiatrov.* Moscow: Shtab Moskovskogo voennogo okruga, 1911.

Droznes, M. Ia. *Osnovy ukhoda za nervno- i dushevnobol'nymi, vyrabotannye v vide opyta dlia sluzhebnogo personala chastnoi lechebnitsy dlia nervno- i dushevnobol'nykh doktora M. Ia. Droznesa v Odesse.* Odessa: Isakovich & Beilenson, 1897.

———. "Vazhneishie zadachi sovremennoi prakticheskoi psikhiatrii." In *Trudy vtorogo s"ezda otechestvennykh psikhiatrov.* Kiev: Kul'zhenko, 1907.

Durkheim, Emile. *Suicide: A Study in Sociology.* London: Routledge & Kegan Paul, 1952. First published 1897.

Edel'shtein, A. O. "L. M. Rozenshtein i Moskovskaia psikhiatricheskaia shkola." In *Problemy nevrastenii i nevrozov,* edited by L. M. Rozenshtein, S. I. Zander, and S. I. Gol'dberg, 17–19. Moscow: GIZ meditsinskoi literatury, 1935.

———. "Psikhiatricheskaia klinika imeni Korsakova za 50 let." In *Piat'desiat let Psikhiatricheskoi kliniki imeni Korsakova,* 9–23. Moscow: Pervyi Moskovskii meditsinskii institut, 1940.

———. *Psikhiatricheskie s"ezdy i obshchestva za polveka (K istorii meditsinskoi obshchestvennosti), 1887–1936.* Moscow: Medgiz, 1948.

Ellis, Henry Havelock. *The Criminal.* 3d ed. London: Walter Scott, 1901.

———. *The Genius of Europe.* Westport, Conn.: Greenwood Press, 1951.

Ermakov, I. D. "Desiatyi Pirogovskii s"ezd v Moskve, 25.IV–2.V.1907." *Zhurnal nevropatologii i psikhiatrii imeni S. S. Korsakova,* 1907, no. 2–3: 544–72.

———. *Ocherki po analizu tvorchestva Gogolia (Organichnost' proizvedenii Gogolia).* Moscow: GIZ, 1922.

———. "Psikhoanaliz u Dostoevskogo." *Rossiiskii psikhoanaliticheskii vestnik,* 1994, no. 3–4: 145–54.

"Evgenicheskie zametki. Russkoe evgenicheskoe obshchestvo v 1923 godu." *Russkii evgenicheskii zhurnal,* 1924, no. 1: 60.

Fel'tsman, O. B. "O psikhoanalyze i psikhoterapii." *Sovremennaia psikhiatriia,* 1909, no. 1: 257–69.

————. "Vpechatleniia o poezdke k Dubois (Pis'mo iz-za granitsy)." *Psikhoterapiia*, 1910, no. 1: 49.

Filipchenko, Iu. A. "Nashi vydaiushchiesia uchenye." *Izvestiia Buro po evgenike*, 1922, no. 1: 22–38.

————. "Rezul'taty obsledovaniia leningradskikh predstavitelei iskusstva." *Izvestiia Buro po evgenike*, 1924, no. 2: 5–28.

————. "Statisticheskie resul'taty ankety po nasledstvennosti sredi uchenykh Peterburga." *Izvestiia Buro po evgenike*, 1922, no. 1: 5–22.

Forel, August. "Europathologie und Eugenik." *Klinicheskii arkhiv genial'nosti i odarennosti*, 1928, no. 1: 51.

Fouillée, Alfred. *Esquisse psychologique des peuples européens.* 4th ed. Paris: Félix Alcan, 1903.

Frank, S. L. "Tolstoi i bol'shevism." In *Russkoe mirovozzrenie*, 455–59. St. Petersburg: Nauka, 1996.

Galach'ian, A. G., and T. I. Iudin. "Opyt nasledstvenno-biologicheskogo analiza odnoi maniakal'no-depressivnoi sem'i." *Russkii evgenicheskii zhurnal*, 1924, no. 3–4: 321–42.

Galant, I. B. "Evroendokrinologiia velikikh russkikh pisatelei i poetov." *Klinicheskii arkhiv genial'nosti i odarennosti*, 1927, no. 1: 19–65; no. 3: 203–42.

————. "O dushevnoi bolezni S. Esenina." *Klinicheskii arkhiv genial'nosti i odarennosti*, 1926, no. 2: 115–32.

————. "O psikhopatologii snovidnoi zhizni (*Traumleben*) Maksima Gor'kogo: O dvukh snakh M. Gor'kogo i tolkovanii ikh L'vom Tolstym." *Klinicheskii arkhiv genial'nosti i odarennosti*, 1925, no. 3: 111–14.

————. "O suitsidomanii Maksima Gor'kogo: Lichnost' M. Gor'kogo v svete sovershennogo im v dekabre 1887 goda pokusheniia na samoubiistvo." *Klinicheskii arkhiv genial'nosti i odarennosti*, 1925, no. 3: 93–109.

————. "Psikhozy v tvorshestve Maksima Gor'kogo." *Klinicheskii arkhiv genial'nosti i odarennosti*, 1928, no. 2: 5–112.

Gannushkin, P. B. *Klinika psikhopatii: ikh statika, dinamika, sistematika.* Moscow: Sever, 1933.

————. "La volupté, la cruauté et la religion." *Annales médico-psychologiques* 14 (1901): 353–75. Translated into Russian as "Sladostrastie, zhestokost' i religiia," in P. B. Gannushkin, *Izbrannye trudy,* edited by O. B. Kerbikov (Moscow: Meditsina, 1964), 80–94.

————. "O psikhoterapii i psikhoanalize." In *Izbrannye trudy,* edited by O. B. Kerbikov, 283–84. Moscow: Meditsina, 1964. Lecture given in the 1920s.

————. "Postanovka voprosa o granitsakh dushevnogo zdorov'ia." In *Izbrannye trudy,* edited by O. B. Kerbikov, 97–108. Moscow: Meditsina, 1964. First published 1908.

Garshin, Vsevolod. *From the Reminiscences of Private Ivanov and Other Stories.* Translated by Peter Henry, Liv Tudge, Donald Rayfield, and Philip Taylor. London: Angel Books, 1988.

―――. "Pis'ma." In *Polnoe sobranie sochinenii v trekh tomakh*. Vol. 3. Moscow: Academia, 1934.

Giliarovskii, V. F. "Lichnost' i deiatel'nost" N. N. Bazhenova (1856–1923) (Nekrolog)." *Zhurnal psikhologii, nevropatologii i psikhiatrii*, 1923, no. 3: 5–14.

Gogol, Nikolai. *Diary of a Madman and Other Stories*. Translated and with an introduction by Ronald Wilks. London: Penguin Books, 1972.

―――. *Selected Passages from Correspondence with Friends*. Translated by Jesse Zeldin. Nashville: Vanderbilt University Press, 1969. First published 1847.

Greidenberg, B. S. "Psikhologicheskie osnovy nervno-psikhicheskoi terapii." In *Trudy Pervogo s"ezda Russkogo soiuza psikhiatrov i nevropatologov, Moskva, 4–11.9.1911*, edited by N. A. Vyrubov et al., 118–41. Moscow: Shtab Moskovskogo voennogo okruga, 1914.

Grinevich, V. S. "Iskusstvo sovremennoi epokhi v svete patologii." *Klinicheskii arkhiv genial'nosti i odarennosti*, 1928, no. 1: 34–50.

―――. "K patografii Esenina." *Klinicheskii arkhiv genial'nosti i odarennosti*, 1927, no. 1: 82–94.

Grombakh, V. A. "Moskovskaia psikhiatricheskaia organizatsiia." *Zhurnal nevropatologii i psikhiatrii imeni S. S. Korsakova*, 1925, no. 1: 105–12.

Gurevich, M. O. "Moskovskaia psikhiatricheskaia klinika v istorii otechestvennoi psikhiatrii." In *Piat'desiat let psikhiatricheskoi klinike imeni Korsakova*, 3–8. Moscow: Pervyi Moskovskii meditsinskii institut, 1940.

Iarotskii, A. I. *Idealizm kak fiziologicheskii faktor*. Iur'ev: K. Matissen, 1908.

Iudin, T. I. "[Review of] *Norm und Entartung der Menschen*, [by] Kurt Hildebrandt." *Russkii evgenicheskii zhurnal*, 1924, no. 1: 72.

Iurman, N. A. "Bolezn' Dostoevskogo." *Klinicheskii arkhiv genial'nosti i odarennosti*, 1928, no. 1: 61–85.

―――. "[Review of] *Vopros o nravstvennom pomeshatel'stve v svete panidealisticheskoi psikhologii sovesti*, [by] K. Ia. Grinberg." *Psikhiatricheskaia gazeta*, 1916, no. 7: 126–27.

Iuzhakov, V. N. "Patografiia kak zabytyi aspekt sotsiokul'turnykh issledovanii v psikhiatrii." *Nezavisimyi psikhiatricheskii zhurnal*, 1994, no. 3: 55–62.

Ivanov-Razumnik, R. V. *Istoriia russkoi obshchestvennoi mysli. Individualizm i meshchanstvo v russkoi literature i zhizni XIX veka*. 3d ed. St. Petersburg: M. M. Stasiulevich, 1911.

"Iz Obshchestva nevropatologov i psikhiatrov v Moskve." *Obozrenie psikhiatrii, nevrologii i eksperimental'noi psikhologii*, 1906, no. 5: 388–89.

Kachenovskii, Dr. *Bolezn' Gogolia. Kriticheskoe issledovanie*. St. Petersburg: Svet, 1906.

Kannabikh, Iu. V. "Zametki o 'normal'nom' i 'nenormal'nom' (skhema)." *Psikhoterapiia*, 1913, no. 2: 7–8.

Kannabikh, Iu. V., L. A. Prozorov, and I. G. Ravkin, "L. M. Rozenshtein, ego nauchnaia i obshchestvennaia deiatel'nost." *Sovetskaia psikhonevrologiia*, 1934, no. 3: 7–14.

Kaplan, Ia. F. "Pliushkin i Starosvetskie pomeshchiki (po povodu stat'i prof. V. F. Chizha 'Znachenie bolezni Pliushkina')." *Voprosy filosofii i psikhologii*, 1903, no. 3: 599–645.

———. "Pliushkin. Psikhologicheskii razbor ego." *Voprosy filosofii i psikhologii*, 1902, no. 3: 796–813.

Kapterev, P. P. "Detstvo Il'i Il'icha Oblomova: Psikhologo-pedagogicheskii etud o prichinakh proiskhozhdeniia i razvitiia leni." *Zhenskoe obrazovanie*, 1891, no. 3: 248–66.

Kapustin, A. A. "O mozge uchenykh v sviazi s problemoi vzaimootnosheniia mezhdu velichinoi mozga i odarennost'iu." *Klinicheskii arkhiv genial'nosti i odarennosti*, 1926, no. 2: 107–14.

Karpov, P. I. *Tvorchestvo dushevnobol'nykh i ego vliianie na razvitie nauki, iskusstva i tekhniki.* Moscow: GIZ, 1926.

Karpov, V. P. *Osnovnye cherty organicheskogo ponimaniia prirody.* Moscow: Put', 1913.

Kashina-Evreinova, A. *Podpol'e geniia (seksual'nye istochniki tvorchestva Dostoevskogo).* Petrograd: Tret'ia strazha, 1923.

Khoroshko, Vas. "Pamiati professora G. I. Rossolimo." *Klinicheskaia meditsina* 22 (1928): 223–25.

"Khronika." *Obozrenie psikhiatrii, nevrologii i eksperimental'noi psikhologii*, 1908, no. 8: 510–11.

"Khronika." *Sovremennaia psikhiatriia*, 1907, no. 6: 191; 1907, no. 10: 383; 1910, no. 8: 242; 1913, no. 10: 836–37; 1915, no. 1: 48.

Kol'tsov, N. K. "O potomstve velikikh ludei." *Russkii evgenicheskii zhurnal*, 1928, no. 4: 164–77.

———. "Rodoslovnye nashikh vydvizhentsev." *Russkii evgenicheskii zhurnal*, 1926, no. 3–4: 103–43.

"Konferentsiia vrachei psikhiatrov i nevropatologov, sozvannaia Pravleniem Soiuza psikhiatrov v Moskve 10–12 aprelia 1917 goda." *Sovremennaia psikhiatriia*, 1917, no. 2: 175–242.

Konorov, M. I. "Don-Kikhot kak tsel'naia patologicheskaia lichnost'." *Vestnik psikhologii, kriminal'noi antropologii i gipnotizma*, 1906, no. 4: 305–18; no. 6: 494–506.

Korolenko, V. G. "Tragediia velikogo iumorista (Neskol'ko myslei o Gogole)." In *N. V. Gogol' v russkoi kritike*, edited by A. K. Kotov and M. Ia. Poliakov, 536–94. Moscow: Khudozhestvennaia literatura, 1953.

"Korrespondentsiia iz sektsii nervnykh i dushevnykh boleznei X-go Pirogovskogo s"ezda, 26.4.1907." *Sovremennaia psikhiatriia*, 1907, no. 3: 138.

Korsakov, S. S. "Ob ustroistve chastnykh lechebnits." *Zhurnal nevropatologii i psikhiatrii imeni S. S. Korsakova*, 1901, no. 5–6: 937–65.

Kovalevskii, P. I. "Genii i sumasshestvie." In *Vyrozhdenie i vozrozhdenie. Sotsial'no-biologicheskii ocherk*, 111–66. St. Petersburg: Akinfiev i Leontiev, 1899.

———. "Ioann Groznyi i ego dushevnoe sostoianie." In *Psikhiatricheskie eskizy iz istorii.* Vol. 2. Khar'kov: Zil'berberg, 1893.

[Kozhevnikov, A]. "O deiatel'nosti Obshchestva nevropatologov i psikhiatrov v

Moskve." *Zhurnal nevropatologii i psikhiatrii imeni S. S. Korsakova,* 1925, no. 1: 123–31.

Kraepelin, Emil. *Memoirs.* Berlin: Springer-Verlag, 1987. First published 1983.

Krasnushkina, M. A. "Preobrazhenskaia bol'nitsa v period rukovodstva N. N. Bazhenovym." In *Sbornik nauchnykh trudov, posviaschennykh 150–letiiu Moskovskoi psikhonevrologicheskoi bol'nitsy N 3,* 440–46. Moscow: Moskovskaia psikhonevrologicheskaia bol'nitsa N 3, 1963.

Kremlev, A. N. "K voprosu o 'bezumii' Gamleta." *Vestnik psikhologii, kriminal'noi antropologii i gipnotizma,* 1905, no. 4: 295–304.

[Kretschmer, Ernst]. "Doklad Kretschmera v Miunkhenskom obshchestve po gigiene ras 11.11.1926 na temu 'genial'nost' i vyrozhdenie.'" *Klinicheskii arkhiv genial'nosti i odarennosti,* 1927, no. 2: 177.

———. *The Psychology of Men of Genius.* Translated by R. B. Cattell. London: Kegan Paul, Trench, & Truber, 1931. First published 1929.

Kropotkin, Peter. *Ideals and Realities in Russian Literature.* New York: Alfred Knopf, 1915.

Kutanin, M. P. "Bred i tvorchestvo." *Klinicheskii arkhiv genial'nosti i odarennosti,* 1929, no. 1: 3–35.

Lakhtin, M. Iu. *Chastnaia lechebnitsa dlia dushevno-bol'nykh voinov: Otchet s 19.5.1905 po 1.1.1906.* Moscow: Russkii trud, 1906.

———. "Patologicheskii al'truizm v literature i zhizni." *Voprosy nevrologii i psikhiatrii,* 1912, no. 7: 289–94.

———. "Stradaniia kak istochnik chelovecheskikh verovanii." *Voprosy nevrologii i psikhiatrii,* 1913, no. 11: 481–92.

Lange, N. N. "O znachenii eksperimenta v sovremennoi psikhologii." *Voprosy filosofii i psikhologii,* 1894, no. 4: 566–78.

Lerner, V. E., E. Vitsum, and G. M. Kotikov. "Bolezn' Gogolia i ego puteshestvie k sviatym mestam." *Nezavisimyi psikhiatricheskii zhurnal,* 1996, no. 1: 63–71.

Lombroso, Cesare. *The Man of Genius.* London: Walter Scott, 1891. First published as *Genio e follia* (Milan, 1863).

Lossky, N. O. *Dostoevsky i ego khristianskoe miroponimanie.* New York: Izdatel'stvo imeni Chekhova, 1953.

———. *History of Russian Philosophy.* London: Allen & Unwin, 1952.

———. "N. E. Osipov kak filosof." In *Zhizn' i smert',* edited by A. L. Bem, F. M. Dosuzhkov, and N. O. Lossky, 46–54. Prague: Petropolis, 1935.

Lourié, Ossip. *La psychologie des romanciers russes du XIXe siècle.* Paris: Félix Alcan, 1905.

L'vov-Rogachevskii, V. L. "V. Veresaev." In *Die Russische Literatur des 20. Jahrhunderts,* edited by S. A. Vengerov, 145–72. Munich: Wilhelm Fink, 1972.

Makovitskii, D. P. "Lev Nikolaevich's departure from Yasnaya Polyana." In *Reminiscence of Lev Tolstoy by His Contemporaries.* Moscow: Foreign Language Publishing House, 1969, 240–58. First published 1938.

Mann, Thomas. "Dostojewski—mit Massen." In *Gesammelte Werke*. Vol. 9: 656–674. Hamburg: S. Fischer, 1974. First published 1945.

Maudsley, Henry. *Fiziologiia i patologiia dushi*. Translated into Russian by I. Isain. St. Petersburg: Bakst, 1871. First published 1867.

Merezhkovskii, D. S. "Gogol." In *Izbrannye stat'i: Simvolizm, Gogol', Lermontov*, 163–286. Munich: Wilhelm Fink, 1972. First published 1909.

———. *L. Tolstoy i Dostoevsky*. 3d ed. St. Petersburg: M. V. Pirozhkov, 1902–3.

Meyer, Adolf. "The Aims of a Psychiatric Clinic." In *The Commonsense Psychiatry of Adolf Meyer: Fifty-two Selected Papers*, edited by Alfred Lief, 359–68. New York: McGraw-Hill, 1948.

Mikhailovsky, N. K. *Dostoevsky: A Cruel Talent*. Translated by Spencer Cadmus. Ann Arbor: Ardis, 1978. First published 1882.

———. *Literaturnye vospominaniia i sovremennaia smuta*. St. Petersburg: Vol'f, 1900.

Mints, Ia. V. "Alexander Blok (patograficheskii ocherk)." *Klinicheskii arkhiv genial'nosti i odarennosti*, 1928, no. 3: 45–53.

———. "Iisus Khristos—kak tip dushevnobol'nogo." *Klinicheskii arkhiv genial'nosti i odarennosti*, 1927, no. 3: 243–52.

Mitskevich, S. I. *Zapiski vracha-obshchestvennika (1888–1918)*. 2d ed. Moscow: Meditsina, 1969.

Möbius, P. J. *Ausgewälte Werke*. 5 vols. Leipzig: Barth, 1909.

Mochul'skii, K. V. *Dukhovnyi put' Gogolia*. Paris: YMCA Press, 1934.

Mukhin, N. I. "Neirasteniia i degeneratsiia." *Arkhiv psikhiatrii, neirologii i sudebnoi psikhologii*, 1888, no. 1: 49–67.

N. Ch. "Psikhopatologicheskie proiavlenia novoi very grafa L'va Tolstogo." *Iuzhnyi krai*, no. 3378, 3381, 3383 (1890).

Nabokov, V. V. *The Defence*. Translated by Michael Scammell in collaboration with the author. Oxford: Oxford University Press, 1986. First published in 1929 as *Zashchita Luzhina*.

Nechaev, A. P. "Otvet Chelpanovu." *Voprosy filosofii i psikhologii*, 1909, no. 5: 805–10.

"Nekrolog V. S. Grinevicha." *Klinicheskii arkhiv genial'nosti i odarennosti*, 1928, no. 3: 79.

Newsholme, Arthur, and John Adam Kingsbury. *Red Medicine: Socialized Health in Soviet Russia*. Garden City, N.Y.: Doubleday, Doran, 1934.

Nietzsche, Friedrich. *Ecce Homo*. Translated by Anthony M. Ludovici. New York: Russell & Russell, 1964. First published 1908.

Nikinin, M. P. "Chekhov kak izobrazitel' bol'noi dushi." *Vestnik psikhologii, kriminal'noi antropologii i gipnotizma*, 1905, no. 1: 1–13.

Nikulin, L. V. *Gody nashei zhizni*. Moscow: Moskovskii rabochii, 1966.

Nitsche, Paul, and Karl Willmans. *The History of the Prison Psychoses*. Translated by Francis M. Barnes and Bernard Glück. New York: Journal of Nervous and Mental Diseases Publishing Company, 1912.

Nordau, Max. *Degeneration*. New York: D. Appleton, 1895. Reprint, Lincoln: University of Nebraska Press, 1993. First published as *Entartung* (Berlin: C. Dunker, 1892).

————. *Psikhofiziologiia geniia i talanta.* St. Petersburg: Vestnik znanii, 1908.

————. "The Psychophysiology of Genius and Talent." In *Paradoxes,* 116–202. Authorized translation from the German. Chicago: L. Schick.

————. *Vyrozhdenie.* Translated by V. Genkevich. Kiev: Ioganson, 1894. First published as *Entartung* (1892).

————. *Vyrozhdenie.* Translated by R. I. Sementkovskii. St. Petersburg: Pavlenkov, 1894. First published as *Entartung* (1892).

Novikov, M. M. *Ot Moskvy do N'iu-Iorka: Moia zhizn' v nauke i politike.* New York: Izdatel'stvo imeni Chekhova, 1952.

Oppengeim, Ia. G. *Rekonstruktsiia zdravookhraneniia i ediny dispanser.* Moscow: Mosobliispolkom, 1930.

Osipov, N. E. "Beseda s Dubois." *Zhurnal nevropatologii i psikhiatrii imeni S. S. Korsakova,* 1910, no. 5–6: 1773.

————. "*Dvoinik:* Peterburgskaia poema Dostoevskogo (Zapiski psikhiatra)." In *O Dostoevskom.* Vol. 1, edited by A. L. Bem, 39–64. Prague: Legiographie, 1929.

————. "Dvulikost' i edinstvo meditsiny." In *Russkii narodnyi universitet v Prage: Nauchnye trudy.* Vol. 2: 175–92. Prague: Russkii narodnyi universitet, 1929.

————. "Eshche o psikhoanalyze." *Psykhoterapiia,* 1910, no. 4–5: 153–72.

————. "Korsakov i Serbskii (Pervye professora psikhiatrii Moskovskogo universiteta)." In *Moskovskii universitet, 1755–1930: Iubileinyi sbornik,* edited by V. B. El'iashevich, A. A. Kizevetter, and M. M. Novikov, 405–26. Paris: Sovremennye zapiski, 1930.

————. "Moskovskii psikhiatricheskii kruzhok 'Malye piatnitsy.'" *Zhurnal nevropatologii i psikhiatrii imeni S. S. Korsakova,* 1912, no. 2–3: 456–87.

————. "Mysli i somneniia po povodu odnogo sluchaia 'degenerativnoi psykhopatii.'" *Psikhoterapiia,* 1911, no. 5: 189–215.

————. "Nevrasteniia." In *Zhizn' i smert',* edited by A. L. Bem, F. M. Dosuzhkov, and N. O. Lossky, 79–106. Prague: Petropolis, 1935.

————. "O bol'noi dushe." *Zhurnal nevropatologii i psikhiatrii imeni S. S. Korsakova,* 1913, no. 5–6: 657–63.

————. "O logike i metodologii psikhiatrii." *Zhurnal nevropatologii i psikhiatrii imeni S. S. Korsakova,* 1912, no. 2–3: 459–65.

————. "O naviazchivoi ulybke." *Zhurnal nevropatologii i psikhiatrii imeni S. S. Korsakova,* 1912, no. 4: 570–78.

————. "O nevroze boiazni (*Ängstneurose*)." *Zhurnal nevropatologii i psikhiatrii imeni S. S. Korsakova,* 1909, no. 5–6: 783–805.

————. "O 'panseksualizme' Freuda." *Zhurnal nevropatologii i psikhiatrii imeni S. S. Korsakova,* 1911, no. 5–6: 749–56.

————. "Psikhologicheskie i psikhopatologicheskie vzgliady Fzeida." *Zhurnal nevropatologii i psikhiatrii imeni S. S. Korsakova,* 1908, no. 3–4: 564–84.

————. "Psikhologiia kompleksov." *Zhurnal nevropatologii i psikhiatrii imeni S. S. Korsakova*, 1908, no. 6: 1021–74.

————. "Psikhoterapiia v literaturnykh proizvedeniiakh L. N. Tolstogo (otryvok iz raboty 'Tolstoy i meditsina')." *Psikhoterapiia*, 1911, no. 1: 1–21.

————. "Revoliutsiia i son." In *Russkii Narodnyi universitet v Prage. Nauchnye trudy.* Vol. 4: 175–203. Prague: Russkii narodnyi universitet, 1931.

————. "Strashnoe u Gogolia i Dostoevskogo." In *Zhizn' i smert'*, edited by A. L. Bem, F. M. Dosuzhkov, and N. O. Lossky, 107–36. Prague: Petropolis, 1935.

————. "Zapiski sumasshedshego, nezakonchennoe proizvedenie L. N. Tolstogo: K voprosy ob emotsii boiazni." *Psikhoterapiia*, 1913, no. 3: 141–58.

————. "Zhizn' i smert'." In *Zhizn' i smert'*, edited by A. L. Bem, F. M. Dosuzhkov, and N. O. Lossky, 67–78. Prague: Petropolis, 1935.

————. Život a smrt." In *Russkii narodnyi universitet v Prage: Nauchnye trudy.* Vol. 1: 138–46. Prague: Russkii narodnyi universitet, 1928.

Ossipoff, N. *Tolstois* Kindheitserinnerungen. *Ein Beitrag zur Freuds Libidotheorie.* Leipzig: Imago-Bücher, II, 1923.

Ovsianiko-Kulikovskii, D. N. "Istoriia russkoi intelligentsii." In *Sobranie sochinenii.* Vol. 8, pt. 2. The Hague and Paris: Mouton, 1969. First published 1903–14.

————. *Literaturno-kriticheskie raboty.* Vol. 2. Moscow: Khudozhestvennaia literatura, 1989.

"P. M. Avtokratov. Nekrolog." *Sovremennaia psikhiatriia*, 1915, no. 3: 153–54.

"Pamiati professora F. F. Erismana." *Voprosy psikhologii*, 1963: no. 2: 189.

"Petr Mikhailovich Zinov'ev. Nekrolog." *Zhurnal nevropatologii i psikhiatrii imeni S. S. Korsakova,* 1966, no. 2: 324–25.

Pisarev, D. N. "L. M. Rozenshtein." *Sovetskaia psikhonevrologiia*, 1934, no. 3: 5–6.

Polosin, M. P. "Doktor meditsiny Nikolai Evgrafovich Osipov (1877–1934)." In *Zhizn' i smert'*, edited by A. L. Bem, F. M. Dosuzhkov, and N. O. Lossky, 3–24. Prague: Petropolis, 1935.

Popov, N. V. "K voprosu o sviazi odarennosti s dushevnoi bolezn'iu (po povodu rabot doktora Segalina i drugikh)." *Russkii evgenicheskii zhurnal*, 1927, no. 3–4: 133–54.

Portugalov, Iu. V. "Po povodu polemiki prof. V. F. Chizh i d-ra Ia. F. Kaplana (Zametki chitatelia-psikhiatra)." *Voprosy filosofii i psikhologii*, 1903, no. 1: 146–55.

Postnikov, S. P. *Russkie v Prage, 1918–1928.* Prague: S. P. Postnikov, 1928.

Prichard, J. C. "Nravstvennoe pomeshatel'stvo." *Arkhiv psikhiatrii, neirologii i sudebnoi psikhologii*, 1893, no. 3: 53–68.

Prozorov, L. A. "Nastoiashchee polozhenie dela psikhiatricheskoi pomoshchi v SSSR." *Zhurnal nevropatologii i psikhiatrii imeni S. S. Korsakova*, 1925, no. 1: 93–104.

————. "Polozhenie dela psikhiatricheskoi pomoshchi v SSSR." *Zhurnal nevropatologii i psikhiatrii imeni S. S. Korsakova*, 1926, no. 2: 97–106.

"Publichnye vystupleniia N. E. Osipova v Prage." In *Zhizn' i smert'. Sbornik rabot v pamiat' N. E. Osipova,* edited by A. L. Bem, F. M. Dosuzhkov, and N. O. Lossky, 60–64. Prague: Petropolis, 1935.

Pushkin, Alexander. *Eugene Onegin.* Translated by Charles Johnston with an introduction by John Bayley. Harmondsworth, U.K.: Penguin Books, 1979. First published 1833.

Richet, Charles. *L'Homme et l'intelligence: fragmentes de physiologie et de psychologie.* Paris: Félix Alcan, 1884.

Riese, Walther. "Bolezn' Vinsenta Van Goga." *Klinicheskii arkhiv genial'nosti i odarennosti,* 1927, no. 2: 137–46.

Rivers, W. H. R. "Experimental Psychology in Relation to Insanity." *Journal of Mental Science* 14 (1895): 591–97.

Rokhlin, L. L. "College of Mental Hygiene in the Ukraine (USSR)." *Mental Hygiene* 3 (1930): 661–71.

———. "O prepodavanii psikhogigieny." *Sovetskaia psikhonevrologiia,* 1934, no. 3: 58–90.

———. "Programma kursa psikhogigieny." *Sovetskaia psikhonevrologiia,* 1934, no. 3: 91–99.

Rossolimo, G. I. *Isskustvo, bol'nye nervy i vospitanie.* Moscow: G. I. Prostakov, 1901.

———. "Metodika massovogo issledovaniia po 'psikhologicheskomu profiliu' i pervonachal'nye dannye." *Zhurnal nevropatologii i psikhiatrii imeni S. S. Korsakova,* 1925, no. 1: 45–58.

———. "Profili psikhologicheski nedostatochnykh detei (opyt eksperimental'no-psikhologicheskogo issledovaniia stepenei odarennosti)." *Sovremennaia psikhiatriia,* 1910, no. 9–10: 377–412.

Rot, V. K. "Obshchestvennoe popechenie o nervno-bol'nykh. Ustroistvo spetsial'nykh sanatorii." In *Trudy Vtorogo s"ezda otechestvennykh psikhiatrov,* 478–99. Kiev: Kul'zhenko, 1907.

Rozanov, V. V. "Pushkin i Gogol." In *Nesovmestimye kontrasty zhitiia: literaturno-esteticheskie raboty raznykh let,* 225–33. Moscow: Iskusstvo, 1990. First published 1891.

———. "Tri momenta v istorii russkoi kritiki." In *Sochineniia,* 154–69. Moscow: Sovetskaia Rossiia, 1990, 154–69. First published 1892.

Rozenshtein, L. M. "The Development of Mental Hygiene in Russia (USSR)." *Mental Hygiene* 3 (1930): 644–47.

———."K voprosu o lechenii alkogolizma (o protivoalkogol'nykh dispanserakh)." *Zhurnal nevropatologii i psikhiatrii imeni S. S. Korsakova,* 1915–16, no. 4–5–6: 519–27.

———. "Moskovskaia psikhiatricheskaia shkola i N. N. Bazhenov." *Klinicheskaia meditsina,* 1924, no. 2: 132–34.

———. "O sovremennykh psikhiatricheskikh techeniiakh v Sovetskoi Rossii." In *Moskovskii Gosudarstvennyi nevro-psikhiatricheskii dispanser: Psikhogigienicheskie i nevrologicheskie issledovaniia,* edited by L. M. Rozenshtein, 115–21. Moscow: Narkomzdrav RSFSR, 1928.

———. "P. B. Gannushkin kak psikhiatr epokhi." In *Trudy Psikhiatricheskoi kliniki Pervogo MMI. Pamiati Gannushkina.* Vol. 4: 13–19. Moscow: Gosizdat, 1934.

————. *Psikhicheskie faktory v etiologii dushevnykh boleznei.* Moscow: Gosizdat, 1923.

————. "Psikhopatologiia myshleniia pri maniakal'no-depressivnom psikhoze i osobye paralogicheskie formy maniakal'nogo sostoianiia." *Zhurnal nevropatologii i psikhiatrii imeni S. S. Korsakova,* 1926, no. 7: 5–28.

————. "Public-Health Service and Mental Hygiene in the USSR." *Mental Hygiene* 4 (1931): 739–43.

————. "[Review of] *Neurasthenie et psychonévroses,* [by] Hippolyte Bernheim." *Psikhoterapiia,* 1910, no. 3: 134–35.

————. "V. P. Serbskii—klassik Moskovskoi psikhiatricheskoi shkoly." *Psikhogigien-icheskie issledovaniia.* Vol. 1, pt 1: 7–16. Moscow: Gos. nauchnyi institut nevro-psikhicheskoi profilaktiki, 1928.

Rozenshtein, L. M., L. Rokhlin, and A. Edel'shtein. "Psikhogigiena." In *Bol'shaia meditsinskaia entsiklopediia.* Vol. 27: 749–62. Moscow: OGIZ, 1933.

Rozental', T. K. "Stradanie i tvorchestvo Dostoevskogo (psikhoanaliticheskoe issle-dovanie." *Voprosy izucheniia i vospitaniia lichnosti,* 1919, no. 1: 88–107.

Rudnev, V. I. "*Zapiski sumasshedshego* L. Tolstogo." *Klinicheskii arkhiv genial'nosti i odarennosti,* 1929, no. 1: 69–71.

Rybakov, F. E. "Alkogolizm i dushevnoe rasstroistvo." In *Otchety Moskovskogo ob-shchestva nevropatologov i psikhiatrov za 1897–1901 gg.* Moscow: G. I. Prostakov, 1901.

————. *Atlas dlia eksperimental'no-psikhologicheskogo issledovaniia lichnosti s podrobnym opisaniem i ob"iasneniem tablits: Sostavlen primenitel'no k tseli pedagogicheskogo i vrachebno-diagnosticheskogo issledovaniia.* Moscow: I. D. Sytin, 1910.

————. "Granitsy sumasshestviia." In *Otchety Moskovskogo obshchestva nevropatologov i psikhiatrov,* 5–6. Moscow: G. I. Prostakov, 1905.

————. *Ob organizatsii ambulatorii dlia alkogolikov.* St. Petersburg: Ia. Trei, 1904.

————. *Sovremennye pisateli i bol'nye nervy. Psikhiatricheskii etud.* Moscow: V. Richter, 1908.

Rybakov, P. V. "Nekrolog N. N. Bazhenova." *Moskovskii meditsinskii zhurnal,* 1923, no. 2: 224–26.

"Sanatorii 'Kriukovo' N. A. Vyrubova." *Sovremennaia psikhiatriia,* 1909, no. 1: inside front cover.

Schweitzer, Albert. *The Psychiatric Study of Jesus: Exposition and Criticism.* Translated and with an introduction by Charles R. Joy and foreword by Winfred Overholser. Boston: Beacon Press, 1948. First published 1911.

Segalin, G. V. "Evropatologiia genial'nykh epileptikov: Formy i kharakter epilepsii u velikikh liudei." *Klinicheskii arkhiv genial'nosti i odarennosti,* 1926, no. 3: 143–87.

————. "Evropatologiia lichnosti i tvorchestva L'va Tolstogo." *Klinicheskii arkhiv genial'nosti i odarennosti,* 1929, no. 3–4: 5–148.

————. "Institut genial'nogo tvorchestva." *Klinicheskii arkhiv genial'nosti i odarennosti,* 1928, no. 1: 53–59.

————. "Izobretateli kak tvorcheskie nevrotiki (evronevrotiki)." *Klinicheskii arkhiv genial'nosti i odarennosti,* 1929, no. 2: 5–73.

————. "K patogenezu leningradskikh uchenykh i deiatelei iskusstv." *Klinicheskii arkhiv genial'nosti i odarennosti*, 1928, no. 3: 3–22.

————. "O zadachakh evropatologii kak otdel'noi otrasli psikhopatologii." *Klinicheskii arkhiv genial'nosti i odarennosti*, 1925, no. 1: 7–23.

————. "Obshchaia simptomatologiia evro-aktivnykh (tvorcheskikh) pristupov." *Klinicheskii arkhiv genial'nosti i odarennosti*, 1926, no. 1: 3–78.

————. "Patogenez i biogenez velikikh liudei." *Klinicheskii arkhiv genial'nosti i odarennosti*, 1925, no. 1: 24–90.

————. "*Zapiski sumasshedshego* L'va Tolstogo kak patograficheskii dokument." *Klinicheskii arkhiv genial'nosti i odarennosti*, 1929, no. 1: 73–78.

Segaloff, Timofei. *Die Krankheit Dostojewskys: Eine ärztlich-psychologische Studie mit einem Bildnis Dostojewskys*. Grenzfragen der Literatur und Medizin in Einzeldarstellungen, vol. 5, edited by S. Ramer. Munich: Ernst Reinhardt, 1907.

Segalov, T. E. "Bolezn' Dostoevskogo." Translated by F. Ge. *Nauchnoe Slovo*, 1929, no. 4: 91–98. First published 1907.

————. "K voprosu o sushchnosti kontuzii sovremennymi artilleriiskimi snariadami (*Morbus decompressionis*)." *Sovremennaia psikhiatriia*, 1915, no. 3: 103–17.

————. "K voprosu ob organicheskikh i funktsional'nykh zabolevaniiakh pri kontuzii artilleriiskimi snariadami: Stat'ia vtoraia." *Sovremennaia psikhiatriia*, 1915, no. 6: 263–70.

"Sektsia nervnykh i dushevnykh boleznei IX-go s"ezda Obshchestva russkikh vrachei v pamiat' N. I. Pirogova." *Zhurnal nevropatologii i psikhiatrii imeni S. S. Korsakova*, 1904, no. 1–2: 196–276.

Semashko, N. A. *Health Protection in the U.S.S.R.* London: Victor Gollancz, 1934.

————. "O zadachakh obshchestvennoi nevrologii i psikhiatrii." *Sotsial'naia gigiena*, 1924, no. 3–4: 93–94.

Serbskii, V. P. "Prestupnye i chestnye liudi." *Voprosy filosofii i psikhologii*, 1896, no. 5: 660–79.

————. "Russkii soiuz psikhiatrov i nevropatologov im. S. S. Korsakova." In *Trudy Pervogo s"ezda Russkogo soiuza nevropatologov i psikhiatrov, 4–11.9.1911*, edited by N. A. Vyrubov et al., 64–83. Moscow: Shtab Moskovskogo voennogo okruga, 1914.

Serebrianikov, V. "Eksperimental'naia psikhologia." In *Entsiklopedicheskii slovar'*. Vol. 40: 285–90. Leipzig: Brockhaus & Efron, 1904.

Shaikevich, M. O. "Eshche o psikhozakh v voiskakh." *Sovremennaia psikhiatriia*, 1913, no. 10: 789–97.

————. *Psikhologiia i literatura*. St. Petersburg: Ts. Kraiz, 1910.

————. "Psikhopatologicheskie cherty geroev Maksima Gor'kogo." *Vestnik psikhologii, kriminal'noi antropologii i gipnotizma*, 1904, no. 1: 55–57; no. 2: 40–50; no. 3: 124–41.

————. "Psikhopatologicheskii metod v russkoi literaturnoi kritike." *Voprosy filosofii i psikhologii*, 1904, no. 3: 309–34.

Shaw, G. B. *The Sanity of Art: An Exposure of the Current Nonsense about Artists Being Degenerate*. London: Constable, 1911.

Shenrok, V. I. "Itogi gogolevskoi iubileinoi literatury." *Vestnik vospitaniia*, 1902, no. 6: 1–31.

———. *Materialy dlia biografii N. V. Gogolia*. 6 vols. Moscow: Lissner & Geshel', 1897.

Shestov, Lev. "Dostoevsky and Nietzsche: The Philosophy of Tragedy." Translated by Spencer Roberts. In *Dostoevsky, Tolstoy, and Nietzsche*, 141–322. Athens, Ohio: Ohio University Press, 1969. First published 1903.

Shuvalov, A. V. "Patograficheskii ocherk o Daniile Kharmse." *Nezavisimyi psikhiatricheskii zhurnal*, 1996, no. 2: 74–78.

Sigerist, Henry E. *Socialized Medicine in the Soviet Union*. New York: Norton, 1937.

Sikorskii, I. A. *Antropologicheskaia i psikhologicheskaia genealogiia Pushkina*. Kiev: Kul'zhenko, 1912.

———. "Biologicheskie voprosy v psikhologii i psikhiatrii." *Voprosy nervno-psikhicheskoi meditsiny*, 1904, no. 1: 79–114.

———. *Ekspertiza po delu ob ubiistve Andriushi Iushchinskogo*. St. Petersburg: A. S. Suvorin, 1913.

———. "Krasnyi tsvetok. Rasskaz Vsevoloda Garshina." *Vestnik klinicheskoi i sudebnoi psikhiatrii i nevropatologii*, 1884, no. 1: 344–48.

———. *O knige V. Veresaeva* Zapiski vracha *(Chto daet eta kniga literature, nauke i zhizni?)*. Kiev: Kushnerev, 1902.

———. "O velikikh uspekhakh i vozrastaiushchem znachenii psikhiatrii i nevrologii sredi nauk i v zhizni." *Voprosy nervno-psikhicheskoi meditsiny*, 1899, no. 1: 1–14.

———. *Psikhologicheskoe napravlenie khudozhestvennogo tvorchestva Gogolia (Rech' v pamiat' 100-letnei godovshchiny Gogolia, [April 10, 1909])*. Kiev: Universitet Sv. Vladimira, 1911.

———. *Psikhopaticheskii etiud*. Kiev: Universitet Sv. Vladimira, 1892.

———. "Russkaia psikhopaticheskaia literatura, kak material dlia ustanovleniia novoi klinicheskoi formy—*Idiophrenia paranoides*." *Voprosy nervno-psikhicheskoi meditsiny*, 1902, no. 1: 5–48.

———. *Sbornik nauchno-literaturnykh trudov*. 5 vols. Kiev: F. A. Ioganson, 1900–1904.

———. "Uspekhi russkogo khudozhestvennogo tvorchestva: Rech' v torzhestvennom zasedanii II-go s"ezda otechestvennykh psikhiatrov v Kieve." *Voprosy nervno-psikhicheskoi meditsiny*, 1905, no. 3: 497–504; no. 4: 608–22.

———. *Vospitanie v vozraste pervogo detstva*. 3d ed. St. Petersburg: A. E. Riabchenko, 1904.

———. *Vseobshchaia psikhologiia s fiziognomikoi*. Kiev: Kul'zhenko, 1904.

———. "Znachenie gigieny vospitaniia v vozraste pervogo detstva." *Vestnik klinicheskoi i sudebnoi psikhiatrii i nevropatologii*, 1899, no. 2: 59–128.

Sleptsov-Teriaevskii, O. N. *Sinestezicheskii sposob izuchenia akkordov*. Petrograd: Sirius, 1915.

Smirnov, V. I., ed. *Sotsialisticheskaia rekonstruktsiia zdravookhraneniia.* Moscow: GIZ, 1930.

Solov'ev, E. Iu. "Biograficheskii analiz kak vid istoriko-filosofskogo issledovaniia." *Voprosy filosofii,* 1981, no. 9: 133–45.

Solov'ev, Vladimir. "Tri rechi v pamiat' Dostoevskogo." In *Literature and National Identity: Nineteenth-Century Russian Critical Essays,* edited by Paul Debreczeny and Jesse Zeldin, 169–79. Lincoln: University of Nebraska Press, 1970. First published 1881–83.

Sorkin, Iu. "Polivalentnyi chelovek." *Nauka Urala,* 1992, no. 12: 4–5.

Stupin, S. S. "K voprosu o narodnykh sanatoriiakh dlia nervno-bol'nykh." *Zhurnal nevropatologii i psikhiatrii imeni S. S. Korsakova,* 1904, no. 3: 360–76.

———. "K voprosu ob obshchestvennom lechenii i prizrenii alkogolikov." *Sovremennaia psikhiatriia,* 1907, no. 11: 385–400.

Sukhotina-Tolstaia, T. L. *Vospominaniia.* Moscow: Khudozhestvennaia literatura, 1976.

Tarnovskaia, P. "Cesare Lombroso." *Vestnik klinicheskoi i sudebnoi psikhiatrii i nevropatologii,* 1885, no. 1: 278–96.

Tchisch, Woldemar von. "Über die Zeitverhältnisse der Apperception einfacher und zusammengesetzter Vorstellungen, untersucht mit Hülfe der Complicationsmethode." *Philosophische Studien,* 1885, no. 2: 603–34.

Tekut'ev, F. S. *Istoricheskii ocherk kafedry i kliniki dushevnykh i nervnykh boleznei pri Imperatorskoi Voenno-Meditsinskoi Akademii.* St. Petersburg: Voennaia tipografiia, 1898.

Tiganova, G. A. "K voprosu o polozhenii invalidov voiny v RSFSR." *Zhurnal nevropatologii i psikhiatrii imeni S. S. Korsakova,* 1927, no. 3: 325–30.

Tokarskii, A. A. "Strakh smerti." *Voprosy filosofii i psikhologii,* 1897, no. 40: 931–78.

———, ed. *Zapiski psikhologicheskoi laboratorii pri psikhiatricheskoi klinike Imperatorskogo Moskovskogo universiteta.* 5 vols. Moscow: Kushnerev, 1895–1901.

Tolstaia, S. A. *Dnevniki, Part 2: 1891–1897.* Moscow: Sabashnikovy, 1929.

Tolstoy, L. N. *Anna Karenina.* Translated by Aylmer Maude. New York: Norton, 1970. First published 1875–76.

———. *The Death of Ivan Ilych.* Translated by Aylmer Maude. New York: New American Library, 1960. First published 1886.

———. "The Memoirs of a Madman." In *Tolstoi Centenary Edition.* Vol. 15: 210–25. London: Humphrey Milford, 1934. First published 1912.

———. "O bezumii." In *Polnoe sobranie sochinenii.* Vol. 38: 395–411. Moscow: Khudozhestvennaia literatura, 1936.

———. *Tolstoy's Diaries.* Edited and translated by R. F. Christian. London: HarperCollins, 1994. First published in Tolstoy's *Complete Works* [*Polnoe sobranie sochinenii*], ed. V. G. Chertkov (Moscow: Khudozhestvennaia literatura, 1937–58), vols. 46–90.

———. *War and Peace.* London: Penguin Books, 1964. First published 1865–69.

———. "What Then Must We Do?" Translated by Aylmer Maude. In *Tolstoi Cente-*

nary Edition. Vol. 30: 1–372. London: Humphrey Milford, 1934. First published 1885.

Tolstoy, S. N. *Ocherki bylogo.* 3d ed. Tula: Priokskoe knizhnoe izdatel'stvo, 1965. First published 1949.

Troshin, G. Ia. "Genii i zdorov'e N. V. Gogolia." *Voprosy filosofii i psikhologii,* 1905, no. 1: 37–82; no. 2: 187–249; no. 3: 333–83.

————. *Pushkin i psikhologiia tvorchestva.* Prague: Society of Russian Physicians in Czechoslovakia, 1937.

————. *Travmaticheskii nevroz po materialam tekushchei voiny.* Moscow: Shtab Moskovskogo voennogo okruga, 1916.

Trotsky, Leon. *Literature and Revolution.* Translated by Rose Strunsky. Ann Arbor: University of Michigan Press, 1975. First published 1923.

Turgenev, I. S. "Gogol." In *N. V. Gogol v russkoi kritike i vospominaniiakh sovremennikov,* edited by S. Mashinskii, 317–23. Moscow: GIZ detskoi literatury, 1951. First published 1869.

————. *Hamlet and Don Quixote: An Essay.* Translated by Robert Nichols. London: Hendersons, 1930. First published 1860.

Tutyshkin, P. P. "Ob ustroistve obshchestvennykh (zemskikh, gorodskikh) lechebnits-pansionatov dlia nervno- i dushevno-bol'nykh, to est' uchrezhdenii dvoiako-smeshannogo tipa." *Zhurnal nevropatologii i psikhiatrii imeni S. S. Korsakova,* 1902, no. 1–2: 206–10.

————. "Sovremennye voprosy pedagogicheskoi psikhologii i psikhiatrii." In *Trudy Pervogo s"ezda Russkogo soiuza psikhiatrov i nevropatologov, 4–11.9.1911,* edited by N. A. Vyrubov et al, 761–72. Moscow: Shtab Moskovskogo voennogo okruga, 1914.

Vavulin, N. *Bezumie, ego smysl i tsennost': Psikhologicheskie ocherki.* St. Petersburg: Vaisberg & Gershunin, 1913.

Vengerov, S. A. *Istochniki slovaria russkikh pisatelei.* St. Petersburg: Imperatorskaia Akademiia Nauk, 1900.

Vereshchaka, Stepan. "Russkii psikhiatricheskii kruzhok v Prage." In *Zhizn' i smert',* edited by A. L. Bem, F. M. Dosuzhkov, and N. O. Lossky, 55–57. Prague: Petropolis, 1935.

Vogüé, Eugène-Melchior de. *Le roman russe.* 3d ed. Paris: Plon-Nourrit, 1892.

Vol'fson, B. Ia. "'Panteon mozga' Bekhtereva i 'Institut genial'nogo tvorchestva' Segalina." *Klinicheskii arkhiv genial'nosti i odarennosti,* 1928, no. 1: 52–60.

Volotskoi, M. V. "O polovoi sterilizatsii nasledstvenno defektivnykh." *Russkii evgenicheskii zhurnal,* 1922–24, no. 2: 201–22.

Vorob'ev, V. V. "Degeneraty i ikh obshchestvennoe znachenie." In *Otchety Moskovskogo Obshchestva nevropatologov i psikhiatrov za 1901–1902 gg.,* 9–10. Moscow: Kushnerev, 1902.

"Vtoroi s"ezd nevropatologov i psikhiatrov." *Obozrenie psikhiatrii, nevrologii i eksperimental'noi psikhologii,* 1906, no. 2: 152.

Vul'fert, A. K. "Vozrazheniia na referat d-ra Bazhenova o s"ezde kriminal'noi antropologii." *Voprosy filosofii i psikhologii*, 1889, no. 2: 41–46.

Vygotsky, L. S., and P. M. Zinov'ev, "Genial'nost'." In *Bol'shaia meditsinskaia entsiklopediia.* Vol. 6: 612–15. Moscow: Sovetskaia entsiklopediia, 1929.

Vyrubov, N. A. "Po psikhiatricheskim bol'nitsam Shotlandii." *Sovremennaia psikhiatriia*, 1913, no. 9: 694–734.

———. "Psikho-analiticheskii metod Freud'a i ego lechebnoe znachenie." *Zhurnal nevropatologii i psikhiatrii imeni S. S. Korsakova*, 1909, no. 1–2: 1–28.

———. "Psikhoterapevticheskie vzgliady S. S. Korsakova." *Psikhoterapiia*, 1910, no. 3: 1–10.

———. *Psikhoterapevticheskie zadachi sanatorii dlia nevrotikov.* Moscow: Kushnerev, 1910.

Williams, Frankwood E. *Russia, Youth and the Present-Day World: Further Studies in Mental Hygiene.* New York: Farrar & Rinehart, 1934.

———. *Soviet Russia Fights Neurosis.* London: Routledge, 1934.

Wulff, Moshe. "Die russische psychoanalytische Literatur bis zum Jahre 1911." *Zentralblatt für Psychoanalyse: Medizinische Monatsschrift für Seelenkunde*, 1911, no. 7–8: 364–71.

Zalkind A. B. "The Fundamentals and the Practice of Mental Hygiene in Adolescence and Youth in Soviet Russia." *Mental Hygiene* 3 (1930): 647–49.

Zalkind, G. G. *P. Kamenev (1772–1803) (Opyt imushchestvennoi kharakteristiki pervogo russkogo romantika).* Kazan', 1926.

Zhukovskii, M. "O vliianii obshchestvennykh sobytii na razvitie dushevnykh zabolevanii." *Vestnik psikhologii, kriminal'noi antropologii i gipnotizma*, 1907, no. 3: 128–64.

Zinov'ev, P. M. *Dushevnye bolezni v kartinakh i obrazakh.* Moscow: Sabashnikovy, 1927.

———. *K voprosu ob organizatsii nevro-psikhiatricheskikh dispanserov (razvitie myslei vtoroi chasti doklada na Vtorom Vserossiiskom soveshchanii po voprosam psikhiatrii i nevrologii, [November 12–17, 1923]).* Moscow, 1924.

———. "O zadachakh patograficheskoi raboty." In *Trudy Psikhiatricheskoi kliniki Pervogo MMI. Pamiati Gannushkina.* Vol. 4: 411–16. Moscow: Gosizdat, 1934.

———. "Privat-dotsent T. E. Segalov." *Klinicheskaia meditsina* 22 (1928): 226.

INDEX